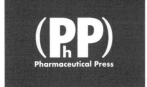

T0173468

Physical Pharmacy

Third Edition

David Attwood
Alexander T Florence

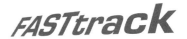

Published by the Pharmaceutical Press
66-68 East Smithfield, London E1W 1AW, UK

© Pharmaceutical Press 2020

(**P.P**) is a trade mark of Pharmaceutical Press
Pharmaceutical Press is the publishing division of the Royal Pharmaceutical Society

First edition published 2008
Second edition published 2012
Third edition published 2020

Printed in Great Britain by TJ International, Padstow, Cornwall

ISBN 978 0 85711 390 0

TABLE OF CONTENTS

Introduction to the *FAST*track series v
Preface vii
About the authors xi

CHAPTER 1. **SOLIDS**.. 13
Crystal structure and external appearance 13
Polymorphism 16
Crystal hydrates and solvates.. 17
Co-crystals 18
Amorphous solids.. 18
Biopharmaceutical importance of particle size... 19
Wetting of solid surfaces and powders 20
Dissolution of drugs.. 23
Sublimation and freeze drying.. 24
Solid solutions and dispersions.. 25
Memory maps 27
Questions 29

CHAPTER 2. **SOLID DOSAGE FORMS**.. 31
Formulation of tablets and capsules 31
Granulation.. 40
Tablet manufacture... 47
Capsule manufacture.. 60
Memory maps 67
Questions 70

CHAPTER 3. **SOLUBILITY AND SOLUTION PROPERTIES OF DRUGS** 71
Concentration units 71
Solvents for pharmaceutical aerosols 73
Factors influencing solubility 75
Ionisation of drugs in solution... 79
pH of drug solutions 82
Buffers... 83
Thermodynamic properties of drugs in solution 86
Osmotic properties of drugs in solution – isotonic solutions 87
Partitioning of drugs between immiscible solvents.. 88
Diffusion of drugs in solution 90
Memory map 91
Questions 92

CHAPTER 4. **DRUG STABILITY** 95
    The chemical breakdown of drugs 95
    Kinetics of chemical decomposition in solution 97
    Factors influencing drug stability of liquid dosage forms 102
    Factors influencing drug stability of solid dosage forms 107
    Stability testing and calculation of shelf-life 108
    Memory maps 110
    Questions 111

CHAPTER 5. **SURFACTANTS** 113
    Types of surfactant 113
    Some typical surfactants 114
    Reduction of surface and interfacial tension 116
    Insoluble monolayers 118
    Lung surfactant monolayers 120
    Adsorption at the solid–liquid interface 121
    Micellisation 124
    Formation of liquid crystals and vesicles 128
    Solubilisation 132
    Memory maps 136
    Questions 138

CHAPTER 6. **EMULSIONS, SUSPENSIONS AND
OTHER DISPERSED SYSTEMS** 141
    Colloid stability 141
    Disperse system flow 147
    Emulsions 153
    Suspensions 161
    Foams and defoamers 165
    Memory maps 165
    Questions 167

CHAPTER 7. **POLYMERS** 169
    Polymer structure 169
    Solution properties of polymers 172
    Properties of polymer gels 174
    Some water-soluble polymers used in pharmacy and medicine 176
    Water-insoluble polymers 179
    Application of polymers in drug delivery 180
    Memory maps 186
    Questions 188

CHAPTER 8. **DRUG ABSORPTION AND DELIVERY** 191
  Biological membranes and drug transport 191
  Routes of administration 197
  Questions 221

CHAPTER 9. **PAEDIATRIC AND GERIATRIC MEDICINES** 223
  Introduction 223
  Paediatric medication.. 225
  The elderly and their medication 232
  Drugs and enteral nutrition (EN) 234
  Memory maps 237
  Questions 239

CHAPTER 10. **PHYSICOCHEMICAL DRUG INTERACTIONS
AND INCOMPATIBILITIES** 241
  Solubility problems 241
  pH effects *in vitro* and *in vivo* 243
  Dilution of mixed solvent systems 244
  Cation–anion interactions.. 245
  Chelation and other forms of complexation.. 246
  Adsorption of drugs.. 249
  Drug interactions with plastics... 250
  Protein binding of drugs 250
  Memory maps 253
  Questions 255

CHAPTER 11. **ADVERSE EVENTS – THE ROLE OF FORMULATIONS
AND DELIVERY SYSTEMS**.. 257
  Adverse events and adverse drug reactions.. 257
  Excipient effects 260
  Influence of dosage form type... 265
  Reactions to impurities.. 268
  Delivery devices and materials 268
  Crystallisation.. 270
  Abnormal bioavailability and adverse events.. 270
  Photochemical reactions and photoinduced reactions..................................... 271
  Nanosystems and new biological entities 273
  Conclusions... 273
  Memory map 275
  Questions 276

CHAPTER 12. PEPTIDES, PROTEINS AND MONOCLONAL ANTIBODIES .. 279
  Structure and solution properties of peptides and proteins 279
  The stability of proteins and peptides 283
  Protein formulation and delivery 287
  Therapeutic proteins and peptides 288
  DNA and oligonucleotides 290
  Monoclonal antibodies 291
  Memory maps 295
  Questions 297

CHAPTER 13. PHARMACEUTICAL NANOTECHNOLOGY 299
  Introduction 299
  Nanoparticles for drug delivery and targeting 301
  Particle structures 302
  Importance of particle size 303
  Preparing nanoparticles 305
  Physicochemical properties determining the fate of nanoparticles 312
  Regulatory challenges: characterisation 314
  Memory maps 316
  Questions 317

CHAPTER 14. *IN VITRO* ASSESSMENT OF DOSAGE FORMS 319
  Dissolution testing of solid dosage forms 319
  In vitro evaluation of non-oral systems 322
  Rheological characteristics of products 323
  Adhesivity of dosage forms 323
  Particle size distribution in aerosols 324
  In vitro–in vivo correlations 327
  In vitro testing of new delivery systems and devices 329
  Memory maps 330
  Questions 332

CHAPTER 15. GENERIC MEDICINES AND BIOSIMILARS 333
  Definitions and characteristics of generic medicines and biosimilars 333
  Regulatory requirements 335
  Bioequivalence of parenteral medicines 338
  Memory maps 343
  Questions 345

Answers 347
Eponymous equations 354
Index 356

Introduction to the *FAST*track series

*FAST*track is a series of revision guides created for undergraduate pharmacy students. The books are intended to be used in conjunction with textbooks and reference books as an aid to revision to help guide students through their exams. They provide essential information required in each particular subject area. The books will also be useful for pre-registration trainees preparing for the General Pharmaceutical Council's (GPhC's) registration assessment, and to practising pharmacists as a quick reference text.

The content of each title focuses on what pharmacy students really need to know in order to pass exams. Features include:*

- concise bulleted information
- key points
- tips for the student
- multiple choice questions (MCQs) and worked examples
- case studies
- simple diagrams.

The titles in the *FAST*track series reflect the full spectrum of modules for the undergraduate pharmacy degree.

Titles include:
- *Applied Pharmaceutical Practice*
- *Chemistry of Drugs*
- *Complementary and Alternative Medicine*
- *Law and Ethics in Pharmacy Practice*
- *Managing Symptoms in the Pharmacy*
- *Pharmaceutical Compounding and Dispensing*
- *Pharmaceutics: Dosage Form and Design*
- *Pharmaceutics: Drug Delivery and Targeting*
- *Pharmacology*
- *Physical Pharmacy (based on Florence & Attwood's Physicochemical Principles of Pharmacy)*
- *Therapeutics*

*Note: not all features are in every title in the series.

Preface

University education is about acquiring knowledge and not about passing examinations. The latter are of course a necessary marker of progress during a course. Our feeling has been that many students do not allot sufficient time to revision. A personal timetable of hours spent revising is a useful aid to realistic study planning. While no textbook can replace a student's own notes, the *FAST*track series is intended to be a guide to revision, providing key points of each topic, questions and memory maps which should help with evaluating the success of revision. We provide several examples of these after each chapter as examples of how you can produce your own.

This third edition of *FAST*track *Physical Pharmacy* is derived unashamedly from our textbook *Physicochemical Principles of Pharmacy*, 6th edition, published by the Pharmaceutical Press in 2016. The book in front of you is not a substitute for the comprehensive text but a version reduced for study purposes. The main text was much enhanced over the 5th edition with chapters which bridge the science to practice. All are included in this edition which has 15 chapters.

Physical pharmacy (pharmaceutics, pharmaceutical technology) comprises one of the fundamental blocks of the unique knowledge base of pharmacists. There have been recent statements from various sources that the future of pharmacy is clinical. More than one senior figure has said, in effect, that the scientific training of pharmacists has had its time. We believe otherwise, given the increasing complexity of medicines. The alternative is to produce graduates in pharmacy with only a vague knowledge of the science underpinning what they do wherever they practice. Knowledge has a half-life so if a topic is treated lightly soon only vague memories remain. Below are some diagrams mapping links between some of the topics of this book to wider practice. We hope that you concur and remember all the ramifications in future years.

1. The underpinning importance of chemistry and its links to pharmaceutics, pharmacology and therapeutics

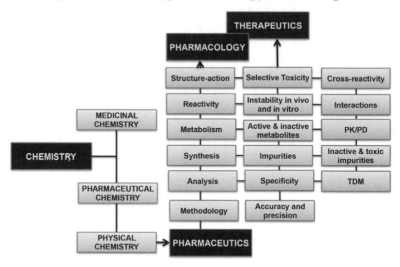

2. The ramifications of surface chemistry

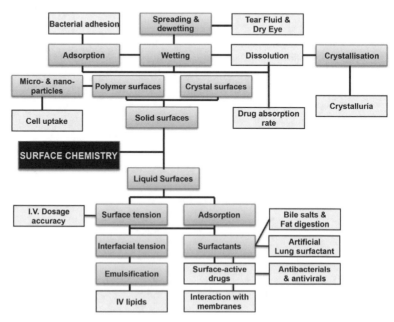

3. The significance of colloid science in understanding conventional and novel systems and situations

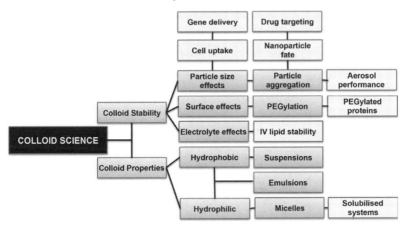

4. Rheology: its importance in physical and biological domains

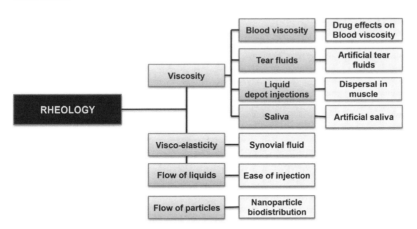

5. The importance of diffusion in understanding the behaviour of systems from drugs in tumours, in the lungs, nanoparticles in tissues

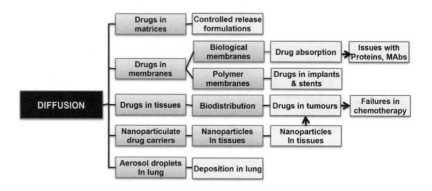

6. Probably thought (by some) to be far from important in pharmacy with its links to drug-receptor interactions, drug uptake in plastics, and wound dressings

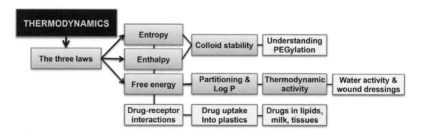

We hope this book will give you a good basis for the practice of the profession in many different areas. Clinical pharmacy needs science as much as science needs application.

David Attwood
Alexander T Florence
July 2020

About the authors

The authors have collaborated in writing texts since the first edition of *Physicochemical Principles of Pharmacy*, which was published by Macmillan in 1981. There followed *Surfactant Systems: their chemistry, pharmacy and biology*, published in 1983 by Chapman & Hall, and successive editions of *Physicochemical Principles of Pharmacy*, the sixth edition of which was published in 2016 by Pharmaceutical Press. The first edition of *FAST*track *Physical Pharmacy* appeared in 2008. Both authors have long experience of research in the field of physical pharmacy and pharmaceutics and have taught these subjects, among others, at Strathclyde, Manchester and London at undergraduate and postgraduate levels.

David Attwood is Professor Emeritus at the School of Pharmacy and Pharmaceutical Sciences, University of Manchester; he previously lectured at the University of Strathclyde.

Alexander Florence is Professor Emeritus, University of London; he was Dean of the School of Pharmacy, University of London, from 1989 to 2006 and previously was James P Todd Professor of Pharmaceutics at the University of Strathclyde.

CHAPTER 1

Solids

LEARNING OBJECTIVES

Upon completion of this chapter you should be able to:
- outline the various types of unit cell from which crystals are constructed and how the crystal lattice may be described using the system of Miller indices
- understand how the external appearance of crystals may be described in terms of their habit and outline the various factors influencing the crystal habit
- describe the formation of polymorphs and crystal hydrates by some drugs and outline the pharmaceutical consequences
- describe the process of wetting of solids and understand the importance of the contact angle in describing wettability
- outline the factors influencing the rate of dissolution of drugs and how drug solubility may be increased by forming eutectic mixtures.

Crystal structure and external appearance

- All crystals are constructed from repeating units called unit cells.
- All unit cells in a specific crystal are the same size and contain the same number of molecules or ions arranged in the same way.
- There are seven primitive unit cells (see *Figure 1.1*): cubic, orthorhombic, monoclinic, hexagonal, tetragonal, triclinic and trigonal. Certain of these may also be end-centred (monoclinic and orthorhombic), body-centred (cubic, tetragonal and orthorhombic) or face-centred (cubic and orthorhombic), making a total of 14 possible unit cells called Bravais lattices (see *Figure 1.2*).
- It is possible to describe the various planes of a crystal using the system of Miller indices (see *Figure 1.3*). The general rules for applying this system are:
  - determine the intercepts of the plane on the a, b, and c axes in terms of unit cell lengths
  - take the reciprocals of the intercepts
  - clear any fractions by multiplying by the lowest common denominator
  - reduce the numbers to the lowest terms
  - replace negative numbers with a bar above the number
  - express the result as three numbers, e.g. 101.

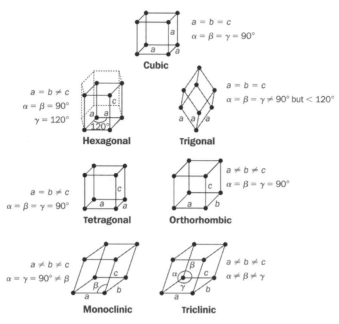

Figure 1.1: *The seven possible primitive unit cells.*

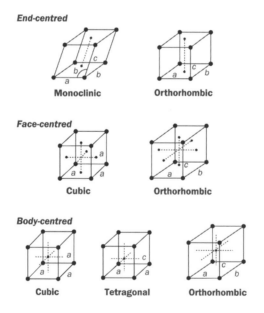

Figure 1.2: *Variations on primitive cells.*

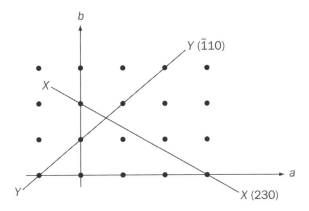

Figure 1.3: *The Miller indices for two planes in a two-dimensional lattice.*

Key points

- The crystal lattice is constructed from repeating units called unit cells, of which there are only 14 possible types.
- The various planes of the crystal lattice can be described using the system of Miller indices.
- The external appearance of a crystal (crystal habit) depends on the conditions of crystallisation and affects the formulation properties of the crystal.

Tips

Notice that:
- the smaller the number in the Miller index for a particular axis, the more parallel is the plane to that axis
- a zero value indicates a plane exactly parallel to that axis
- the larger a Miller index, the more nearly perpendicular a plane is to that axis.

- The external appearance of a crystal is described by its overall shape or habit, for example, acicular (needle-like), prismatic or tabular. The crystal habit affects:
  - the ability to inject a suspension containing a drug in crystal form – plate-like crystals are easier to inject through a fine needle than needle-like crystals
  - the flow properties of the drug in the solid state – equidimensional crystals have better flow properties and compaction characteristics than needle-like crystals, making them more suitable for tableting.
- The crystal habit depends on the conditions of crystallisation, such as solvent used, the temperature, and the concentration and presence of impurities. Surfactants in the

solvent medium used for crystal growth can alter crystal form by adsorbing onto growing faces during crystal growth.

> **Tip**
>
> The habit describes the overall shape of the crystal in general terms and so, for example, acicular crystals can have a large number of faces or can be very simple.

Polymorphism

- When polymorphism occurs, the molecules arrange themselves in two or more different ways in the crystal; either they may be packed differently in the crystal lattice or there may be differences in the orientation or conformation of the molecules at the lattice sites.
- Polymorphs of the same drug have different X-ray diffraction patterns, they may have different melting points and solubilities and they also usually exist in different habits.
- Certain classes of drug are particularly susceptible to polymorphism; for example, about 65% of the commercial sulfonamides and 70% of the barbiturates used medicinally are known to exist in several polymorphic forms.
- The particular polymorph formed by a drug depends on the conditions of crystallisation, for example, the solvent used, the rate of crystallisation and the temperature.
- Under a given set of conditions the polymorphic form with the lowest free energy will be the most stable, and other polymorphs will tend to transform into it.
- Polymorphism has the following pharmaceutical implications:

Formulation problems

- Polymorphs with certain crystal habits may be difficult to inject in suspension form or to formulate as tablets (see before).
- Transformation between polymorphic forms during storage can cause changes in crystal size in suspensions and their eventual caking.
- Crystal growth in creams as a result of phase transformation can cause the cream to become gritty.
- Changes in polymorphic forms of vehicles such as theobroma oil, used to make suppositories, could cause products with different and unacceptable melting characteristics.

Analytical issues

- Difficulties in identification arise when samples that are thought to be the same substance give different infrared spectra in the solid state because they exist in different polymorphic forms.

- Change in polymorphic form can be caused by grinding with KBr (potassium bromide) when samples are being prepared for infrared analysis.
- Changes in crystal form can also be induced by solvent extraction methods used for isolation of drugs from formulations prior to examination by infrared spectroscopy — these can be avoided by converting both samples and reference material into the same form by recrystallisation from the same solvent.

Bioavailability differences

- The difference in the bioavailability of different polymorphic forms of a drug is often insignificant but is a problem in the case of the chloramphenicol palmitate, one (form A) of the three polymorphic forms of which is poorly absorbed.

Tip

It is not possible to predict whether a particular drug will exist as several polymorphic forms and hence caution should always be applied when handling drugs to avoid possible changes in polymorphic form and hence of their properties.

Key points

- The crystals of some drugs can exist in more than one polymorphic form or as different solvates.
- Polymorphs and solvates of the same drug have different properties and this may cause problems in their formulation, analysis and absorption.

Crystal hydrates and solvates

- When some compounds crystallise they may entrap solvent in the crystal. Crystals that contain solvent of crystallisation are called crystal solvates, or crystal hydrates when water is the solvent of crystallisation. Crystals that contain no water of crystallisation are termed anhydrates.
- There are two main types of crystal solvate:
  1. Polymorphic solvates are very stable and are difficult to desolvate because the solvent plays a key role in holding the crystal together. When these crystals lose their solvent they collapse and recrystallise in a new crystal form.
  2. Pseudopolymorphic solvates lose their solvent more readily and desolvation does not destroy the crystal lattice. In these solvates the solvent is not part of the crystal bonding and merely occupies voids in the crystal.
- The particular solvate formed by a drug depends on the conditions of crystallisation, particularly the solvent used.

- The solvated forms of a drug have different physicochemical properties to the anhydrous form:
  - The melting point of the anhydrous crystal is usually higher than that of the hydrate.
  - Anhydrous crystals usually have higher aqueous solubilities than hydrates.
  - The rates of dissolution of various solvated forms of a drug differ but are generally higher than that of the anhydrous form.
  - There may be measurable differences in bioavailabilities of the solvates of a particular drug; for example, the monoethanol solvate of prednisolone tertiary butyl acetate has an absorption rate *in vivo* which is nearly five times greater than that of the anhydrous form of this drug.

Co-crystals

- Pharmaceutical co-crystals are composed of the drug and another molecule (the coformer) which is a pharmaceutically acceptable compound that is a solid at ambient temperatures and to which it is usually hydrogen-bonded. For example, carbamazepine can be co-crystallised with saccharin; caffeine and theophylline both form co-crystals with a range of dicarboxylic acids.
- The aim of co-crystallisation is to alter the physical properties of the drug, for example to increase solubility or reduce hygroscopicity, without covalent modification of its molecular structure. It can achieve improvements in solubility and dissolution profile similar to that which can be achieved by forming more soluble salts of the drug.
- Co-crystal formation also provides an opportunity to alter the pH-solubility profile of the drug through the choice of a suitable ionisable coformer. For example, co-crystallisation of carbamazepine with a diprotic coformer such as succinic acid leads to an increase of solubility with pH; an amphoteric coformer such as 4-aminobenzoic acid will, however, result in a U-shaped curve with a solubility minimum in a pH range between the two pK_a values.
- Despite the successful application of co-crystallisation in manipulation of the physical properties of a drug, there are currently no marketed products utilising co-crystals. A possible reason for this may be a concern that these metastable crystal forms may change their form during storage, necessitating recall of the product.

Amorphous solids

- Unlike crystals, amorphous solids do not have long-range ordering of their molecules and differ in solubility, stability, dissolution properties and compression characteristics from their crystalline counterparts, which can make them useful alternatives in drug delivery formulations.
- In principle, most classes of material can be prepared in the amorphous state if the

rate at which they are solidified is faster than the rate at which their molecules can align themselves into a crystal lattice with three-dimensional order.

- Crystalline material can inadvertently be converted to amorphous powders when supplying mechanical or thermal energy, for example during grinding, compression and milling the solid or during drying processes.
- Some materials, notably polymers such as poly(lactic acid), polyvinylpyrrolidone and polyethylene glycol, are inherently amorphous because even at slow solidification rates these large molecules are unable to arrange their flexible chains in an ordered manner; such materials are frequently semicrystalline with areas of a crystalline nature surrounded by amorphous regions.
- Amorphous or semicrystalline materials do not have sharp melting points but instead there is a change in the properties of the material at a characteristic temperature, called the glass transition temperature, T_g. Below T_g the material is said to be in its glassy state and is brittle; as the temperature is increased above T_g, the molecules become more mobile and the material is said to become rubbery. The transition temperature may be lowered by the addition of plasticisers, for example water is used as a plasticiser for a wide range of polymers used in film coating.

Key points

The types of multicomponent crystals include:
- Crystal hydrates and solvates in which the crystal contains not only the drug but also some of the solvent of crystallisation whether water (crystal hydrates) or solvent (crystal solvates). They can be polymorphic solvates, which are very stable and difficult to desolvate, or pseudopolymorphic solvates, which readily lose their solvent without loss of crystal lattice structure, depending on the conditions of crystallisation.
- Co-crystals which are composed of the drug and another molecule (the coformer) to which it is usually hydrogen-bonded. The aim of forming co-crystals is to increase solubility, reduce hygroscopicity or alter the pH-solubility characteristics of the drug.

Biopharmaceutical importance of particle size

- Although most drugs are transported across the intestinal wall in their molecular form and absorbed into the systemic circulation, there is evidence showing that very small particles (in nanometre size range) can also be transported through enterocytes by pinocytosis.
- If the solubility of a drug substance is less than about 0.3% then the dissolution rate *in vivo* may be the rate-controlling step in absorption. The particle size of a drug is therefore of importance if the substance in question has a low solubility because the rate at which the drug dissolves is proportional to the surface area exposed to the

solvent (see the Noyes–Whitney equation, further) which increases as the particle size is reduced.

- Reduction of particle size below 0.1 μm, for example by milling, may increase the dissolution rate because these very small particles will interact more readily with solvent to produce higher degrees of solubility. For example, similar blood levels of griseofulvin were obtained with half the dose of micronised drug compared to non-micronised drug.
- Adverse side-effects of drugs can sometimes be reduced by manipulation of particle size. For example, increase of particle size of nitrofurantoin (as in Macrodantin) reduced the high incidence of nausea in patients that was observed after administration of tablets in which the drug was present as fine particulate material.
- The particle size of drugs administered by pulmonary delivery must be carefully controlled because only very fine particles are able to penetrate the alveolar regions of the respiratory tract (see **Chapter 8**).

Wetting of solid surfaces and powders

Spreading wetting

- The wetting of a solid when a liquid spreads over its surface is referred to as spreading wetting.
- The forces acting on a drop on the solid surface (*Figure 1.4a*) are represented by Young's equation:

$$\gamma_{S/A} = \gamma_{S/L} + \gamma_{L/A}\cos\theta$$

where $\gamma_{S/A}$ is the surface tension of the solid, $\gamma_{S/L}$ is the solid–liquid interfacial tension, $\gamma_{L/A}$ is the surface tension of the liquid and θ is the contact angle.

- The tendency for wetting is expressed by the spreading coefficient, S, as:

$$S = \gamma_{L/A}(\cos\theta - 1)$$

- For complete spreading of the liquid over the solid surface, S should have a zero or positive value.
- If the contact angle is larger than 0°, the term $(\cos\theta - 1)$ will be negative, as will the value of S.
- The condition for complete, spontaneous wetting is thus a zero value for the contact angle.

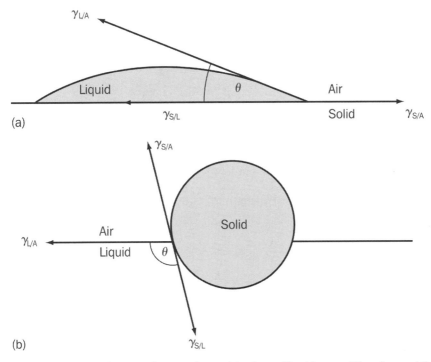

Figure 1.4: *Equilibrium between forces acting on (a) a drop of liquid on a solid surface and (b) a partially immersed solid.*

- A useful indicator of the wettability of a solid surface is its critical surface tension for spreading, γ_c.
  - This is determined from measurements of the contact angle θ of drops of a series of liquids of known surface tension when placed on a flat non-porous surface of the chosen solid.
  - Extrapolation of a plot of $\cos\theta$ against surface tension (a Zisman plot) to a value of $\cos\theta = 1$ (i.e. to $\theta = 0$) (see *Figure 1.5*) provides a value of γ_c.
  - Only those liquids or solutions having a surface tension less than γ_c will wet the surface, hence solids such as solid hydrocarbons and waxes that have a low critical surface tension will be wetted only by solutions of low surface tension. More polar solids such as those of nylon and cellulose have higher γ_c values and consequently are more easily wetted.
  - Human skin has a γ_c of 22–30 mN m^{-1} and it is usual to add surfactants to lotions for application to the skin to ensure adequate wetting.

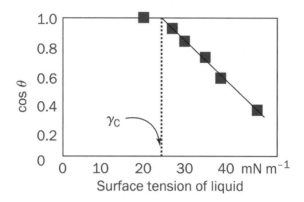

Figure 1.5: *Determination of critical surface tension for wetting, γ_c, from a plot of cosine contact angle against surface tension.*

Immersional wetting

- The wetting of a powder when it is initially immersed in a liquid is referred to as immersional wetting (once it has submerged, the process of spreading wetting becomes important).
- The effectiveness of immersional wetting may be related to the contact angle which the solid makes with the liquid–air interface (*Figure 1.4b*).
- Contact angles of greater than 90° indicate wetting problems, for example when compounds are formulated as suspensions.
- Examples of very hydrophobic (non-wetting) drugs include magnesium and aluminium stearates, salicylic acid, phenylbutazone and chloramphenicol palmitate.
- The normal method of improving wettability is by inclusion of surfactants in the formulation. The surfactants not only reduce $\gamma_{L/A}$ but also adsorb onto the surface of the powder, thus reducing $\gamma_{S/L}$. Both of these effects reduce the contact angle and improve the dispersibility of the powder.

Key points

- The wettability of a solid surface is described by the contact angle; complete wetting occurs when the contact angle is zero.
- The wetting of a powder when it is brought into contact with water is difficult if the contact angle is greater than 90°.

Dissolution of drugs

The rate of dissolution of solids is described by the Noyes-Whitney equation:

$$\frac{dw}{dt} = \frac{DA}{\delta}(c_s - c)$$

where dw/dt is the rate of increase of the amount of material in solution dissolving from a solid; c_s is the saturation solubility of the drug in solution in the diffusion layer; c is the concentration of the drug in the bulk solution; A is the area of the solvate particles exposed to the solvent; δ is the thickness of the diffusion layer; and D is the diffusion coefficient of the dissolved solute. *Figure 1.6* is a diagrammatic representation of dissolution from a solid particle into the gastrointestinal tract. The Noyes–Whitney equation predicts:

- a decrease of dissolution rate because of a decrease of D when the viscosity of the medium is increased
- an increase of dissolution rate if the particle size is reduced by micronisation because of an increase in A
- an increase of dissolution rate by agitation in the gut or in a flask because of a decrease in δ
- an increase of dissolution rate when the concentration of drug is decreased by intake of fluid, and by removal of drug by partition or absorption
- a change of dissolution rate when c_s is changed by alteration of pH (if the drug is a weak electrolyte).

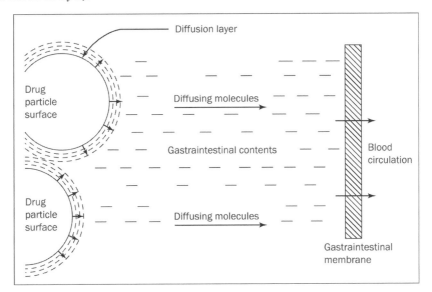

Figure 1.6: *Schematic diagram of dissolution from a solid surface.*

Sublimation and freeze drying

- The process by which solids pass directly from the solid phase to the vapour phase is referred to as sublimation.
- Sublimation forms the basis of the technique of freeze drying for the drying of thermolabile materials.
- In the process of freeze drying an aqueous solution of the heat-sensitive material is frozen and its pressure reduced to below the triple point (see *Figure 1.7*); a small amount of heat is then supplied to increase the temperature to the sublimation curve, at which the ice changes directly to vapour without passing through the liquid phase. Removal of water, i.e. drying, is therefore achieved at temperatures well below room temperature, so preventing decomposition of the thermolabile product.
- Sublimation can cause weight loss of some drugs when they are stored in the solid state. The rate of weight loss increases with temperature, according to the Clausius–Clapeyron equation.
- Sublimation of some toxic drugs during handling can present safety problems.

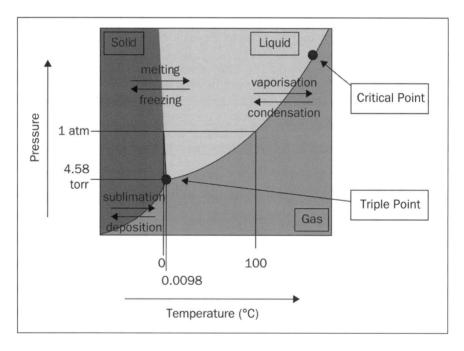

Figure 1.7: *Phase diagram of water (not to scale) showing the boundaries between liquid, solid and vapour phases.*

Solid solutions and dispersions

Solid solutions and dispersions are designed to improve the biopharmaceutical properties of drugs that are poorly soluble or difficult to wet by altering the crystallinity of the drug to increase its solubility and rate of solution and surrounding it intimately with water-soluble material.

Solid dispersions

- In solid dispersions the solute is dispersed as fine particles in another solid (referred to as the solvent) as, for example, in eutectic mixtures.
- In *Figure 1.8*, the melting temperature of mixtures of A and B is plotted against mixture composition. On addition of B to A or of A to B, melting points are reduced. At a particular composition the eutectic point is reached, the eutectic mixture (the composition at that point) having the lowest melting point of any mixture of A and B. When the mixture is cooled to below the eutectic temperature the remaining solution crystallises out, forming a microcrystalline mixture of pure A and pure B.
- This has obvious pharmaceutical possibilities. This method of obtaining microcrystalline dispersions for administration of drugs involves the formation of a eutectic mixture composed of drug and a substance readily soluble in water. On administration, the soluble carrier dissolves leaving a dispersion of the drug, which because of the reduction of its crystalline size (and hence an increase in surface area), rapidly dissolves.
- Examples of eutectic mixtures include griseofulvin–succinic acid, chloramphenicol–urea, sulfathiazole–urea, and niacinamide–ascorbic acid.

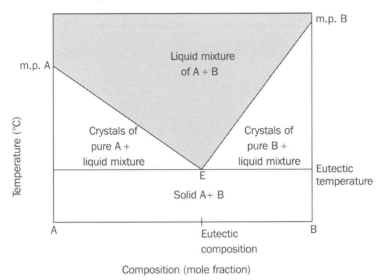

Figure 1.8: *Phase diagram showing eutectic point, E.*

Solid solutions

- Solid solutions comprise molecules (rather than fine particles) of the drug dispersed in a very soluble solid solvent (the carrier).
- Because the drug is in molecular form the dissolution rate is determined solely by that of the carrier and can be increased by up to several orders of magnitude. For example, a solid solution of griseofulvin–succinic acid dissolves 6–7 times faster than pure griseofulvin and significantly faster than its eutectic mixture.
- Solid solutions are also termed mixed crystals because the two components crystallise together in a homogeneous one-phase system. They should, however, be distinguished from co-crystals (see before) which are single crystalline forms consisting of two types of molecule.
- In a development of these solid solution formulations, carriers were used in an amorphous state resulting in improved dissolution characteristics.
- In an amorphous solid solution, the drug molecules are dispersed irregularly within the amorphous solid rather than locating regularly within the crystal lattice of the carrier. Polymers such as polyvinylpyrrolidone (PVP), polyethylene glycol (PEG) and various cellulose derivatives have been utilised as amorphous carriers.
- More recently, it has been shown that the dissolution profile can be improved if the carrier has surface active or self-emulsifying properties leading to the development of solid dispersions containing a surfactant carrier or a mixture of amorphous polymers and surfactants as carriers.

Memory maps

Important factors relating to the solid state of crystalline drugs

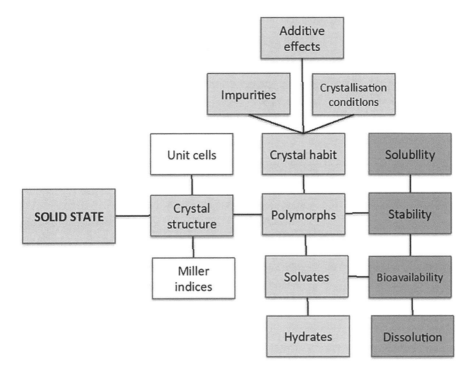

Importance of particle size of solid drugs

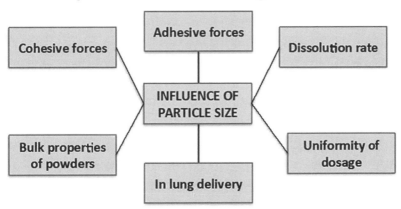

Formulation issues with crystalline drugs

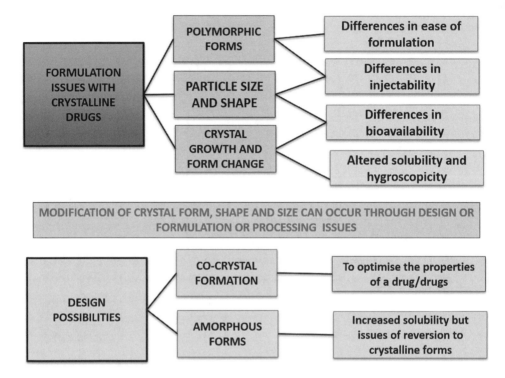

Questions

1. Which unit cell is characterised by the following parameters?

$$\begin{cases} a \neq b \neq c \\ \alpha = \gamma = 90^{\circ} \\ \beta \neq 90^{\circ} \end{cases}$$

   A: Triclinic
   B: Monoclinic
   C: Orthorhombic
   D: Tetragonal
   E: Hexagonal

2. From the list below, select which of the statements may be correctly applied to an orthorhombic unit cell.
   A: The angles $\alpha = \beta = \gamma = 90^{\circ}$
   B: The angles $\alpha \neq \beta \neq \gamma \neq 90^{\circ}$
   C: The angles $\alpha = \beta = 90^{\circ}$; $\gamma = 120^{\circ}$
   D: The lengths $a \neq b \neq c$
   E: The lengths $a = b \neq c$

3. The Miller indices of a plane which intersects the a, b and c axes at a = 3, b = 2 and c = ∞ are:
   A: 320
   B: 460
   C: 230
   D: $\bar{2}30$
   E: $\bar{3}20$

4. From the list below, select which of the statements may be correctly applied to a pseudopolymorphic solvate.
   A: The solvent is strongly bound
   B: Desolvation does not destroy the crystal lattice
   C: Desolvation leads to collapse and recrystallisation in a different form
   D: The solvent is easily removed
   E: The solvent plays a key role in holding together the crystal lattice

5. From the list below, select which of the statements may be correctly applied to the wetting of a flat solid surface by a liquid.
   A: The wetting is referred to as spreading wetting
   B: Complete, spontaneous wetting of the surface will occur when the contact angle is greater than 90°
   C: The condition for spontaneous wetting is a zero contact angle
   D: Spreading occurs more readily if the surface tension of the liquid is high
   E: Spreading will occur if the spreading coefficient is negative

6. **From the list below, select which of the statements may be correctly applied to the wetting of a powder when immersed in a liquid.**
   A: Complete, spontaneous wetting of the powder will occur when the contact angle is greater than 90°
   B: Wetting will only occur if the contact angle is zero
   C: The wetting is referred to as spreading wetting
   D: Wettability may be improved by reducing the surface tension of the liquid
   E: Wettability may be improved by reducing the hydrophobicity of the solid surface

7. **Indicate which of the following statements are true. The Noyes–Whitney equation predicts an increase of dissolution rate when:**
   A: The viscosity of the medium is increased
   B: The particle size is reduced
   C: The liquid medium is agitated
   D: The saturated solubility of solid is decreased
   E: Dissolved drug is removed from solution

8. **Two components A and B (the melting point of component A is lower than that of component B) form solid dispersions. Indicate which of the following statements are true.**
   A: Below the eutectic temperature the system consists of microcrystals of A dissolved in liquid B
   B: Below the eutectic temperature the system consists of microcrystals of B dissolved in liquid A
   C: Below the eutectic temperature the system consists of a mixture of microcrystals of A and B in solid form
   D: On cooling a solution of A and B, which is richer in A than B, crystals of B will appear
   E: The eutectic mixture has the lowest melting point of any mixture

CHAPTER 2

Solid dosage forms

LEARNING OBJECTIVES

Upon completion of this chapter you should be able to:
- describe the many physicochemical factors which come into play during the formulation and production of tablets and capsules
- outline the role of the excipients incorporated in typical tablet and capsule formulations
- understand the influence of particle size on the flow, mixing and compression of a powder during tablet manufacture
- outline the mechanisms of bonding of particles during both wet and dry granulation
- outline the events that occur in the process of tablet compression
- outline the reasons for applying coatings to tablets and the methods by which this is achieved using film coating and dry coating techniques
- outline the processes for the formulation and manufacture of hard and soft capsules.

Formulation of tablets and capsules

- Oral dosage forms are the predominant means of administering medication and by far the most common solid dosage forms for oral administration are tablets.
- Many of the processes involved in the formulation and manufacture of tablets are common to other solid dosage forms, particularly capsules which may be filled with powders, granules and tablets.
- Most tablets are manufactured by compression of granules prepared from a powder mix: a typical tableting process involves the following stages:
  - blending of the active drug with excipients in a powder mix
  - wet granulation of the powder mix
  - drying
  - milling
  - blending
  - compression into tablets
  - coating the tablets.
- When it is necessary to avoid contact with water or other solvents an alternative method in which the powder mix itself is directly compressed into tablets may be preferable.

Excipients

Fillers
- Added to increase the bulk volume of the powder.
- Are inert, inexpensive materials with an acceptable taste.

- Should have good compression properties.
- Examples include:
  - Lactose used in its anhydrous crystalline form when wet and dry granulation processes are employed and as an amorphous form produced by spray drying when direct compaction methods of tableting are employed. Other sugars, particularly mannitol, are used as fillers in chewable tablets because of their sweet taste.
  - Microcrystalline cellulose is available in several grades with different degrees of crystallinity and physicochemical properties.
  - Dicalcium phosphate is water-insoluble but easily wetted by water. Used in fine powder form when granulation processes are involved and as an aggregated form when tablets are produced by direct compression.

Disintegrants

- Included in tablet formulations to ensure that the tablet breaks down into smaller fragments when in contact with liquids.
- Main mechanisms of disintegrant action:
  - may increase the porosity and wettability of the tablet allowing liquid to readily penetrate the matrix and cause its breakdown, e.g. a surface active agent, or
  - may swell in the presence of liquid so increasing the pressure within the matrix resulting in its disintegration. The most widely used examples are starch, or modified starches such as sodium starch glycolate or pregelatinised starch, and modified celluloses such as cross-linked sodium carboxymethylcellulose.
- The disintegrant used in effervescent tablets is usually a bicarbonate or carbonate salt which liberates carbon dioxide in an acidic aqueous environment and causes the rapid disruption of the tablet matrix.

Binders

- Binders are added to increase the mechanical strength of the tablet. They may be:
  - added as a dry powder to the powder mix and subsequently dissolve in the liquid added during the granulation process;
  - added as a solution during granulation (solution binders); or
  - mixed as a dry powder with the other excipients before compaction (dry binders).
- Solution binders are usually polymers such as polyvinylpyrrolidone and hydroxypropylcellulose; dry binders include microcrystalline cellulose and crosslinked polyvinylpyrrolidone.

Lubricants

- Lubricants are added to almost all tablet formulations and act by reducing the friction between the tablet surface and the face of the die during the ejection of the tablet.
- Without adequate lubrication, capping may occur or tablets having pitted or scratched surfaces may be produced leading to rejection of the batch.
- They may be either:

— insoluble, particulate solids such as stearic acid or stearic acid salts, e.g. magnesium stearate, or
— soluble lubricants such as polyethylene glycols or sodium lauryl sulfate.

Glidants

- Glidants are included in the formulation to improve the flow of the powder by reducing the friction between the powder and hopper surface and also between the particles themselves.
- Glidant particles need to be hydrophobic and sufficiently small to locate at the surfaces of the particles or granules.
- Talc (hydrated magnesium silicate, $Mg_3Si_4O_{10}(OH)_2$) has traditionally been used as a glidant but is now usually replaced by colloidal silicon dioxide which typically has a particle size of <15 nm.

Flavouring agents and colourants

- Flavouring and sweetening agents are added to the formulation to give the tablet a more pleasant taste, particularly when the tablet contains a bitter tasting drug or when the tablet is a chewable tablet. Typical sweetening agents include sorbitol, glycerol, sucrose and aspartame. The calorie free molecule sucralose is now available for pharmaceutical use.
- Tablets are coloured as a means of identification and/or to improve their appearance, particularly if the drug itself is coloured giving an otherwise speckled appearance to the tablet. The required colour can be incorporated into the film coating or can be included in the formulation prior to compaction.

Tip

The active ingredient constitutes often only a small fraction of the total weight of the tablet. Other ingredients are added to increase the bulk of the tablet, to ensure that it can be successfully manufactured, and will break up satisfactorily after administration.

Key points

Tablet formulations typically contain several ingredients to optimise their manufacture and disintegration including:
- fillers to add bulk to low dose tablets;
- binders to enhance the cohesion of particles of the powder mix during granulation and compression;
- disintegrants to aid the break-up of tablets in contact with aqueous media;
- lubricants to reduce friction between particles during compression;
- glidants to enhance the flow of powders;
- flavouring agents to give the tablet a more pleasant taste, and colourants to aid identification and improve the appearance of tablets.

Flow properties of powder mix

- It is important that powders or granules are able to flow freely into storage containers or hoppers of tablet- and capsule-filling equipment so that a uniform packing of the particles and hence a uniform tablet or capsule weight is achieved.
- Uneven particle flow can increase the possibility of the jamming of particles as they flow out of the hopper into the tablet die and may also cause excessive entrapment of air within the powders which may promote capping of tablets.
- Particle size influences the flow properties of powders mainly through its effect on the cohesivity of the particles and the adhesivity of the particles to a surface in contact with the powder.
- Cohesive and adhesive forces between particles arise from short-range van der Waals forces, electrostatic forces from frictional charging during handling, or surface tensional forces between adsorbed liquid layers on the particle surface. These are all related to the surface area of the particle and increase as the particle size decreases, as follows:
  - particles larger than about 250 μm are usually relatively free flowing
  - flow problems are likely to be observed when the size falls below 100 μm because of cohesion
  - very fine particles (below 10 μm) are usually extremely cohesive and have a high resistance to flow.
- Flow properties are also influenced by particle shape: particles of similar sizes but different shapes can have markedly different flow properties because of differences in interparticulate contact areas. Spherical particles for example have minimum area of contact with each other compared to more irregular particles and as a consequence have better flow properties.
- The extent of cohesion of particles or the adhesion of particles to a substrate can be determined by a variety of experimental methods including the measurement of the following:
  - The angle of repose assumed by a cone-like pile of the powder formed on a horizontal surface when the powder is allowed to fall under gravity from a nozzle. An angle of about 25° is indicative of a powder with suitable flow properties for use in manufacturing processes.
  - The shear strength, which is the resistance to flow of a powder bed caused by cohesional or adhesional forces. This can be determined using a simple shear cell such as the Jenike shear cell shown in *Figure 2.1*. Shear stress measured using a range of applied normal forces is plotted against the applied normal stress. Extrapolation back to zero normal force gives a value for the cohesion of the powder; the higher the intercept, the higher is the cohesion, a graph for a completely non-cohesive powder would pass through the origin.
- The bulk density of the powder relates particle flow to packing characteristics; the more tightly a powder is able to pack the more resistant it will be to flow. Packing volume may be simply measured by mechanically tapping a measuring cylinder containing a mass, m, of the powder until it decreases from an initial value, V_0, to a stable final volume, V_f,

as the void space decreases. The initial bulk density (also referred to as the fluff density), $\rho B_{min} = m/V_0$, and final bulk density (also called the tapped density), $\rho B_{max} = m/V_f$. The cohesivity of the powder is given by the Hausner ratio, $(\rho B_{max}/\rho B_{min}) \times 100$. Ratios of less than 1.25 are indicative of low cohesive forces and good flow characteristics. Alternatively, the Carr's index or % compressibility may be derived from bulk densities using

$$\% \text{ compressibility} = \frac{\rho B_{max} - \rho B_{min}}{\rho B_{max}} \times 100$$

- The lower the value of percentage compressibility the better the flow properties, values above about 25 are indicative of poor flow characteristics.
- Measurement of the powder flow through an orifice is the most direct method of assessing flow rate. Complete emptying of a hopper filled with powder is timed and the mass flow rate is calculated by dividing the mass of discharged powder by this time. Flow rates obtained are not absolute values because they depend on, for example, the orifice diameter, nevertheless they are useful in comparing different powders using the same hopper.

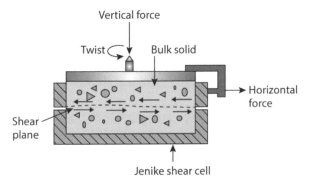

Figure 2.1: *The Jenike cell for measurement of the shear strength of a powder. A vertical (normal) force is applied to the lid of the assembled cell by the application of weights and a shear force is applied by the slow, steady movement of the upper half of the cell.*

Tip

Tablets are manufactured commercially by compressing the powder mix in a die by the action of a punch under high pressure and at high speed. The powder mix is not, however, weighed into the die but flows into it from a hopper. It is therefore essential that there is an even flow of powder and this is achieved by careful control of the properties of the powder and in particular the particle size.

Key points

- Particle size has an important influence on the flow properties of powders and granules; uneven flow can cause non-uniform tablet weight, jamming in tablet hoppers, and entrapment of air causing tablet capping.
- Particles larger than about 250 μm are usually relatively free flowing but flow problems are likely to be observed when the size falls below 100 μm because of cohesion. Very fine particles (below 10 μm) are usually extremely cohesive and have a high resistance to flow.
- The extent of cohesion of particles or the adhesion of particles to a substrate can be determined by a variety of experimental methods including indirect methods such as the measurement of the angle of repose, the shear strength, and the bulk density, and more direct measurements of flow through an orifice.
- The cohesivity of the powder may be expressed using the Hausner ratio or the Carr's index (percentage compressibility). Hausner ratios of less than 1.25 are indicative of low cohesive forces, whereas values greater than 1.5 are obtained when the powder has poorer flow characteristics; the lower the Carr's index the better the flow properties, values above about 25 are indicative of poor flow characteristics.

Particle size reduction

- It is unlikely that raw material will be of a suitable particle size specification for use as an excipient in tablet manufacture and milling of the material is usually required.
- The mechanism by which particle size reduction (comminution) occurs in non-crystalline material is through the propagation of localised cracks in the material produced during the comminution process through regions of the material that have most flaws and discontinuities, setting up new cracks by a cascade effect. Crack propagation is rapid causing almost instantaneous fracture of the material.
- Comminution is a most inefficient process with only a very small percentage (possibly as low as 2%) of the energy input actually involved in the process of size reduction, the remainder is lost through elastic deformation of the particles, friction between particles themselves and between particles and the walls of the equipment, and the usual energy losses associated with machine processes-heat, vibration, sound etc.
- A variety of industrial equipment is available for particle size reduction, the selection largely depending on the initial particle size and the degree of size reduction required:
  - Cutting methods are suitable when coarse particles are involved, for example in reducing the size of granules prior to tabletting. In cutter mills, size reduction is achieved by a series of rotating knives which act against stationary knives in the metal casing of the mill at a clearance of a few millimetres, so fracturing the particles (see *Figure 2.2a*).
  - Compression methods, for example in roller mills, achieve a similar degree of size reduction. Here the particles are compressed between two horizontal rollers which can rotate about their long axes. One of the rollers is driven directly, the other rotates by friction as the powder is passed through the narrow gap between them.

- Impact methods are considered more suitable in cases where finer particles of narrower size distributions are required. Several designs of mill cause size reduction by impact, including hammer mills in which size reduction is achieved by a series of swinging hammers hinged on a central rotating shaft, and vibration mills in which size reduction is achieved by the vibration of stainless steel or porcelain balls.
- A combination of impact and attrition methods is generally used to achieve the finest particles. The two main types of mill are the ball mill and the fluid energy mill. Particles in the ball mill are subjected to impact forces through their collision with the balls during the rotation of the mill and shear forces (attrition forces) as they move between the cascading balls which are travelling at different velocities (see *Figure 2.2b*). Impact, and to a lesser extent attrition, forces in the fluid energy mill arise from repeated high momentum collisions of the particles with each other and with the walls as they travel through a region of high turbulence created in the mill.

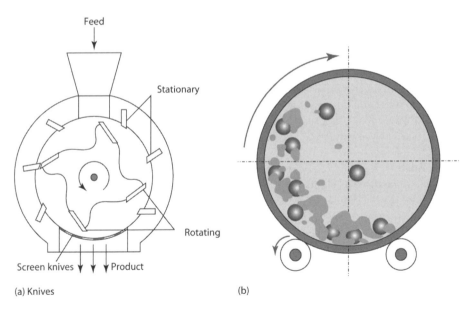

Figure 2.2: *Schematic representation of (a) cutter mill and (b) ball mill.*

Key points

- Particle size reduction (comminution) in non-crystalline materials occurs by the propagation of localised cracks in the material causing almost instantaneous fracture of the material.
- Comminution can be achieved industrially using:
  - cutting methods using cutter mills
  - compression methods using roller mills
  - impact methods to produce finer particles using hammer mills and vibration mills
  - a combination of impact and attrition methods for the finest particles using ball mills and fluid energy mills.

Powder mixing and demixing

Mixing

- The process of mixing the powdered excipients and drug(s) is a complex process involving three main mechanisms:
  - Convective mixing is the movement of groups of particles from one region to another rather than the movement of individual particles within the mix.
  - Shear mixing occurs when layers of material moving at different speeds flow over each other and mix at the layer interface.
  - Diffusive mixing in which there is movement of individual particles through voids created as a consequence of expansion of the powder bed during some types of mixing.
- The efficiency of mixing is influenced by the flow characteristics of the particles and their relative sizes, and the type of mixer and processing conditions. The contribution of each of the three mechanisms of mixing varies with the design of the mixer. The principle types of industrial mixers are:
  - Planetary bowl mixers (*Figure 2.3*) in which the powders are mixed in a bowl by a rotating blade attached to a rotating shaft which is offset rather than centrally placed so that the blade rotates around the circumference of the bowl as well as on its own axis. The main mixing mechanism is convective.
  - Tumbling drum mixers (*Figure 2.3*) in which the drum containing the powders is attached to a drive shaft and rotated by the action of a motor. Shear mixing occurs as layers within the powder move relative to each other. In addition, the powder bed expands or dilates as it tumbles, allowing particles to move downwards under gravity, and diffusive mixing occurs.
  - High-speed mixers which have excellent powder-mixing properties and have the added advantage that the mixing process can be followed by wet granulation in the same equipment if required. The powders are contained in a mixing bowl on the bottom of which is an impeller capable of high-speed rotation. During the mixing process the material is thrown towards the wall of the bowl by centrifugal force and then forced upwards before finally falling down to the centre of the

mixer. Expansion of the powder bed during this highly efficient mixing process allows diffusive mixing to occur.
- With each type of mixer, the processing variables, particularly the mixer load and the speed and time of mixing, are carefully controlled to ensure that a homogeneous mixture is produced, that is, one in which the concentration of each component in each region of the mixture is identical.

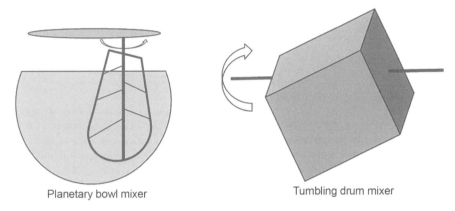

Planetary bowl mixer   Tumbling drum mixer

Figure 2.3: *Diagrammatic representations of planetary bowl and tumbling drum mixers.*

Demixing
- It is important that the particle size of the powder mix is controlled and unaffected by processing so that consistent blood levels and absorption of the drug are achieved.
- Separation of the components of the mixture is referred to as segregation or demixing. It usually arises because of large differences in the characteristics of the components of the mixture, particularly variations in the size, shape, density and surface properties of the particles. Such events can cause variability in the drug dose between individual dosage units.
- The two main types of demixing are:
  - trajectory segregation, in which particles with similar characteristics congregate together, and
  - percolation segregation, in which smaller particles fall through voids created when the powder bed dilates on being disturbed by, for example, vibration or pouring.
- Since demixing arises mainly as a consequence of differences in particle size and density, attempts may be made to achieve a narrower size range of ingredients, for example:
  - by sieving the ingredients to remove clumps or fines,
  - by milling components to reduce their size range, or
  - by controlled crystallisation of the ingredients to give components of similar size range.

- A mixture containing both very small and very much larger particles, contrary to expectations does not readily segregate. This is because the very small particles tend to adsorb onto the larger particles which act as 'carrier particles', resulting in minimal segregation and good flow properties. This phenomenon, referred to as ordered mixing, is utilised, for example, in the production of dry powder inhalations for delivery to the lungs. Here the drug needs to be in a micronised form to reach its site of action and is usually formulated in combination with lactose as the carrier particle to which it becomes adsorbed.

Key points

- The process of mixing the powdered excipients and drug(s) is a complex process involving three main mechanisms:
  - Convective mixing refers to the movement of groups of particles from one region to another and is the predominant type of mixing in planetary bowl mixers.
  - Shear mixing occurs when layers of material moving at different speeds flow over each other and mix at the layer interface; it occurs in tumbling drum mixers.
  - Diffusive mixing involves the movement of individual particles through voids created as a consequence of expansion of the powder bed and occurs in high speed mixers and to some extent in tumbling drum mixers.
- The two main types of demixing are trajectory segregation, in which particles with similar characteristics congregate together, and percolation segregation, in which smaller particles fall through voids created when the powder bed dilates on being disturbed by, for example, vibration or pouring.
- Demixing may be minimised by sieving the ingredients to remove clumps or fines; by milling components to reduce their size range; or by controlled crystallisation of the ingredients to give components of similar size range.

Granulation

- Granulation is the process whereby the dry powder mix of active ingredient and suitable excipients (excluding the lubricant) are aggregated into larger particles either by mixing with a suitable fluid (wet granulation) or by the application of high stresses without solvent addition (dry granulation).
- The granules may constitute a dosage form in their own right, in which case they are usually produced with a size range of between 1 and 4 mm, but more usually they are an intermediate stage in the production of tablets or capsules and are between 0.2 and 0.5 mm in size.
- There are several reasons for the use of granules in the production of tablets:
  - To prevent demixing (segregation) of the constituents of the powder mix during tablet manufacture leading to an unacceptable variation of composition within a batch of tablets. Each granule formed in the granulation process will contain roughly the same proportion of each ingredient so producing tablets of a uniform composition.

- To produce particles of an appropriate size to avoid potential problems arising from the poor flow properties associated with small, irregularly shaped particles ('jamming').
- To improve the compaction properties. In general, granules are more easily compacted than powder mixes mainly because of the presence of binder on the granule surface which improves the adhesion between granules and leads to a stronger tablet on compression.
- To minimise dust production during handling, particularly important when toxic drugs are being processed.

Wet granulation

The essential stages in the wet granulation process are as follows:

1. A suitable liquid, usually water, ethanol or isopropanol (or mixtures of these solvents), is added to the powder mixture. To ensure efficient binding of the granules, a binder is either included in the powder mix or dissolved in the granulating fluid. The wet mass is forced through a sieve producing granules.
1. The wet granules are dried, milled to break down large agglomerates, screened to remove fine material and finally mixed with the lubricant in readiness for the compression process.

Stage 1: Granule formation

- In most modern industrial processes the powder mixing and wet granulation stages are carried out in a single operation using a high speed mixer/granulator. This equipment is based on the planetary bowl mixer shown diagrammatically in *Figure 2.3*. After mixing the dry ingredients, the granulating fluid is added and mixed with the impeller blades to form a wet mass, which is then broken up into granules by the action of a rotating chopper located in the mixer bowl. Once granules of a suitable size have been produced, they are passed through a wire mesh (screen) to break down any large agglomerates and transferred to the drying equipment.
- An alternative technique employs a fluidised bed granulator. The process is shown diagrammatically and explained in *Figure 2.4*.
- For certain applications, particularly where it is required to control the release rate, spherical particles of uniform size (pellets) are required which can be filled into hard gelatin capsule shells or compacted into tablets. These are produced by extrusion or spheronisation. In this process:
  - Granulation fluid is added to the mix of drug and excipients using a mixer/granulator, but then transferred to extrusion equipment designed to produce rod-shaped particles of uniform diameter.
  - The extrudate particles which emerge break at similar lengths under their own weight into the rod-shaped particles of uniform size.
  - If spherical particles are required, the rods are transferred to a spheroniser which consists of a bowl having a rapidly rotating bottom plate which rounds off the particles by frictional forces as they collide with each other.

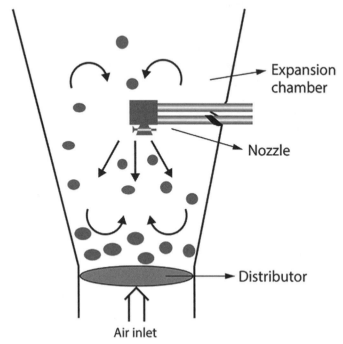

Figure 2.4: *Diagrammatic representation of a fluidised bed granulator. The dry powders are suspended (fluidised) by a vertical stream of warm air entering the base of the equipment and the granulating fluid sprayed through a nozzle located near the top on to the dispersed particles. When granules of the required size have been formed, the spraying process is terminated but the air flow is continued to dry the suspended granules.*

Stage 2: Drying and milling

The objective of these two unit operations is to produce dried granules of a size suitable for processing into tablets by compression or for filling into hard gelatin capsules.

Drying

A variety of equipment is available for drying the wet granules; the choice of method depends on factors including the stability of the material to heat, the nature of the liquid to be removed and the physical characteristics of the material.

- In shelf or tray driers heat transfer is mainly by conduction; the wet granules are placed on a series of horizontal shelves, hot air is passed across the surface of the granules and moisture is removed through an outlet.
- Greater efficiency is achieved if drying is carried out using a specially-designed oven connected via a condenser (to remove the moisture released) to a vacuum pump. The use of vacuum ovens is mainly restricted to the drying of thermolabile materials as much lower drying temperatures can be used, or those subject to oxidation since little air is present.

- When granulation is carried out in a fluidsed bed granulator the granules are usually dried as part of the process using a current of warm air as described before (see *Figure 2.4*); efficient convective drying is achieved because of the excellent transfer of heat to the suspended granules and removal of moisture released. Because of the efficiency of the process drying times are generally short, which is not only an economic advantage but also minimises the exposure of thermolabile material to high temperatures.

One of the problems associated with granule drying is that of solvent migration:

- The movement of solvent either through individual granules (intragranular migration) or from granule to granule (intergranular migration) during the drying process, carries with it any dissolved solutes to the surface of the granule or the granule bed where they are deposited when the solvent evaporates.
- As a consequence, there may be variability in the concentration of both drug and excipients leading to an unacceptable variation of drug content in the finished tablets.
- Intergranular migration is a particular problem when drying is carried out in static beds, as in tray driers, and leads to a deposit of solute on the top surface of the bed. Contact between granules is minimised in fluidised bed driers and hence intergranular migration is less of a problem although intragranular migration may still occur.

Milling

- The main reason for milling the granules is to achieve the particle size required for smooth flow of the dried granules into the tablet die, which is an important factor affecting the uniformity of weight of the tablet.
- The chosen size of the granules is determined by the size of the tablet; smaller tablets require proportionally smaller granules for efficient filling of the smaller dies used for their manufacture.
- Particle size reduction may be achieved by, for example, a cutter mill as described before (see *Figure 2.2*).
- Before final compaction into tablets, the granules are dry mixed with lubricant, which as discussed above, reduces the friction between the tablet surface and the face of the die during the ejection of the tablet from the die. Other excipients such as glidants, and disintegrants may be added at this stage.

Bonding mechanisms in wet granulation

Several bonding mechanisms operate during the various stages from the initial cohesion of the particles to the final formation of granules, as follows:

- Adhesion and cohesion forces in the stationary films between particles. The presence of the thin stationary liquid film around and between the powder particles brings them closer together and increases the area of contact between them. As a consequence, there will be increased particle cohesion and small agglomerates are formed.
- Interfacial forces in mobile liquid films within the granules. The quantity of granulating fluid added to the dry powder mix is usually more than that required to coat the powder particles and the excess forms mobile films between the particles

within the granules. The forces acting between particles are dependent on the amount of water present in the mix:

— when insufficient fluid has been added to displace all of the air originally present, the particles within the granules are held together by surface tension forces at the air/liquid interface of liquid bridges formed between the particles; this is referred to as the pendular state (see *Figure 2.5a*);

— in the presence of larger amounts of fluid, the liquid bridges become thicker, (the funicular state, *Figure 2.5b*) and finally,

— the capillary state (*Figure 2.5c*) is reached when the amount of water is sufficient to displace all of the entrapped air or this has been removed by an extended mixing process. The particles are now held together by capillary forces at the liquid/air interface which now exists only at the granule surface. These small agglomerates grow to form larger granules either by addition of single particles via pendular bridges or by combining together to form larger units, which become reshaped during the mixing process;

— further addition of water (overwetting) and continued agitation can produce large granules (depicted in *Figure 2.5d*) that are unsuitable for pharmaceutical use, mainly because individual granules are not produced on drying, but also because of problems of tablet disintegration and dissolution due to an excessive amount of binder.

● Solid bridge formation between particles. A binder is usually dissolved in the granulating fluid which, during the drying process, solidifies the liquid bridges so binding the particles together to form a granule with suitable mechanical strength for processing into tablets or capsules (see *Figure 2.6*). As discussed above, binders are usually polymeric (e.g. polyvinylpyrrolidone and hydroxypropylcellulose) and the solid bridges resemble a polymeric network holding the particles together in the granule. In some instances, the solvent used for granulation may partially dissolve one of the powdered excipients, which then crystallises out during drying and acts as a hardening agent.

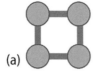 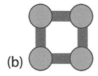 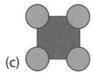 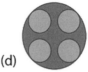

(a)   (b)   (c)   (d)

Figure 2.5: *Diagrammatic representation of interfacial forces between granules during granulation showing: (a) pendular; (b) funicular; (c) capillary; and (d) overwetted states.*

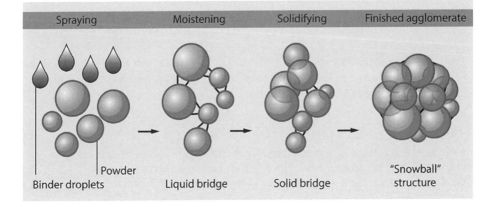

| Spraying | Moistening | Solidifying | Finished agglomerate |

Powder

Binder droplets | Liquid bridge | Solid bridge | "Snowball" structure

Figure 2.6: *Processes occurring in wet granulation, using a liquid binder that forms liquid bridges between the particles, which then solidify on drying to provide a quasi-spherical granule suitable for processing.*

Dry granulation

- In the process of dry granulation the powder mix is converted to granules by the application of high pressure.
- Unlike wet granulation, no solvent is added to the powder, so avoiding issues with chemical degradation or solubility of drug in the granulation fluid, and consequently heating to remove solvent is not necessary, which is an advantage if the active ingredients are thermolabile.
- Despite these potential advantages, dry granulation is not as widely used as wet granulation and has, to some extent, been superseded by direct compression methods, as discussed in the following section.
- There are two stages involved in dry granulation:
  1. Compression of the powder into a compact. This may be carried out either by slugging or by roller compaction. In the slugging technique large tablets (usually about 25 mm diameter) are produced in a tableting press capable of applying a high stress. In roller compaction the powder is fed via a hopper on to a moving belt to pass between two rollers rotating in opposite directions, which compress the powder into a thin sheet.
  2. Milling to produce the granules. Conventional milling equipment is employed to breakdown the tablet or compressed sheet into granules of the required size which are then mixed with lubricant ready for compression into tablets.

Bonding mechanisms in dry granulation

Three types of particle-particle interaction may be involved in the dry granulation process:

- Increased van der Waals interactions between particles of the powder mix as a consequence of the high stresses applied in this method which forces them into close contact. This is a major contributor to the overall particle-particle attraction.

- Electrostatic forces between powder particles contribute to the initial cohesion of the particles.
- Partial melting of low melting point excipients of the powder mix may occur as a result of the high shear stresses involved in compression; solidification on cooling may increase the interaction between particles.

Tip

Most tablets are made by the compression of granules prepared from the powder mix rather than the powder itself. Granulation minimises separation of the constituents of the mix and improves the flow and compaction properties.

Key points

- Granulation is the process whereby the dry powder mix is aggregated into larger particles. It is carried out to prevent segregation of the constituents of the powder mix, to enhance the flow properties of the mix, to improve the compaction properties, and to minimise dust production during handling.
- There are two types of granulation: wet granulation in which a solvent is added to the powder mix to aggregate the particles, and dry granulation in which a high stress is applied to form granules without adding solvent.
- Wet granulation may be performed using:
  - a high speed mixer/granulator or a fluidised bed granulator;
  - for certain applications, uniformly sized pellets are produced using extrusion or spheronisation techniques.
- There are two stages involved in dry granulation:
  - Compression of the powder into large tablets by slugging under high stress, or compression of the powder into thin films by roller compaction.
  - Milling the tablets or films to produce granules of the required size which are then mixed with lubricant ready for compression into tablets.
- The bonding mechanisms which operate during the two types of granulation are as follows:
  - Wet granulation. The types of bonds involved include adhesion and cohesion forces in the stationary films between particles; interfacial forces in mobile liquid films within the granules; formation of solid bridges between particles.
  - Dry granulation. Cohesion of the particles of the powder mix in the dry granulation process is mainly due to van der Waals interactions and electrostatic forces, but increased interaction may arise from the partial melting and subsequent solidification of low melting point excipients.

Tablet manufacture

The compression process

- Tablets may be manufactured by two processes:
  - by forming granules and compressing these into tablets in the die of the tablet press (most usual method), or
  - by a direct compression method which involves compressing the powder mix itself without forming granules.
- The direct compression method has the advantages that:
  - fewer steps are involved making this a less expensive process, and
  - no water or other solvents are used, which is an advantage when the excipients or drugs are susceptible to hydrolysis (or solvolysis).
- However, there are many potential problems associated with the direct compression method:
  - The excipients have usually to be specially processed and their physical properties such as morphology, particle size and density, should be similar to avoid demixing.
  - The tablets produced by this method tend to be softer than those formed by compression of granules and are consequently more difficult to film-coat.
  - It is not always possible to manipulate the properties of the drug to be suitable for successful direct compression; this may cause problems if the drug is present in amounts exceeding about 10% of the final formulation.
  - Direct compression is not usually suitable for the manufacture of coloured tablets because of the mottled appearance of the resulting tablet.
- The three stages of basic tablet formation are shown in *Figure 2.7*:
  1. A measured amount of granules/powder is filled into the tablet die under gravity from the hopper shoe which moves backwards and forwards over the top of the die.
  2. Tablets are formed by the action of two punches; the lower punch seals the bottom of the die and the upper punch descends to compact the granules (or powder) under high pressure.
  3. The tablet is ejected as the lower punch is pushed upwards and is pushed away by the hopper shoe, which then refills the die to repeat the operation. You can see an animation showing this process at *https://www.youtube.com/watch?v=g4rrGMJqEdk*.
- High speed tablet manufacture is achieved using rotary presses operating with a large number of dies and sets of punches. You can see a high speed tablet machine in action at *https://www.youtube.com/watch?v=oXEKVuucxbg*. Such machines are capable of producing 10 000 tablets per min.
- A common problem that occurs during ejection of the tablets is the mechanical splitting of the tablets. This is referred to as capping, when the top of the tablet is fractured, and lamination when fracture occurs in the body of the tablet. This defect can be a consequence of the application of excessive stress during compression or an intricate punch geometry.

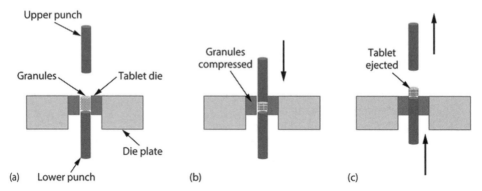

Figure 2.7: *Events occurring in the manufacture of tablets in a tablet press: (a) measured amount of granules/powder filled into tablet die from shoe; (b) granules compressed into tablet as upper punch descends; and (c) tablet ejected as lower punch is pushed upwards.*

Compression forces

The particles of drug and excipients are subject to changing forces, often at high speed, during the manufacturing process, as follows:

1. Transitional repacking. After application of the initial stress as the upper punch descends into the die, there is a small movement of the granules as they rearrange within the space between the two punches. In the direct compression process the extent of the rearrangement is usually greater and depends on the size of the particles and the frictional forces between them.

2. Deformation under the applied stress. At a certain load, the granules can no longer continue to rearrange because of reduced space and an increase of interparticulate friction. Reduction of the volume of the die contents is now associated with changes in the shape of the particles, by:

   — Elastic deformation: this is reversible, i.e. the particles can regain their shape when the loading is removed. The loading applied in tablet manufacture is generally greater than that required for elastic deformation to avoid the possibility of tablet failure associated with low stress levels.

   — Plastic deformation: this results in a permanent change of particle shape. Successful achievement of plastic deformation necessitates the inclusion of excipients that can themselves undergo plastic deformation, otherwise the quality of the compressed tablet will be adversely affected. Following plastic deformation, the granules retain their structure, but the applied stress causes changes in both granule shape and porosity because of the movement of individual particles within the granule.

   — Particle fragmentation: this is an additional type of deformation when tablets are produced by the direct compression method. In this, the intraparticle bonds are broken and the particle is fractured into a number of smaller discrete particles, which repack to further reduce the volume of the powder bed. These smaller particles may then undergo further deformation with increase of the applied stress.

3. Bonding. The compressional forces involved in the production of the tablet are sufficient to overcome repulsive forces between adjacent particles and these are forced together into close proximity, causing the formation of intergranule or interparticle bonds which are responsible for the mechanical strength of the tablet. The two main mechanisms involved in tablets produced by both granulation and direct compression techniques are:
   — adsorption bonding in which the particles or granules are held together by van der Waals forces between component molecules at the surface, and
   — the formation of solid bridges (or diffusion bonding). The interaction forces are a consequence of the temporary increased mobility of molecules at the particle surface due to melting of components or induced rubbery properties under compression; as a consequence there is the possibility of molecular diffusion and mixing at the surfaces of adjacent particles to form a continuous solid phase (bridge) which bonds them together. Granules formed by the wet granulation process usually include a binder which plays an important role in the cohesion of the tablet through the formation of binder bridges between adjacent granules.

4. Stress relaxation. After the release of the compaction forces on ejection of tablets from the tablet press, there may be a continuing viscous deformation of particles, referred to as stress relaxation, which occurs for a limited time following compaction and leads to a significant increase of tablet strength without any noticeable changes in the physical appearance. Such increases of mechanical strength are reliant on careful control of the conditions, particularly relative humidity and temperature, under which tablets are stored. For example, the condensation of water in the pores of the tablet under conditions of high relative humidity can drastically reduce the tablet strength, eventually leading to the collapse of the tablet.

Tip

Tablets are usually manufactured industrially using rotary tablet presses having a large number of punches and producing up to about 10 000 tablets per minute.

Key points

- Tablets are usually manufactured by compression of the granulated powder mix. In an alternative method (direct compression) the granulation stage is omitted and the powder mix itself is compressed; this method is advantageous when the ingredients are susceptible to hydrolysis but is less frequently used because of the potential problems associated with it.
- The process of compression takes place in the die of the tablet press and involves three steps: filling of the die from the hopper, compression by the upper punch, and ejection of the tablet as the lower punch is pushed upwards.
- The events that occur in the process of compression include: transitional repacking of the granules after application of the initial stress; deformation under the applied stress; formation of intergranule or interparticle bonds during compaction; stress relaxation after the release of the compaction forces on ejection of tablets.

Tablet coating

- Coatings are applied to tablets and capsules for a variety of decorative, protective and functional purposes including:
  - to improve the aesthetic appearance of the product and aid identification by healthcare professionals and patients
  - to enhance the chemical stability of a drug by protecting it from the environment particularly light, oxygen and moisture
  - to mask the bitter taste or unpleasant odour of certain drugs
  - to modify drug-release profiles, for example to provide controlled release of drug throughout the gastrointestinal tract or target release of drug at a specific site
  - to protect the drug from degradation in the stomach (enteric coating)
- The earliest compound applied to tablets was sucrose, which was traditionally used for coating confectionery products, but this has now been mostly replaced by polymeric materials, which are able to form rate-controlling barriers to drug release.
- Conventional technologies for the application of film coatings usually involve the atomisation of the polymeric material dispersed as a solution or suspension, which is then sprayed on to a rotating or fluidised mass of tablets. Subsequent drying to remove the solvent leaves a thin deposit of the coating material on the tablet surface.
- Several alternative techniques have been developed in order to reduce the use of water or organic solvents, which involve the compaction of dry material around the tablet cores, a process referred to as dry or compression coating.

Film coating process

- Most solid dosage forms are coated using either a pan (drum) coating or fluidised bed technique; the underlying principle of the film coating process is the same in both.
- Conceptually, the process involves the repeated exposure of the tablets to a spray containing the polymeric coating material dissolved or suspended in a suitable solvent. As the tablet moves through the spray zone it receives a partial coating which is then solidified by heating to evaporate the solvent. This cycle of spraying and drying is repeated until the desired coating mass and uniformity is achieved (see *Figure 2.8*).
- The mechanism by which films are formed is dependent on whether the polymer is dissolved or dispersed in the spray liquid as follows:
  - When the polymer is dissolved in an organic solvent the process of film formation is relatively straightforward. The droplets of the atomised spray spread over the surface of the tablets to form a film of liquid, which becomes a gel when the polymer concentration increases during evaporation of the solvent and the polymer chains interact to form a three-dimensional network. Finally, a film is formed when more solvent is lost during the drying process. Adhesion between the polymer chains and the tablet surface, which increases with polymer chain length, secures the film to the surface.
  - When the polymer is dispersed in an aqueous solvent the mechanism of film formation is more complex. The atomised droplets initially remain as discrete droplets on the surface rather than spreading over it. Before a film can form, these droplets must first coalesce; this occurs as the water is evaporated. The polymer spheres first deform to fill the void spaces left by the evaporating water and eventually, with continued drying, they coalesce to form the film.
- Operational parameters important in ensuring efficient film formation differ depending on whether the polymer is dissolved or dispersed in the spray liquid:
  - When the polymer is dissolved in the spray liquid the droplet size of the atomised spray and the rate of solvent evaporation have to be carefully controlled. Large droplets caused by inadequate atomisation of the spray liquid or a slow solvent evaporation rate may overwet the tablet surface, possibly causing dissolution of the surface materials, whereas fine droplets, arising when the solvent evaporates too rapidly, may dry before reaching the tablet or spreading over its surface, resulting in rougher surfaces and high loss of material.
  - When the polymer is dispersed in an aqueous solvent processing variables such as spray rate and temperature have to be adjusted to allow for the higher latent

heat of water compared to organic solvents. In addition, unlike films formed from solutions, it is often necessary to store the film coated tablets in an oven at a controlled temperature and humidity to ensure complete coalescence of the polymer spheres, a procedure often referred to as curing.

- The specific requirements for the formulated spray solution also vary depending on whether the polymer is dissolved or dispersed in the spray liquid:
  - When the polymer is dissolved in the spray liquid. The ability of the sprayed polymer solution to wet the surface in the initial stages of the coating process (but not when the surface is already covered by a film) is related to the nature of the solid surface, particularly its hydrophobicity, and the surface tension of the polymer solution. Improvement of the wetting capabilities of the polymer solutions can be achieved by reduction of the surface tension of the spray formulation by the inclusion of an appropriate surfactant. The viscosity of the formulation is also important in coating operations involving solutions. The viscosity generally increases with chain length of the polymer and the concentration of its solution. Higher solution viscosities require more energy to atomise the solution and this is a limiting factor restricting the concentration of polymer that can be used. Viscosity also influences the spreading of the droplets; more viscous solutions do not readily spread across the tablet surface and spreading will become increasingly difficult due to an increase of viscosity as the concentration increases during drying.
  - When the polymer is dispersed in an aqueous solvent. There are different requirements for the formulated spray solutions compared to those when the polymer is in solution. Although the viscosity of the spray formulation is important in determining the ease of atomisation, it does not influence the spreading since the polymer is present as discrete droplets rather than a solution. Consequently, it is possible to use higher polymer concentrations in the coating process.
- An important variable in the coating process is temperature, which influences the ability of the polymer spheres to deform and fuse together to form a continuous film. For each system there is a minimum film forming temperature (MFFT) below which the polymeric dispersion will form an opaque discontinuous material upon solvent evaporation rather than the desired clear continuous film. In contrast, there is no MFFT for polymer solutions which form films at room temperature. The inclusion of plasticisers in the formulation affects the MFFT as they soften the polymer spheres (lower the T_g), allowing coalescence at lower temperatures.

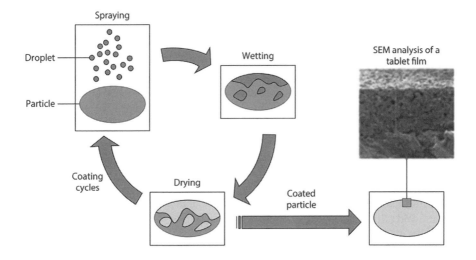

Figure 2.8: *General principles of a film-coating process showing repeated spraying and drying cycles. SEM, scanning electron microscopy. Reproduced with permission from Suzzi D et al. Local analysis of the tablet coating process: impact of operation conditions on film quality. Chem Eng Sci 2010;65:5699–5715. Copyright Elsevier 2010.*

Film-coating formulation

The spray liquid typically comprises a solvent, a polymer, a plasticiser, a surfactant, and a colourant or opacifier.

Solvent

- The use of an aqueous solvent to disperse or dissolve the polymer is preferred to dissolving the polymer in a volatile organic solvent even though this latter process is much more rapid. This is because of the absence of solvent toxicity, increased process safety and lower manufacturing costs when aqueous solvents are used. However, as discussed before, film formation is more complicated when the polymer is dispersed in an aqueous medium, because the dispersed polymer spheres must also coalesce to form a uniform film. This generally necessitates post-coating storage at elevated temperatures.
- Aqueous solvents are inappropriate when the active ingredient is sensitive to water and in these cases organic solvents such as methanol/dichloromethane combinations are used to dissolve the polymer in the spray liquid.

Polymer

Polymers that have been used in film coating include the Eudragit polymers (polymethylmethacrylates) and cellulose acetate phthalate (CAP). The choice of film-forming polymer is determined by:

- The proposed use of the dosage form: rapidly dissolving polymers are required when immediate release of active ingredient is intended, whereas film coatings for sustained or controlled release products should have limited or no solubility in aqueous media. The latter polymers are usually applied in organic solvents or as aqueous dispersions.
- Their influence on the physical properties of the film-coating liquid. As discussed before, this liquid should have low viscosity to aid atomisation to form the spray, and its surface tension should facilitate spreading of the film to cover the tablet surface. The polymer should have good adhesive properties and should be able to pack within the film to provide the desired permeability of the coating.

Plasticiser

- Plasticisers are generally substances that exhibit little or no tendency for evaporation or volatilisation. Commonly used plasticisers include polyols (e.g. polyethylene glycols and propylene glycol), oils (e.g. fractionated coconut oil), citrate esters (e.g. triethyl citrate) and phthalate esters (e.g. diethyl phthalate).
- The functions of the plasticiser are to:
  - increase the flexibility of the film by intercalating between the polymer molecules allowing increased motion within the film; this reduces problems as the film shrinks and tends to become brittle during the drying process, and
  - facilitate coalescence of the discrete polymer spheres of aqueous-based dispersed systems in the film formation process.
- The plasticiser must be miscible with the polymer and, for aqueous-based dispersed systems must also partition into the polymer phase. Water-soluble polymer plasticisers partition into the polymer quite rapidly, whereas longer mixing times are required for uptake of the water-insoluble plasticisers.
- A commonly-used method of evaluating the effectiveness of a plasticiser is to determine changes in the glass transition temperature (T_g) of the polymer as the concentration of added plasticiser is increased. A more effective plasticiser will cause a greater decrease in T_g of the film.

Colourant

- Although water-soluble dyes may be used as colourants, it is more usual to select water-insoluble pigments such as titanium dioxide and the iron oxides which tend to be more stable to light and also do not readily migrate within the film as do some water-soluble dyes – a process that produces mottled tablets.
- Pigments can significantly affect the mechanical and permeability properties of the film. For example, large pigment particles are thought to disrupt the interfacial bonding between the polymer and the tablet surface, and the extent of polymer-pigment interaction may influence the elastic modulus of polymer films.
- The maximum pigment concentration that can be incorporated into a film without compromising film properties is denoted by the critical pigment volume concentration (CPVC). When this concentration is exceeded there will be insufficient polymer to

surround all the insoluble particles and there will be a consequent deterioration in the mechanical and permeability characteristics of the film.

Surfactant
Surfactants may be included in the film-coating formulation in low concentration in order to:
- emulsify water-insoluble plasticisers
- stabilise suspensions (when the polymer is dispersed in the formulation)
- improve the wettability of the tablet surface and facilitate spreading of the sprayed droplets over the tablet surface.

Film-coating techniques
The most commonly used processes for film coating are pan (or drum) coating and fluidised bed coating. Differences between these two methods primarily relate to the way particles move between the spray and drying zones and the method used to remove the solvent.
- Drum or pan coating. In the usual pan coating method the tablet cores are placed in a round drum that rotates on an inclined axis (see *Figure 2.9*). The tablets cascade down the top of the bed, some passing through the atomised spray from one or more nozzles mounted at the top of the drum. Large scale equipment for pan coating is shown in operation at *https://www.youtube.com/watch?v=FotaiI38NXA*.
- Fluidised bed coating. This technique is commonly used for multiparticulates rather than larger particles such as tablets. In this method particles are suspended and circulated within a cylinder by heated air introduced from below. The air flow mixes and dries the particles which are constantly recirculated making multiple passes through the spray zone. The high level of air flow makes this coating method more efficient at water removal than the pan coating technique. The coating liquid is sprayed onto the particles from a nozzle located above or, as shown in *Figure 2.10*, below the fluidised bed. The top spray method tends to produce less uniform film coats and is used mainly for taste and odour masking purposes. You can see equipment for fluidised bed coating in action at *https://www.youtube.com/watch?v=snLEMu1NAdM*.

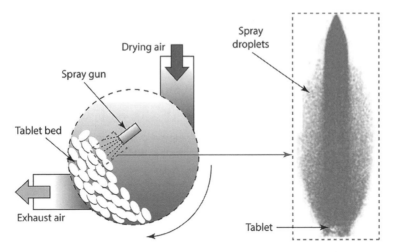

Figure 2.9: *Schematic of a modern pan coater (side-vented) and domain for the spray analysis. Reproduced with permission from Suzzi D et al. Local analysis of the tablet coating process: impact of operation conditions on film quality. Chem Eng Sci 2010;65:5699–5715. Copyright Elsevier 2010.*

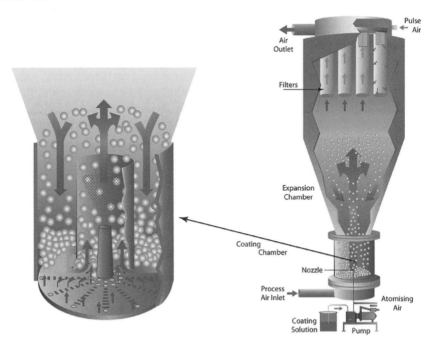

Figure 2.10: *Schematic representation of a fluidised bed film coater in which particles are suspended and circulated in a cylinder by heated air introduced from below. The air flow mixes and dries the particles, which are constantly recirculated, making multiple passes through the spray zone. The coating liquid is sprayed on to the particles from a nozzle located in this case below the fluidised bed.*

Dry coating

- Although film coating using dispersions of polymers in aqueous based systems remains the preferred method of coating tablets and particles, there are disadvantages associated with both this method and also the alternative film coating technique in which the polymer is dissolved in an organic solvent. In particular:
    - Organic solvents may be toxic and there are high processing costs arising from ensuring operating safety and safe solvent recovery.
    - The coating process in aqueous-based systems uses large amounts of water and requires considerable energy to evaporate off the water during the drying stages. There will also be special problems with this method when the ingredients are susceptible to degradation in an aqueous environment or when the drug product is formulated as an amorphous solid dispersion.
- For these reasons, alternative methods of coating in which the use of water or organic solvents is reduced to a minimum, so-called dry coating techniques, may be considered.
- Essentially, the process of dry powder coating follows similar steps to those of the film coating methods outlined before, i.e. the coating material is applied to the surface, it then coalescences and spreads over the surface to form an adhesive film. However, because of the minimal amount of solvent (if any) used in applying the film coating material there is no evaporation stage in the process, as there is with the film coating technique.
- The mechanism of film formation of the powders layered onto the solid may be summarised as shown in the schematic of *Figure 2.11*. The polymeric coating powder deposited on the substrate surface partially coalesces to form a film that then undergoes a levelling process in which it becomes more dense and smoother as the empty spaces are removed. Finally, the film is cooled and hardened.
- There are several important differences in the formulation of the coating materials for this type of coating process compared with those for film coating.
    - To ensure uniformity of the material on the substrate surface and to improve adhesion and processing times, the particle size of the powder should be less than about 1% of the size of the substrate on which it is coated. In general, powders having a particle size below 100 µm are suitable.
    - To ensure adequate spreading of the polymeric coating material in the absence of any significant amount of solvent, it is important that a polymer with a lower T_g than the processing temperature is used so that the polymer is more 'liquid-like' and more susceptible to plastic deformation. By reducing the viscosity in this way there will be adequate capillary forces to aid the spreading of this semi-molten material and to ensure its adherence to the substrate surface. The choice of a polymeric coating material with a low T_g avoids the need to operate at high temperatures which might accelerate degradation of materials. Where polymers with high glass transition temperatures ($T_g > 60°C$) are selected, plasticisers can be mixed with the polymeric materials during production to reduce the value of T_g.
- Dry coating techniques may be classified into three major types depending on the layer formation process:

1. Liquid assisted coating.
   - These techniques rely on the interfacial capillary action of liquid components of the formulation to aid adhesion of the coating layer to the core surface.
   - The quantity of liquid included in the formulation is very much less than that utilised in more conventional film coating methods and this liquid is often intended to remain in the drug product.
   - Similar equipment to that used for conventional strategies (particularly fluidised beds), with slight modifications, may be used for coating, although longer processing times and additional curing steps may be required.
   - The choice of excipients will be governed by the need to ensure sufficient softening at moderate temperatures, often necessitating larger amounts of plasticiser to facilitate adequate film formation than used for liquid based coating techniques, and polymers with a lower glass transition temperature. In addition, a much smaller particle size, often as low as 10 µm is required.
2. Thermal adhesion.
   - In this method of dry coating no liquid is included in the formulation and adhesion relies entirely on the thermal properties of the coating powder. Removal of the liquid, however, places more exacting requirements on the formulation to ensure adequate adhesion and film formation. In particular:
     » The amount of plasticiser becomes a critical factor in ensuring effective processing: higher levels of plasticiser than in conventional methods are usually required.
     » A polymer with a suitable glass transition temperature is required to ensure spreading and adhesion of the coating.
     » It may be necessary to include anti-sticking agents such as talc to prevent the agglomeration of the powder particles during storage and during the distribution of the powders on the cores; an additional coating of talc after the curing step may be required to reduce the tackiness of the final coated tablet, particularly when the T_g of the polymer is low.
3. Electrostatic coating.
   - This technique involves the deposition of charged coating powder on to the core surface and consequently it is essential that charge can be induced into the powder components so that there is an electrostatic attraction between the powder and tablet core which promotes adhesion.
   - The process can be carried out using specialised equipment similar to that used for the deposition of ink toner in photocopying; the essential steps in this process are shown diagrammatically in *Figure 2.12*. Each side of the tablet is coated and cured separately. With this technique, the coating material can be deposited with sufficient precision to create intricate patterns on the tablet surface for brand identification purposes.

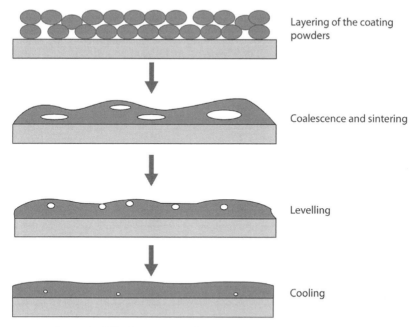

Figure 2.11: *Schematic of film formation in dry-powder coating systems. Reproduced with permission from Felton LA, Porter SC. An update on pharmaceutical film coating for drug delivery. Expert Opin Drug Deliv 2013;10:421–435.*

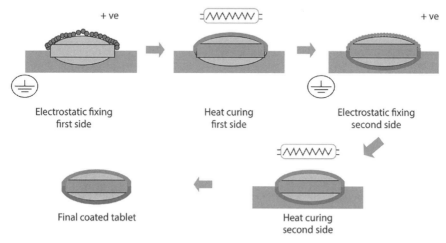

Figure 2.12: *Schematic diagram of the electrostatic dry-coating process. Reproduced with permission from Sauer D et al. Dry powder coating of pharmaceuticals: a review. Int J Pharm 2013;457:488–502. Copyright Elsevier 2013.*

Key points

- Coatings may be applied to tablets to improve their appearance, to enhance chemical stability, to mask a bitter taste or unpleasant odour, to modify drug-release profiles, and to protect the drug from degradation in the stomach (enteric coating).
- Tablets may be coated by film coating (most frequently used) or dry coating techniques.
- The film coating process involves the repeated exposure of the tablets to a spray containing the polymeric coating material dissolved or suspended in a suitable solvent, the coating is then solidified by heating to evaporate the solvent. The mechanism by which films are formed and the processing variables are dependent on whether the polymer is dissolved or dispersed in the spray liquid. The most commonly used processes for film coating are pan (or drum) coating and fluidised bed coating.
- In dry coating techniques the use of water or organic solvents is reduced to a minimum and the polymeric coating material is deposited on the substrate surface as a dry (or almost dry) powder rather than a spray. Dry coating techniques may be classified into three major types depending on the layer formation process: liquid assisted, thermal adhesion and electrostatic coating.

Capsule manufacture

Types of capsule

Two types of capsules are produced as solid dosage forms – hard and soft capsules – which differ in their design and mechanical properties.

- Hard capsules are constructed from two cylindrical pieces sealed at one end; the shorter piece (the cap) fits over the open end of the longer piece (the body). They are generally used to deliver powders but other materials such as pellets, granules, tablets, semisolids, and non-aqueous liquids may be filled into the hard capsules providing they do not react chemically with the gelatin or hydroxypropylmethylcellulose shells or contain free water which causes the shells to soften or distort.
- Soft capsules are composed of a one-piece capsule shell and are more flexible than hard capsules; they are usually filled with non-aqueous liquids in which the active ingredient is dissolved or dispersed.
- Both hard and soft capsules are usually composed of gelatin or less commonly hydroxypropylmethylcellulose (hypromellose).

Gelatin
- Gelatin possesses many desirable properties making it the material of choice for the manufacture of capsules:
  - it is non-toxic and widely used in foodstuffs

- it is capable of forming a strong flexible film
- it has gelation characteristics which make it suitable for the manufacture of capsules: concentrated aqueous solutions of gelatin are mobile liquids above about 45°C and undergo a reversible transition to the rigid gel state on cooling (similar in behaviour to the Type II gels)
- it is readily soluble in biological fluids at body temperature.
- Gelatin is a heterogeneous mixture of single or multi-stranded polypeptides, each containing between 50–1000 amino acids joined together by amide linkages to form linear polymers varying in molecular weight from 15 000 to 250 000.
- Gelatin is prepared by the hydrolysis of collagen which is extracted from animal skin and bones. There are two types of gelatin depending on whether the method of extraction involves an acid or alkaline pre-treatment:
  - Type A gelatin is obtained by immersing pigskin in dilute mineral acid (pH 1–3) for approximately 24 h, the pH is then adjusted to between 3.5 and 4.0 and the gelatin extracted by a series of hot-water washes.
  - Type B gelatin is derived from immersion of cattle hides and bones in a calcium hydroxide (lime) slurry over a period of several months, after which time the stock is washed with cold water to remove as much of the lime as possible and then neutralised with acid before extraction with hot water as in the acid process. In both processes the gelatin solutions are cooled to form gel sheets, which are dried and then ground to the required particle size.
- The two types of gelatin have differing physicochemical properties:
  - their isoelectric points are 7–9 (Type A) and 4.7–5.3 (Type B)
  - 1% w/v aqueous solutions at 25°C have pHs of 3.8–6.0 (Type A) and 5.0–7.4 (Type B)
  - there is a difference in the pH dependence of solubility (because of their differing isoelectric points), but both types are poorly soluble in water at 25°C and gradually swell and soften as water is absorbed. In gastric fluid the gelatin capsules swell to rapidly release their contents.
- The grade of gelatin is indicated by its Bloom strength which is a measure of gel rigidity; it is defined as the load in grams required to push a standard plunger (diameter 12.7 mm) 4 mm into a 6.66% w/w gelatin gel that has been prepared in water and allowed to mature at 10°C. Gelatin used in the manufacture of hard capsules has a Bloom strength of 200–250 g: that suitable for soft gelatin capsules has a lower Bloom strength (150 g) because a less rigid gel is required.

Tip

There are two types of capsules: hard capsules which are generally used mainly to deliver powders, pellets and granules, and soft capsules which are used to deliver non-aqueous liquids in which the active ingredient is dissolved or dispersed.

Hard capsule manufacture and filling

Manufacture

- The manufacture of hard gelatin capsules makes use of the sol-gel transition occurring at about 40°C, and involves the following steps:
    1. A concentrated solution of gelatin (35–40%) is prepared in demineralised hot water (60–70°C) and any entrapped air is removed under vacuum.
    2. Excipients are then added including dyes or pigments to colour the capsules for identification and aesthetic purposes, and, if necessary, wetting agents such as sodium lauryl sulfate to enhance the wetting of the shell on contact with an aqueous solution.
    3. The viscosity is now reduced to a target value by the addition of hot water. Viscosity regulates the thickness of the capsule shell during production: the higher the viscosity, the thicker is the shell.
- Hydroxypropylmethylcellulose solutions do not gel and gelling agents such as carrageenan together with a co-gelling agent such as potassium chloride, have to be added to their solutions when used to manufacture hard capsules.
- Commercial equipment for manufacturing hard gelatin capsules consists of upper and lower sets of metal strips (bars) each containing a series of stainless steel moulds (pins) mounted in rows: one set for the production of the cap, the other for the body of the capsule. Hydroxypropylmethylcellulose hard capsules are manufactured in a similar manner, except that the gelling step is slower necessitating a lower machine output. *Figure 2.13* shows diagrammatically the sequence of processes involved.
    1. The lubricated pins at room temperature are dipped into a hopper containing a fixed quantity of the gelatin solution at about 45°C, which coats each pin with a gel formed when the warm gelatin solution is cooled below the gel point on contact with the colder pins.
    2. The bar containing the pins is slowly removed from the solution and rotated to form a film of uniform thickness.
    3. The pins are then passed through a series of driers in which air at controlled humidity is blown over them to remove moisture. At this stage the water level is reduced to about 13–16% w/w, to ensure that the capsule shell is not too brittle (too low water content), or easily deformed as a result of plastic flow (too high water content).
    4. Finally, the dried films are removed from the pins, cut to size and the two halves joined together to form the complete capsules.

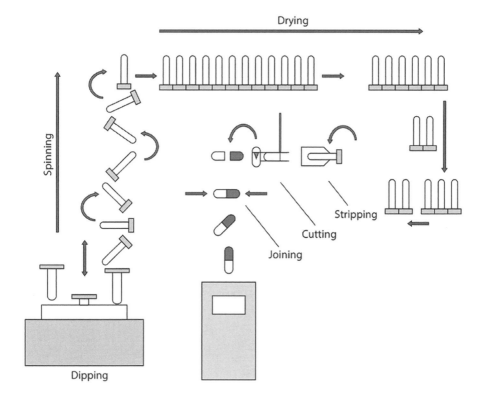

Figure 2.13: *Sequence of procedures involved in the manufacture of hard gelatin capsules.*

Formulation of powder mixes

- Many of the excipients used in the formulation of powder mixes for filling into hard capsules are similar to those used in the formulation of tablets, since the two dosage forms require the powder mix to have similar general properties.
- The powder blend should have reproducible flow properties to ensure uniformity of filling and contain components of similar size distribution to ensure homogeneous mixing within the powder blend. These requirements necessitate the use of free-flowing diluents with good plug-forming properties such as lactose, starch and microcrystalline cellulose.
- The flow and packing properties of the powders are assessed using techniques described above. Suitable flow and cohesive properties are associated with an angle of repose of approximately 25° and a Hausner ratio preferably of about 1.2 but certainly not exceeding 1.6.
- In addition, glidants, for example colloidal silicon dioxide, and lubricants particularly magnesium stearate, may be added to reduce interparticulate friction and adhesion of powder to metal surfaces.

- Other excipients including disintegrants, to break up the powder mass when released in the stomach, and surfactants, to ensure powder wetting following release, may be included in the powder mix.

Filling of powder formulations

The hard capsules are filled by either of two main methods: a dependent dosing and the more widely used independent dosing method.

- In the dependent dosing method:
  - The lower half of the capsule is placed in slots in a turntable which rotates at a range of speeds under a hopper containing the powder formulation.
  - After filling, the upper halves of the capsules, contained in a similar turntable, are brought together with the capsule bodies and the two halves sealed.
  - In this method, the mass of powder filled into the capsule is dependent primarily by the time that the capsule body remains under the hopper which itself is determined by the speed of rotation of the turntable.
- In the independent dosing method:
  - A plug of powder is formed when the open end of a dosing tube fitted with a spring loaded piston is lowered into the powder mix.
  - The tube containing the plug of powder is then raised from the powder bed, rotated and positioned over the lower half of the capsule, and the plug ejected into the capsule body by lowering the piston.
  - The volume of powder filled into the capsule may be controlled by altering the position of the piston within the tube.

Filling of pellets and tablets

- Pellets and granules are filled using equipment adapted from powder use and utilise a dosing system based on a chamber with an adjustable volume.
- Tablets are filled from hoppers into the capsule body via a gate device that controls the number of tablets allowed to pass.

Filling of liquids and semisolids

- Filling of hard gelatin capsules with semisolids is usually performed using a volumetric dosing device. Where possible, semisolids are filled in the liquid state, either by heating, in the case of thermosoftening mixtures, or by stirring, in the case of thixotropic mixtures. After filling, these formulations revert to the solid state to form a plug.
- An important consideration when liquids are filled into capsules is the prevention of leakage; this may be achieved by applying a gelatin solution around the junction between the two halves of the capsule, which dries to form a hermetic seal preventing liquid leakage.
- The liquids in which the therapeutic agent is dissolved or dispersed must be non-aqueous and must be carefully selected to avoid any adverse effect on the stability of the capsule. Of particular concern when water-miscible liquids are used as vehicles

is their effect on the moisture content of the capsule, which for optimum mechanical properties should be maintained between 13 and 16%. Suitable water-miscible liquids with low moisture uptake are higher molecular weight polyethylene glycols and liquid polyoxyethylene-polyoxypropylene block copolymers. Suitable lipophilic liquids or oils are the vegetable oils such as sunflower oil and fatty acid esters such as glyceryl monostearate.

- It is important that the viscosity of liquid fill formulations is within a suitable range (between 0.1 and 25 Pa/s) for optimum filling properties; liquids with high viscosities are difficult to pump when using the volumetric dosing devise, whereas liquids with very low viscosities may splash from the capsule during filling. It may be necessary when viscosities are outside these acceptable limits to include viscosity-modifying agents in the liquid formulation.
- Other excipients that may be required include surface active agents for solubilisation of poorly soluble drugs or as suspending agents for suspensions, and antioxidants to stabilise the liquid formulation.

Soft gelatin (softgel) capsule manufacture and filling

Manufacture
- It is necessary to manipulate the properties of gelatin to produce a capsule shell with a greater degree of flexibility than that of a hard capsule.
  - Type B gelatin is most commonly used and this is modified by the addition of plasticisers to impart a greater pliability.
  - Plasticisers are selected depending on their compatability with the capsule fill; they are usually polyhydric alcohols such as glycerol or sorbitol or their mixtures, sometimes in combination with glycerol.
  - The amount of plasticiser incorporated affects the mechanical properties of the soft gelatin capsule and is usually within the range 20–30% of the wet mass of the mixture. At levels above this the capsules are too flexible, whereas lower concentrations produce capsules that are too brittle.
  - The other additive influencing the flexibility of the capsule is water, which constitutes between 30–40% of the wet formulation, but reduces to an equilibrium concentration in the final capsule of 5–8% as a result of the drying process during capsule manufacture.
  - Other excipients that may be included in the wet gel formulation include colourants, such as soluble dyes, and opacifiers, usually titanium dioxide, which are used to produce an opaque shell.
- The manufacture of the capsules generally involves the following steps:
  - Hot gel liquid containing the additives described above is fed into the encapsulation machine where it is cooled to the gel state and cast into two ribbons each of which forms one half of the capsule. So again, as with the manufacture of hard gelatin capsules, an essential stage of the process is the sol-gel transition as the hot gelatin mass is cooled below the gel point.

- — The two ribbons are fed between two rotary dies to form pockets into which a metered dose of the liquid fill is simultaneously dispensed as shown diagrammatically in *Figure 2.14*.
- — Finally, the two halves are sealed together by the application of heat and pressure and cut automatically from the gelatin ribbon by raised rims on each die.
- — After collection the capsules are washed in a tumbler dryer, spread onto trays and dried with air at 20% humidity until the water level is reduced to the required equilibrium value.
- Filling of the capsules.
  - — Liquid-based vehicles in which the active ingredient is dissolved or dispersed are used as the capsule fill of soft gelatin capsules.
  - — For the reasons discussed earlier, water must be avoided because of its effect on the capsule integrity.
  - — Lipophilic liquids, particularly vegetable oils such as soyabean oil, are widely used as fill materials, although, because of their limited capacity to dissolve drugs, it may be necessary to also include cosolvents, unless the formulation is intended as a suspension, in which case a viscosity-modifying agent is included.
  - — Water-miscible liquids such as the polyethylene glycols PEG 400 and PEG 600 are commonly used and, to a lesser extent, non-ionic surfactants, such as Tweens, and liquid polyoxyethylene-polyoxypropylene block copolymers.

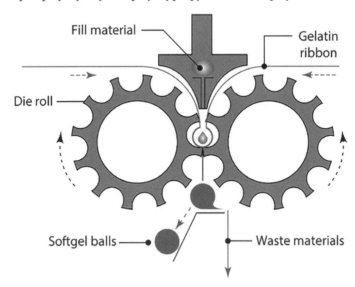

Figure 2.14: *Mechanism for the manufacture of soft gelatin (softgel) capsules. Two ribbons of gelatin are fed between the rotary dies to form pockets into which a metered dose of the liquid fill is simultaneously dispensed. The two halves are then sealed together and cut from the gelatin ribbon.*

Key points

- Two types of capsules are produced as solid dosage forms: hard capsules which are generally used mainly to deliver powders, pellets and granules, and soft capsules which are used to deliver non-aqueous liquids in which the active ingredient is dissolved or dispersed. The shells of both types are usually composed of gelatin, although hydroxypropylmethylcellulose has also been used.
- In commercial equipment, the two halves of hard gelatin capsules are formed separately when gelatin solution at about 45°C, is cooled below the gel point to form a film-coating on a series of lubricated pins. The films are dried, removed from the pins, cut to size and the two halves joined together to form the complete capsules.
- Soft gelatin capsules are prepared from gelatin modified by the addition of plasticisers (20–30%) to impart a greater pliability. Gelatin solution containing 30–40% water is cooled to the gel state and cast into two ribbons each of which forms one half of the capsule. The two ribbons are fed between two rotary dies to form pockets into which a metered dose of the liquid fill (a lipophilic liquid containing dissolved or dispersed drug) is dispensed. The two halves are sealed together by the application of heat and pressure and cut automatically from the gelatin ribbon.

Memory maps

Components of tablets

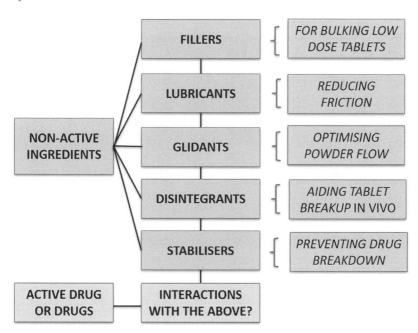

Some features of process optimisation

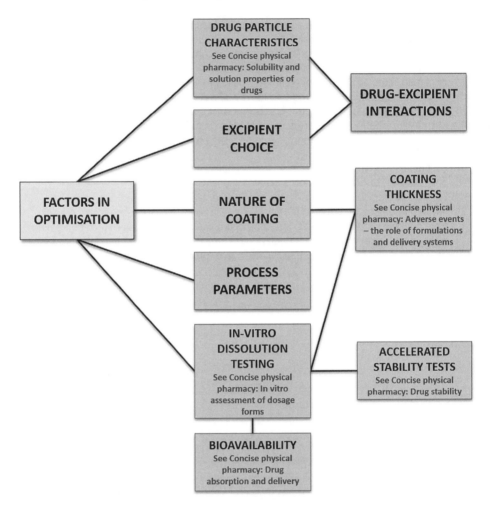

Why granulation?

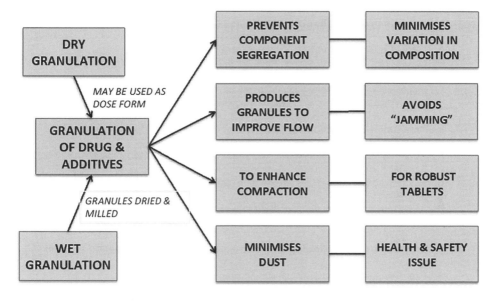

Questions

1. Indicate which of the following statements concerning the formulation of tablets are true.
   - **A:** Lactose is commonly used to increase the bulk volume of the powder mix
   - **B:** Sorbitol may be used to ensure tablet breakdown on contact with liquids
   - **C:** Colloidal silicon dioxide may be used to improve powder flow
   - **D:** Magnesium stearate may be used to reduce friction during compression
   - **E:** Starch may be added to improve the mechanical strength of the tablet

2. Indicate which of the following statements concerning the flow properties of powders are true.
   - **A:** Cohesive forces between particles decrease as the particle size increases
   - **B:** Spherical particles have better flow properties than irregular shaped particles
   - **C:** Particles should have a size smaller than about 100 μm to ensure free flowing properties
   - **D:** A Hausner ratio higher than 1.5 is indicative of good flow properties
   - **E:** The lower the Carr's index the better are the flow properties

3. Indicate which of the following statements concerning the granulation process are true.
   - **A:** Granules are more easily compacted than powder mixes and produce stronger tablets
   - **B:** Granules used for the manufacture of tablets are generally larger than 4 mm
   - **C:** The size of granules is determined by the size of the tablets
   - **D:** Alcohol may be used as a granulating liquid in wet granulation
   - **E:** Dry granulation is not suitable for thermolabile materials

4. Indicate which of the following statements concerning the direct compression method of tablet manufacture rather than granulation are true.
   - **A:** Tablets produced by direct compression are stronger and easier to film-coat
   - **B:** Direct compression is suitable when the tablet constituents are susceptible to hydrolysis
   - **C:** Direct compression is preferred for the manufacture of coloured tablets
   - **D:** Tablets produced by direct compression are more prone to undergo particle fragmentation
   - **E:** The main mechanisms involved in direct compression are adsorption bonding and diffusion bonding

5. Indicate which of the following statements concerning the manufacture of capsules are true.
   - **A:** Soft gelatin capsules are usually used to deliver pellets and granules
   - **B:** Gelatin used in the manufacture of hard capsules usually has a Bloom strength higher than that used for soft gelatin capsules
   - **C:** Plasticisers are usually added to gelatin during the manufacture of hard gelatin capsules
   - **D:** The method used for the extraction of Type A gelatin involves the alkaline pre-treatment of cattle hides and bones
   - **E:** When hydroxypropylmethylcellulose is used to form hard capsules it is necessary to add a gelling agent

CHAPTER 3

Solubility and solution properties of drugs

LEARNING OBJECTIVES

Upon completion of this chapter you should be able to:
- outline the properties of liquefied gases (propellants) used as solvents for drugs delivered in aerosol devices and in particular consider the factors influencing the vapour pressure in these devices
- outline the factors controlling the solubility of drugs in solution, in particular the nature of the drug molecule and the crystalline form in which it exists, its hydrophobicity, its shape, its surface area, its state of ionisation, the influence of pH of the medium and the importance of the pK_a of the drug
- understand the effect of pH on the ionisation of drugs in aqueous solution, calculate the pH of solutions of drugs from a knowledge of their pK_a and understand how to prepare buffer solutions to control pH
- outline some thermodynamic properties of drugs in solution such as activity and chemical potential
- outline the partitioning of drugs between two immiscible phases and their diffusional properties in solution.

Concentration units

Weight or volume concentration

- Concentration is often expressed as the weight of solute in a unit volume of solution, for example as g dm^{-3} or as % w/v, which is the number of grams of solute in 100 mL of solution.
- When the solute is a liquid, the concentration may also be expressed as the volume of solute in a unit volume of solution, for example as % v/v, which is the number of mL of solute in 100 mL of solution.
- When very dilute solutions are involved the concentration may be expressed as parts per million (or ppm). This is the number of grams in 10^6 grams of solution (which equals the number of mg per kg of solution) or, if the solute is a liquid, the number of mL in 10^6 mL (1000 litres) of solution. As the density of very dilute aqueous solutions at room temperature approximates to 1 g mL^{-1}, then 1 ppm is approximately 1 mg of solute per litre of solution (i.e. 1 g in 10^6 mL).

Molarity and molality

- The molarity of a solution is the number of moles of solute in 1 litre (1 dm^3) of solution. For example, a 0.9% w/v solution of sodium chloride (mol wt = 58.5 Da) contains 9 g dm^{-3} which equals 0.154 mol dm^{-3}.
- The molality is the number of moles of solute in 1 kg of solvent. For example, a 0.9% w/v solution of sodium chloride contains 9 g of sodium chloride dissolved in 991 g of water (assuming density = 1 g cm^{-3}). Therefore 1000 g of water contains 9.08 g of sodium chloride which equals 0.155 moles, i.e. molality = 0.155 mol kg^{-1}.

Milliequivalents

- In a clinical situation the concentration of an ion in solution is often expressed as the number of milliequivalents of the ion in a given volume of solution, for example as mEq per litre.
- The equivalent weight of an ion is equal to the molecular weight divided by its valency, so when monovalent ions are considered, the equivalent weight = molecular weight and therefore a 1 molar solution of sodium bicarbonate, $NaHCO_3$, contains 1 mol or 1 Eq of Na^+ and 1 mol or 1 Eq of HCO_3^- per litre of solution.
- With multivalent ions, attention must be paid to the valency of each ion and the numbers of each ion in the molecule. For example, 10% w/v $CaCl_2.2H_2O$ contains 1 g of $CaCl_2.2H_2O$ (mol wt = 147.0 Da) in 10 cm^3 and therefore 6.8 mmol or 13.6 mEq of Ca^{2+} in 10 cm^3. In calculating the number of equivalents of Cl^- you should note that each molecule of $CaCl_2.2H_2O$ ionises to give 2 Cl^- ions so that, although the valency of the chloride ion is 1, the number of milliequivalents in 10 cm^3 of solution is also 13.6.

Mole fraction

- The mole fraction of a component of a solution is the number of moles of that component divided by the total number of moles present in solution.
- In a two-component (i.e. solute + solvent) solution, the mole fraction of solvent, x_1, is given by $x_1 = n_1/(n_1 + n_2)$, where n_1 and n_2, are respectively the number of moles of solvent and solute present in solution. Similarly, the mole fraction of solute, x_2, is given by $x_2 = n_2/(n_1 + n_2)$. For example, in 1 litre of a 0.9% w/v solution of sodium chloride (mol wt = 58.5 Da) there are 9/58.5 = 0.154 moles of solute and 991/18 = 55.06 moles of water (mol wt = 18.0 Da); the mole fraction of sodium chloride is therefore $0.154/(0.154 + 55.06) = 2.79 \times 10^{-3}$.
- The sum of the mole fractions of all components in a solution is equal to 1, i.e. for a binary solution, $x_1 + x_2 = 1$; the mole fraction of water in the above solution is therefore 0.997.

Tips

Conversion into SI units:
- Volume is commonly expressed in litres (L) and millilitres (mL) rather than the SI unit of cubic metres (m^3).
  $1 L = 1 dm^3 = 10^{-3} m^3$
  $1 mL = 1 cm^3 = 10^{-6} m^3$
- Concentration is often given in grams per litre ($g L^{-1}$) rather than kilograms per cubic metre ($kg m^{-3}$).
  $1 g L^{-1} = 1 g dm^{-3} = 1 kg m^{-3}$
  Note also that $1 mg mL^{-1}$ is therefore also equal to $1 kg m^{-3}$
- Molarity is commonly expressed as $mol litre^{-1}$ and often written using the symbol M. Its conversion to SI units is:
  $1 mol litre^{-1}$ (or $1 M$) $= 1 mol dm^{-3} = 10^3 mol m^{-3}$

Solvents for pharmaceutical aerosols

- Liquefied gases under pressure in aerosol devices revert to the gaseous state when the device is activated and the liquid reaches atmospheric pressure. The drug is suspended or dissolved in the liquefied gas (propellant) and the drug–propellant mixture is expelled when the device is activated.
- Hydrofluoroalkanes (HFAs) now replace chlorofluorocarbon (CFC) propellants in pressurised metered-dose inhalers because of the ozone-depleting properties of CFCs (Montreal Protocol 1989).
- There is an equilibrium between a liquefied propellant and its vapour and there is a vapour pressure above the liquid, the value of which is determined by the propellants used and the presence of dissolved solutes.
- The vapour pressure above the aerosol mixture determines the aerosol droplet size. In metered-dose inhalers, for example, this has an important influence on the efficiency of deposition in the lungs.

Key points

- A solution can be defined as a system in which molecules of a solute (such as a drug or protein) are dissolved in a solvent vehicle.
- If the solvent is volatile there will be a vapour pressure above the solution which depends on the solvent's properties, the presence of solute and the temperature.
- When a solution contains a solute at the limit of its solubility at any given temperature and pressure it is said to be saturated.
- If the solubility limit is exceeded, solid particles of solute may be present and the solution phase will be in equilibrium with the solid, although under certain circumstances supersaturated solutions may be prepared, where the drug exists in solution above its normal solubility limit.
- The maximum equilibrium solubility of a drug dictates the rate of solution (dissolution) of the drug; the higher the solubility, the more rapid is the rate of solution.

- The vapour pressure above a liquid propellant is constant at constant temperature and this property is exploited in the design of implantable infusion pumps (see **Chapter 8**):
- Raoult's law is important because it allows the calculation of vapour pressure above an aerosol mixture from a knowledge of the composition of the solution:
  - It gives the relationship between the partial vapour pressure of a component i in the vapour phase, p_i, and the mole fraction of that component in solution, x_i, (assuming ideal behaviour) as:

$$p_i = p_i^{\ominus} x_i$$

where $p_i^{\ominus}$ is the vapour pressure of the pure component.

- Binary mixtures of hydrofluoroalkanes show behaviour which approaches ideality.
- There may be large positive deviations from Raoult's law when cosolvents such as alcohol are included in the aerosol formulation to enhance its solvent power.
- Raoult's law can be used to calculate the lowering of vapour pressure following the addition of a non-volatile solute to a solvent. The equation is,

$$\frac{p_1^{\ominus} - p_1}{p_1^{\ominus}} = x_2$$

which shows that the relative lowering of the vapour pressure is equal to the mole fraction x_2 of the solute.

Tips

When calculating the total vapour pressure above an aerosol mixture you will need to:
- Apply Raoult's law to calculate the partial pressures of each component from the mole fraction of each in the mixture.
- Calculate the total vapour pressure P using Dalton's law of partial pressures, which states that P is the sum of the partial pressures of the component gases, assuming ideal behaviour.
- Convert the pressure (if required) from Pa to pounds per square inch gauge (psig) using 1 Pa = (1/6894.76) – 14.7 psig.

Factors influencing solubility

- The solution process can be considered in three stages (*Figure 3.1*):
  1. A solute (drug) molecule is 'removed' from its crystal.
  2. A cavity for the molecule is created in the solvent.
  3. The solute molecule is inserted into this cavity.
- The surface area of the drug molecule affects solubility because placing the solute molecule in the solvent cavity (step 3) requires a number of solute–solvent contacts; the larger the solute molecule, the larger the cavity required (step 2) and the greater the number of contacts created. For simple molecules solubility decreases with increase of molecular surface area.
- The boiling point of liquids and the melting point of solids both reflect the strengths of interactions between the molecules in the pure liquid or the solid state (step 1). In general, aqueous solubility decreases with increasing boiling point and melting point.
- The influence of substituents on the solubility of molecules in water can be due to their effect on the properties of the solid or liquid (for example, on its molecular cohesion, step 1) or to the effect of the substituent on its interaction with water molecules (step 3). Substituents can be classified as either hydrophobic or hydrophilic, depending on their polarity:
  - Polar groups such as $-OH$ capable of hydrogen bonding with water molecules impart high solubility.
  - Non-polar groups such as $-CH_3$ and $-Cl$ are hydrophobic and impart low solubility.
  - Ionisation of the substituent increases solubility, e.g. $-COOH$ and $-NH_2$ are slightly hydrophilic whereas $-COO^-$ and $-NH_3^+$ are very hydrophilic.
  - The position of the substituent on the molecule can influence its effect on solubility, for example the aqueous solubilities of o-, m- and p-dihydroxybenzenes are 4, 9 and 0.6 mol dm^{-3}, respectively.
- The solubility of inorganic electrolytes is influenced by their crystal properties and the interaction of their ions with water (hydration). If the heat of hydration is sufficient to provide the energy needed to overcome the lattice forces, the salt will be freely soluble at a given temperature and the ions will readily dislodge from the crystal lattice.
- Additives may either increase or decrease the solubility of a solute in a given solvent; their effect on the solubility of sparingly soluble solutes may be evaluated using the solubility product (see below). Salts that increase solubility are said to 'salt in' the solute and those that decrease solubility 'salt out' the solute. The effect that they have will depend on several factors:
  - the effect the additive has on the structure of water
  - the interaction of the additive with the solute
  - the interaction of the additive with the solvent.

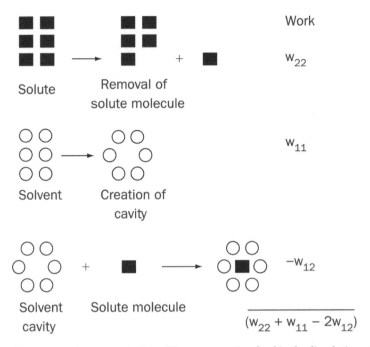

Figure 3.1: *Diagrammatic representation of the processes involved in the dissolution of a crystalline solute.*

pH is one of the primary influences on the solubility of most drugs that contain ionisable groups (*Figure 3.2*):
- Acidic drugs, such as the non-steroidal anti-inflammatory agents, are less soluble in acidic solutions than in alkaline solutions because the predominant undissociated species cannot interact with water molecules to the same extent as the ionised form which is readily hydrated. The equation relating the solubility, S, of an acidic drug to the pH of the solution is:

$$\text{pH} - pK_a = \log\left(\frac{S - S_0}{S_0}\right)$$

where S_0 is the solubility of the undissociated form of the drug.
- Basic drugs such as ranitidine are more soluble in acidic solutions where the ionised form of the drug is predominant. The equation relating the solubility, S, of a basic drug to the pH of the solution is:

$$\text{pH} - pK_a = \log\left(\frac{S_0}{S - S_0}\right)$$

- Amphoteric drugs such as the sulfonamides and tetracyclines display both basic and acidic characteristics. The zwitterion has the lowest solubility, S_0, and the variation of solubility with pH is given by:

$$pH - pK_a = \log \left(\frac{S_0}{S - S_0} \right) \text{ at pH values below the isoelectric point and}$$

$$pH - pK_a = \log \left(\frac{S - S_0}{S_0} \right) \text{ at pH values above the isoelectric point.}$$

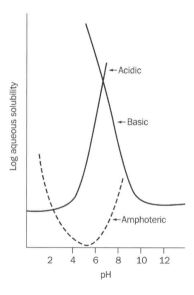

Figure 3.2: *Solubility of acidic, basic and amphoteric drugs as a function of pH.*

Tip

The solubility product, K_{sp}, of a sparingly soluble solute such as silver chloride is written as:

$$K_{sp} = [Ag^+][Cl^-]$$

Therefore, if either $[Ag^+]$ or $[Cl^-]$ is increased by adding an Ag^+ or Cl^- ion to the solution then because the value of the solubility constant cannot change, some of the sparingly soluble salt will precipitate, i.e. the solubility of the sparingly soluble solute is decreased by adding a common ion (referred to as the common ion effect).

Tip

At a particular pH, known as the isoelectric point, pH_i, the effective net charge on the amphoteric molecule is zero. pH_i can be calculated from:

$$pH_i = (pK_a^{acidic} + pK_a^{basic})/2$$

where pK_a^{acidic} and pK_a^{basic} are the pK_as of the acidic and basic groups respectively.

Tip

As a rough guide, the solubility of drugs in which the un-ionised species has a low solubility varies by a factor of 10 for each pH unit change.

Key points

- Many drugs are weak organic acids (for example, acetylsalicylic acid) or weak organic bases (for example, procaine) or their salts (for example, ephedrine hydrochloride).
- A weak acid or base is only slightly ionised in solution, unlike a strong acid or base, which is completely ionised.
- The degree to which weak acids and bases are ionised in solution is highly dependent on the pH.
- The exceptions to this general statement are the non-electrolytes, such as the majority of steroids, and the quaternary ammonium compounds, which are completely ionised at all pH values and in this respect behave as strong electrolytes.
- The extent of ionisation of a drug has an important effect on its absorption, distribution and elimination.

Methods to increase solubility

- Mixed solvents (cosolvents): mixed solvents such as glycerol–water, ethanol–water and ethanol–glycerol are often used as a means of increasing drug solubility. For example, the solubility of phenobarbital is increased from 0.125% w/v in water to about 16% w/v in ethanol–glycerol mixtures containing 85% ethanol, and 13% w/v in ethanol–water mixtures containing 90% ethanol.
- Solubilising agents: surfactant micelles may be used to solubilise poorly water-soluble drugs (see **Chapter 5**).
- Cyclodextrins may be used to encapsulate poorly water-soluble drugs. Cyclodextrins are enzymatically modified starches available as α-, β- and γ-cyclodextrins and a

range of their derivatives including, for example, hydroxypropyl-β-cyclodextrin (Encapsin HPB). Their glucopyranose units form a ring: α-CD is a ring of six units, β-CD a ring of seven units and γ-CD a ring of eight units The 'ring' is cylindrical, the outer surface being hydrophilic and the internal surface of the cavity being non-polar. Appropriately sized lipophilic molecules can be accommodated wholly or partially in the complex, so increasing their solubility. For example, the solubility of betametasone is increased 118 times, diazepam 21 times and ibuprofen 55 times by 10% w/v hydroxypropyl-β-cyclodextrin.

- Choice of drug salt: the solubility of a drug in aqueous solution may be markedly dependent on the salt form. For example, the solubility of chlorhexidine in water is 0.08 mg cm^{-3} whereas the solubility of its digluconate salt is greater than 700 mg cm^{-3}.

Ionisation of drugs in solution

Ionisation of weakly acidic drugs and their salts

- If the weak acid is represented by HA, its ionisation in water may be represented by the equilibrium:

$$HA + H_2O \rightleftharpoons A^- + H_3O^+$$

- The equilibrium constant, K_a, is referred to as the ionisation constant, dissociation constant or acidity constant and is given by:

$$K_a = \frac{[H_3O^+][A^-]}{[HA]}$$

- The negative logarithm of K_a is referred to as pK_a, i.e. $pK_a = -\log K_a$.
- When the pH of an aqueous solution of the weakly acidic drug approaches to within 2 pH units of the pK_a there is a very pronounced change in the ionisation of that drug (*Figure 3.3*).
- The percentage ionisation at a given pH can be calculated from:

$$\text{percentage ionisation} = \frac{100}{1 + \text{antilog}(pK_a - pH)}$$

- Weakly acidic drugs are virtually completely un-ionised at pHs up to 2 units below their pK_a and virtually completely ionised at pHs greater than 2 units above their pK_a. They are exactly 50% ionised at their pK_a values.
- Salts of weak acids are essentially completely ionised in solution, for example when sodium salicylate (salt of the weak acid, salicylic acid, and the strong base NaOH) is dissolved in water, it ionises almost entirely into the conjugate base of salicylic acid, $HOC_6H_5COO^-$, and Na^+ ions. The conjugate acids formed in this way are subject to acid–base equilibria described by the general equations before.

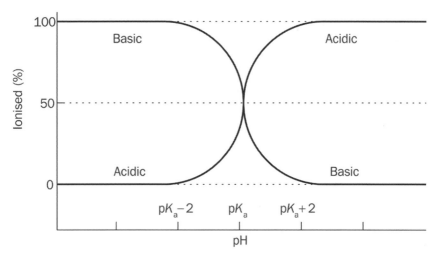

Figure 3.3: *Percentage ionisation of weakly acidic and weakly basic drugs as a function of pH.*

Ionisation of weakly basic drugs and their salts

- If the weak acid is represented by B, its ionisation in water may be represented by the equilibrium:

$$B + H_2O \rightleftharpoons BH^+ + OH^-$$

- The equilibrium constant, K_b, is referred to as the ionisation constant, dissociation constant or basicity constant and is given by:

$$K_b = \frac{[OH^-][BH^+]}{[B]}$$

- The negative logarithm of K_b is referred to as pK_b, i.e. $pK_b = -\log K_b$.
- The percentage ionisation at a given pH can be calculated from:

$$\text{percentage ionisation} = \frac{100}{1 + \text{antilog}(pH - pK_w + pK_b)}$$

where pK_w is the negative logarithm of the dissociation constant for water, K_w.
- Weakly basic drugs are virtually completely ionised at pHs up to 2 units below their pK_a and virtually completely un-ionised at pHs greater than 2 units above their pK_a. They are exactly 50% ionised at pHs equal to their pK_a values (*Figure 3.3*).
- Salts of weak bases are essentially completely ionised in solution; for example, ephedrine hydrochloride (salt of the weak base, ephedrine, and the strong acid HCl) exists in aqueous solution in the form of the conjugate acid of the weak base, $C_6H_5CH(OH)CH(CH_3)N^+H_2CH_3$, together with its Cl^- counterions. The conjugate

bases formed in this way are subject to acid–base equilibria described by the general equations before.

Tips

- It is usual to use only pK_a values when referring to both weak acids and bases.
- pK_a and pK_b values of conjugate acid–base pairs are linked by the expression:

$$pK_a + pK_b = pK_w$$

- $pK_w = 14.00$ at 25°C (but decreases with temperature increase) and hence a value of pK_b can easily be calculated if required.
- pK_a and pK_b values provide a convenient means of comparing the strengths of weak acids and bases. The lower the pK_a, the stronger the acid; the lower the pK_b, the stronger is the base (but note they are still weak acids or bases).

Ionisation of amphoteric drugs

- These can function as either weak acids or weak bases in aqueous solution depending on the pH and have pK_a values corresponding to the ionisation of each group.
- If the pK_a of the acidic group, pK_a^{acidic}, is higher than that of the basic group, pK_a^{basic}, they are referred to as ordinary ampholytes and exist in solution as a cation, an un-ionised form, and an anion depending on the pH of the solution. For example, the ionisation of m -aminophenol ($pK_a^{acidic} = 9.8$ and $pK_a^{basic} = 4.4$) changes as the pH increases as follows:

$$NH_3^+C_6H_4OH \rightleftarrows NH_2C_6H_4OH \rightleftarrows NH_2C_6H_5O^-$$

- If $pK_a^{acidic} < pK_a^{basic}$ the compounds are referred to as zwitterionic ampholytes and exist in solution as a cation, a zwitterion (having both positive and negative charges), and an anion depending on the pH of the solution. Examples of this type of compound include the amino acids, peptides and proteins. Glycine ($pK_a^{acidic} = 2.3$ and $pK_a^{basic} = 9.6$) ionises as follows:

$$HOOCCH_2NH_3^+ \rightleftarrows {}^-OOCCH_2NH_3^+ \rightleftarrows {}^-OOCCH_2NH_2$$

- The ionisation pattern of both types is more complex, however, with drugs in which the difference in pK_a of the two groups is much smaller (<2 pH units), this is because of the overlap of the two equilibria.

Ionisation of polyprotic drugs

- Several acids, for example citric, phosphoric and tartaric acid, are capable of donating more than one proton and these compounds are referred to as polyprotic or polybasic acids. Similarly, polyprotic bases are capable of accepting two or more protons. Examples of polyprotic drugs include the polybasic acids amoxicillin and fluorouracil,

and the polyacidic bases pilocarpine, doxorubicin and aciclovir.
- Each stage of the dissociation of the drug may be represented by an equilibrium expression and hence each stage has a distinct pK_a or pK_b value. For example, the ionisation of phosphoric acid occurs in three stages:

$$H_3PO_4 + H_2O \rightleftharpoons H_2PO_4^- + H_3O^+ \qquad pK_1 = 2.1$$

$$H_2PO_4^- + H_2O \rightleftharpoons HPO_4^{2-} + H_3O^+ \qquad pK_2 = 7.2$$

$$HPO_4^{2-} + H_2O \rightleftharpoons PO_4^{3-} + H_3O^+ \qquad pK_3 = 12.7$$

- If the pK_a values for each stage of dissociation are far apart it is usually possible to assign them to the ionisation of specific groups, but if they are within about 2 pH units of each other this is not possible. For a more complete picture of the dissociation it is necessary to take into account all possible ways in which the molecule may be ionised and all the possible species present in solution. In this case the constants are called microdissociation constants.

pH of drug solutions

The pH of a strong acid such as HCl is given by $pH = -\log[H^+]$. This is because strong acids are completely ionised in solution. However, as seen above, weak acids and bases are only slightly ionised in solution and the extent of their ionisation changes with pH and so therefore does their pH. The pH at any particular concentration, c, can be calculated from the pK_a value.
- Weakly acidic drugs: $pH = \frac{1}{2} pK_a - \frac{1}{2} \log c$
- Weakly basic drugs: $pH = \frac{1}{2} pK_w + \frac{1}{2} pK_a + \frac{1}{2} \log c$
- Drug salts:
  - Salts of a weak acid and a strong base:
    $pH = \frac{1}{2} pK_w + \frac{1}{2} pK_a + \frac{1}{2} \log c$
  - Salts of a weak base and a strong acid:
    $pH = \frac{1}{2} pK_a - \frac{1}{2} \log c$
  - Salts of a weak acid and a weak base:
    $pH = \frac{1}{2} pK_w + \frac{1}{2} pK_a - \frac{1}{2} pK_b$
    (note that there is no concentration term in this equation, meaning that the pH does not vary with concentration).

Tips

You can usually tell the type of drug salt from the drug name. For example:
- The sodium of sodium salicylate means that it is the salt of the strong base sodium hydroxide and the weak acid salicylic acid, i.e. sodium (or potassium) in the drug name implies the salt of a strong base.
- The hydrochloride of ephedrine hydrochloride means that it is the salt of a strong acid (hydrochloric acid) and a weak base (ephedrine), i.e. hydrochloride (or bromide, nitrate, sulfate, etc.) in the drug name implies the salt of a strong acid.
- Codeine phosphate is the salt of a weak base (codeine) and a weak acid (phosphoric acid). Other weak acid salts include, for example, butyrates, propionates, palmitates, tartrates, maleates and citrates.

Buffers

- Buffers are usually mixtures of a weak acid and its salt (that is, a conjugate base), or a weak base and its conjugate acid.
- A mixture of a weak acid HA and its ionised salt (for example, NaA) acts as a buffer because the A⁻ ions from the salt combine with the added H⁺ ions, removing them from solution as undissociated weak acid:

$$A^- + H_3O^+ \rightleftarrows H_2O + HA$$

Added OH⁻ ions are removed by combination with the weak acid to form undissociated water molecules:

$$HA + OH^- \rightleftarrows H_2O + A^-$$

- A mixture of a weak base and its salt acts as a buffer because added H⁺ ions are removed by the base B to form the salt and OH⁻ ions are removed by the salt to form undissociated water:

$$B + H_3O^+ \rightleftarrows H_2O + BH^+$$
$$BH^+ + OH^- \rightleftarrows H_2O + B$$

- The concentration of buffer components required to maintain a solution at the required pH may be calculated from the Henderson–Hasselbalch equations:
  - Weak acid and its salt:

$$pH = pK_a + \log \frac{[salt]}{[acid]}$$

— Weak base and its salt:

$$pH = pK_w - pK_b + \log \frac{[base]}{[salt]}$$

- The effectiveness of a buffer in minimising pH change is expressed as the buffer capacity, β, calculated from:

$$\beta = \frac{2.303c_0K_a\,[H_3O^+]}{([H_3O^+] + K_a)^2}$$

where c_0 is the total initial buffer concentration. A plot of β against pH (*Figure 3.4*) shows that:
— the buffer capacity is maximum when pH = pK_a
— maximum buffer capacity, β_{max} = 0.576c_0.

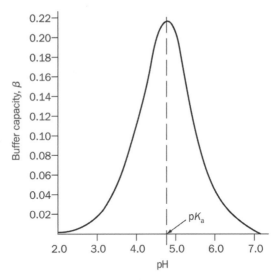

Figure 3.4: *Buffer capacity of a weak acid/salt buffer (initial concentration = 0.3754 mol dm^{-3}) as a function of pH, showing maximum buffer capacity at pK$_a$.*

Universal buffers

- If, instead of using a single weak monobasic acid, which has a maximum buffering capacity at pH = pK_a, you use a suitable mixture of polybasic and monobasic acids, it is possible to produce a buffer which is effective over a wide pH range because each stage of the ionisation of the polybasic acid has its own β_{max} value. Such solutions are referred to as universal buffers.

- A typical example is a mixture of citric acid (pK_{a1} = 3.06, pK_{a2} = 4.78 and pK_{a3} = 5.40), Na_2HPO_4 (pK_a of conjugate acid, $H_2PO_4^-$ = 7.2), diethylbarbituric acid (pK_{a1} = 7.43) and boric acid (pK_{a1} = 9.24). This buffer is effective over a pH range 2.4 to 12.

Physiological buffers

There are three major chemical buffers that maintain the blood pH at 7.4:

1. The bicarbonate buffer system consists of a solution of the weak acid carbonic acid (pK_a 6.1) and its salt sodium bicarbonate:

$$H_2CO_3 \rightleftharpoons HCO_3^- + H^+$$

An acidic substance added to the blood would be neutralised by the bicarbonate ions and the carbon dioxide produced excreted by the lungs:

$$HCO_3^- + H^+ \rightleftharpoons H_2CO_3 \rightleftharpoons H_2O + CO_2$$

A base added to the blood would be neutralised by the reaction:

$$H_2CO_3 + OH^- \rightleftharpoons HCO_3^- + H_2O$$

The buffer system is extremely efficient because it is self-regulating; carbonic acid is replenished by carbon dioxide from respiration, and bicarbonate ions by the kidneys.

2. The phosphate buffer system operates in the internal fluid of all cells and consists of dihydrogen phosphate ions ($H_2PO_4^-$) as hydrogen-ion donor (acid) and hydrogen phosphate ions (HPO_4^{2-}) as hydrogen-ion acceptor (base). These two ions are in equilibrium:

$$H_2PO_4^- \rightleftharpoons H^+ + HPO_4^{2-}$$

If additional hydrogen ions enter the cellular fluid, they are consumed in the reaction with HPO_4^{2-}, and the equilibrium shifts to the left. If additional hydroxide ions enter the cellular fluid, they react with $H_2PO_4^-$, producing HPO_4^{2-}, and shifting the equilibrium to the right.

3. The protein buffer system accounts for about 75% of all chemical buffering ability of the body fluids. The buffering ability of proteins is due to the dissociation of the acidic $-COOH$ groups of the amino acid residues to $-COO^-$ and H^+, and the dissociation of the basic $-NH_3 OH$ groups of the amino acids into $-NH_3$ and OH^-. Furthermore, the pK_a values of the amino acids are not far from 7.4, making the protein-buffering systems by far the most powerful of the body.

In addition there are two physiological buffer mechanisms:

1. The basis of the buffering action of the respiratory system is an immediate alteration of the rate of pulmonary ventilation and consequently the rate of removal of carbon dioxide from the body fluids – a process that takes 2–3 minutes to restore the pH to normal.

2. The urinary buffer system operates differently from the other buffering systems in that the hydrogen ions are actually expelled from the body in the urine, thereby readjusting their concentration in body fluids to normal; the process is slow, taking several hours to readjust the hydrogen ion concentration.

Thermodynamic properties of drugs in solution

Activity and activity coefficient

- In any real solution, interactions occur between the components which reduce the effective concentration of the solution. The activity is a way of describing this effective concentration.
- The ratio of the activity to the concentration is called the activity coefficient, γ, that is, γ = activity/concentration. Therefore, for an ideal solution $\gamma = 1$.
- When drugs are salts they ionise in solution and the activity of each ion is the product of its activity coefficient and its molar concentration, that is, $a_+ = \gamma_+ m_+$ and $a_- = \gamma_- m_-$. However, because it is not possible to measure ionic activities separately we use mean ionic parameters, i.e. $\gamma_\pm = a_\pm / m_\pm$.
- The mean ion activity coefficient $\gamma_\pm$ can be calculated using the Debye–Hückel equation:

$$-\log \gamma_\pm = z_+ \, z_- \, A\sqrt{I}$$

where z_+ and z_- are the valencies of the ions, A is a constant ($A = 0.509$ in water at 298 K) and I is the total ionic strength. For a 1:1 electrolyte, $I = m$, for a 1:2 electrolyte $I = 3m$ and for a 2:2 electrolyte, $I = 4m$.

Tips

- Salts such as ephedrine hydrochloride ($C_6H_5CH(OH)CH(NHCH_3)CH_3HCl$) are 1:1 (or uni-univalent) electrolytes; that is, on dissociation each mole yields one cation $C_6H_5CH(OH)CH(N^+H_2CH_3)CH_3$, and one anion, Cl^-.
- Other salts are more complex in their ionisation behaviour; for example, ephedrine sulfate is a 1:2 electrolyte, each mole giving two moles of the cation and one mole of SO_4^{2-} ions.

Chemical potential

- Chemical potential is the effective free energy per mole of each component in the mixture and is always less than the free energy of the pure substance.
- The chemical potential of a component in a two-phase system (for example, oil and water) at equilibrium at a fixed temperature and pressure is identical in both phases. A substance in a two-phase system which is not at equilibrium will have a tendency to

diffuse spontaneously from a phase in which it has a high chemical potential to another in which it has a low chemical potential. The difference in chemical potential is the driving force for diffusion between the two phases.

- The chemical potential, μ_2, of a non-ionised component in dilute solution is given by:

$$\mu_2 = \mu_2^{\ominus} + RT\ln\ M_1 - RT\ln 1000 + RT\ln m$$

where $\mu_2^{\ominus}$ is the chemical potential of the component in its standard state and M_1 = molecular weight of the solvent.

- The chemical potential of a 1:1 electrolyte is given by:

$$\mu_2 = \mu_2^{\ominus} + 2RT\ln\ m\gamma_{\pm}$$

Osmotic properties of drugs in solution – isotonic solutions

- Whenever a solution is separated from a solvent by a membrane that is only permeable to solvent molecules (referred to as a semipermeable membrane), there is a passage of solvent across the membrane into the solution. This is the phenomenon of osmosis.
- Solvent passes through the membrane because the chemical potentials on either side of the membrane are not equal. Since the chemical potential of a solvent molecule in solution is less than that in pure solvent, solvent will spontaneously enter the solution until the chemical potentials are the same.
- If the solution is totally confined by a semipermeable membrane and immersed in the solvent, then a pressure differential develops across the membrane: this is referred to as the osmotic pressure.
- The equation which relates the osmotic pressure of the solution, Π, to the solution concentration is the van't Hoff equation:

$$\Pi V = n_2 RT$$

where V is the molar volume of the solute and n_2 is the number of moles of solute.

- Osmotic pressure is a colligative property, which means that its value depends on the number of ions in solution. Therefore, if the drug is ionised you need to include the contribution of the counterions to the total number of ions in solution. Note, however, that the extent of ionisation changes as the solution is diluted and is only complete in very dilute solution.
- Because the red blood cell membrane acts as a semipermeable membrane it is important to ensure that the osmotic pressure of solutions for injection is approximately the same as that of blood serum. Such solutions are said to be isotonic with blood. Solutions with a higher osmotic pressure are hypertonic and those with

a lower osmotic pressure are termed hypotonic solutions. Similarly, in order to avoid discomfort on administration of solutions to the delicate membranes of the body, such as the eyes, these solutions are made isotonic with the relevant tissues.

- Osmotic pressure is not a readily measurable quantity and it is usual to use the freezing-point depression (which is also a colligative property) when calculating the quantities required to make a solution isotonic. A solution which is isotonic with blood has a freezing-point depression, ΔT_f, of $0.52°C$. Therefore the freezing point of the drug solution has to be adjusted to this value by adding sodium chloride to make the solution isotonic. The amount of the adjusting substance required can be calculated from:

$$w = \frac{0.52 - a}{b}$$

where w is the weight in grams of adjusting substance to be added to $100\,cm^3$ of drug solution to achieve isotonicity, a is the number of grams of drug in $100\,mL$ of solution multiplied by ΔT_f of a 1% drug solution, and b is ΔT_f of 1% adjusting substance.

Key point

Parenteral solutions should be of approximately the same tonicity as blood serum; the amount of adjusting substance which must be added to a formulation to achieve isotonicity can be calculated using the freezing point depressions of the drug and the adjusting substance.

Tip

Note that, although the freezing point of blood serum is -0.52°C, the freezing-point depression is +0.52°C because the word 'depression' implies a decrease in value. This is a common source of error in isotonicity calculations.

Partitioning of drugs between immiscible solvents

- Examples of partitioning include:
  - drugs partitioning between aqueous phases and lipid biophases
  - preservative molecules in emulsions partitioning between the aqueous and oil phases
  - antibiotics partitioning into microorganisms
  - drugs and preservative molecules partitioning into the plastic of containers or giving sets.
- If two immiscible phases are placed in contact, one containing a solute soluble to some

extent in both phases, the solute will distribute itself until the chemical potential of the solute in one phase is equal to its chemical potential in the other phase.

- The distribution of the solute between the two phases is represented by the partition coefficient or distribution coefficient, P, defined as the ratio of the solubility in the non-aqueous (oily) phase, C_o, to that in the aqueous phase, C_w, i.e. $P = C_o/C_w$
- It is usual to express the partitioning as log P. The greater the value of log P, the higher the lipid solubility of the solute.
- Octanol is usually used as the non-aqueous phase in experiments to measure the partition coefficient of drugs. Other non-aqueous solvents, for example isobutanol and hexane, have also been used.
- In many systems the ionisation of the solute in one or both phases or the association of the solute in one of the solvents complicates the calculation of partition coefficient:
  - For example, if the solute associates to form dimers in phase 2 then $K = \sqrt{C_2}/C_1$, where K is a constant combining the partition coefficient and the association constant and C_1 is the concentration in phase 1.
  - Many drugs will ionise in at least one phase, usually the aqueous phase. It is generally accepted that only the non-ionised species partitions from the aqueous phase into the non-aqueous phase. Ionised species, being hydrated and highly soluble in the aqueous phase, disfavour the organic phase because transfer of such a hydrated species involves dehydration. In addition, organic solvents of low polarity do not favour the existence of free ions.
  - If ionisation and its consequences are neglected, an apparent partition coefficient, P_{app}, is obtained simply by assay of both phases, which will provide information on how much of the drug is present in each phase, regardless of status. The relationship between the true thermodynamic P and P_{app} is given by the following equations:
    - » For acidic drugs:

$$\log P = \log P_{app} - \log \frac{1}{1 + 10^{pH - pK_a}}$$

    - » For basic drugs:

$$\log P = \log P_{app} - \log \frac{1}{1 + 10^{pK_a - pH}}$$

    - » For amphoteric compounds such as the tetracyclines, the pH dependence of the partition coefficient is more complex than for most drugs. For slightly simpler amphoteric compounds, such as p- aminobenzoic acid and sulfonamides, the apparent partition coefficient is maximal at the isoelectric point.

- Correlations between partition coefficients and biological activity are expressed by Ferguson's principle which states that, within reasonable limits, substances present at approximately the same proportional saturation (that is, with the same

thermodynamic activity) in a given medium have the same biological potency.
- Other examples of partitioning of pharmaceutical importance include the permeation of antimicrobial agents into rubber stoppers and other closures, the partitioning of glyceryl trinitrate (volatile drug with a chloroform/water partition coefficient of 109) from simple tablet bases into the walls of plastic bottles and into plastic liners used in packaging tablets, and the permeation of drugs into polyvinyl chloride infusion bags.

Diffusion of drugs in solution

- Drug molecules in solution will spontaneously diffuse from a region of high chemical potential to one of low chemical potential.
- Although the driving force for diffusion is the gradient of chemical potential, it is more usual to think of the diffusion process in terms of the concentration gradient.
- The rate of diffusion may be calculated from Fick's first law:

$$J = -D \, (dc/dx)$$

where J is the flux of a component across a plane of unit area, dc/dx is the concentration gradient and D is the diffusion coefficient (or diffusivity). The negative sign indicates that the flux is in the direction of decreasing concentration. J is in mol m^{-2}s^{-1}, c is in mol m^{-3} and x is in m; therefore, the units of D are m^2 s^{-1}.
- The relationship between the radius, a, of the diffusing molecule and its diffusion coefficient (assuming spherical particles or molecules) is given by the Stokes–Einstein equation as:

$$D = \frac{RT}{6\pi\eta a N_A}$$

where η is the viscosity of the drug solution and N_A is Avogadro's constant.
- The diffusional properties of a drug have relevance in pharmaceutical systems in a consideration of such processes as the dissolution of the drug and transport through artificial (e.g. polymer) or biological membranes, and diffusion in tissues such as the skin or in tumours (see **Chapter 13**).

Memory map

Properties of solutions

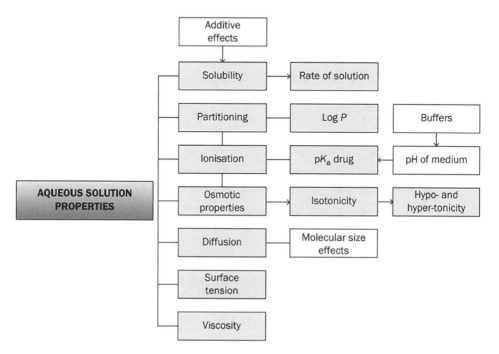

Questions

1. Calculate the molarity of a $50\,mg\,cm^{-3}$ aqueous solution of ascorbic acid (mol wt = 176.1 Da):
   A: $2.839\,mol\,dm^{-3}$
   B: $0.2839\,mol\,dm^{-3}$
   C: $0.0028\,mol\,dm^{-3}$

2. Calculate the molality of a 0.833% w/v aqueous solution of codeine monohydrate (mol wt = 317.4 Da). Assume density of water = $1\,g\,cm^{-3}$.
   A: $0.0026\,mol\,kg^{-1}$
   B: $0.0262\,mol\,kg^{-1}$
   C: $0.0265\,mol\,kg^{-1}$
   D: $0.2646\,mol\,kg^{-1}$

3. What is the mole fraction of oxycodone hydrochloride (mol wt = 405.9 Da) in a 5% w/v aqueous solution of this drug? Assume density of water = $1\,g\,cm^{-3}$; mol wt water = 18.0 Da.
   A: 0.1232
   B: 2.213×10^{-3}
   C: 2.329×10^{-3}
   D: 2.333×10^{-4}

4. Calculate the vapour pressure in Pa and psig above an aerosol mixture consisting of 30% w/w of a propellant (molecular weight 170.9 Da) with a vapour pressure of 1.90×10^5 Pa and 70% w/w of a second propellant (molecular weight 120.9 Da) with a vapour pressure of 5.85×10^5 Pa. Assume ideal behaviour.
   A: 4.67×10^5 Pa
   B: 4.49×10^5 Pa
   C: 7.75×10^5 Pa
   D: 50.42 psig
   E: 65.12 psig

5. Indicate which of the following molecular characteristics will be expected to increase the solubility of a simple solute in an aqueous solution.
   A: A low melting point
   B: The presence of a polar group
   C: A high molecular surface area
   D: The presence of an ionised group
   E: A high boiling point

6. Indicate which of the following general statements are true.
   A: Acidic drugs are less soluble in acidic solutions than in alkaline solutions
   B: Basic drugs are more soluble in alkaline solutions than in acid solutions
   C: The zwitterion of an amphoteric drug has a higher solubility than the acidic or basic forms of the drug
   D: The effective net charge on the zwitterion is zero at the isoelectric point

7. **Indicate which of the following general statements are true.**
   A: A weakly acidic drug is un-ionised when the pH of the solution is at least 2 pH units below its pK_a
   B: A weakly basic drug is fully ionised when the pH of the solution is at least 2 pH units greater than its pK_a
   C: Quaternary ammonium compounds are fully ionised at all pHs
   D: Weakly acidic drugs are 50% ionised when the pH of the solution is equal to their pK_a
   E: Salts of weak acids are fully ionised in solution
   F: The higher the pK_a of a weak acid, the stronger is the acid
   G: The sum of pK_a and pK_b is greater than 14.00 at 15°C

8. **Indicate which of the following drugs are salts of a weak acid and strong base.**
   A: Chlorpromazine hydrochloride
   B: Sodium salicylate
   C: Acetylsalicylic acid
   D: Flucloxacillin sodium
   E: Chlorpheniramine maleate

9. **The solubility of the weakly acidic drug benzylpenicillin (pK_a = 2.76) at pH 8.0 and 20°C is 0.174 mol dm^{-3}. Calculate the solubility when the pH is so low that only the undissociated form of the drug is present in solution. Answer in mol dm^{-3} is:**
   A: 0.174×10^{-6}
   B: 1.00×10^{-6}
   C: 3.024×10^{4}
   D: 3.024×10^{-4}
   E: 1.00×10^{6}

10. **What is the pH of a solution of ascorbic acid (pK_a = 4.17) of concentration 0.284 mol dm^{-3}?**
    A: 1.82
    B: 2.64
    C: 2.36
    D: 1.54
    E: 9.36

11. **What is the percentage of promethazine (pK_a = 9.1) existing as free base (i.e. un-ionised) in a solution of promethazine hydrochloride at pH 7.4?**
    A: 98.04
    B: 1.96
    C: 0.32
    D: 99.68

12. **What is the pH of a buffer solution containing 0.025 mol of ethanoic acid (pK_a = 4.76) and 0.035 mol of sodium ethanoate in 1 litre of water?**
    A: 6.14
    B: 4.59
    C: 4.89
    D: 2.37

13. **Indicate which of the following statements are correct.**
    A: When a solution is contained within a semipermeable membrane and separated from the solvent, the solvent will pass across the membrane into the solution
    B: The chemical potential of the solvent molecule in the solution is greater than that in pure solvent
    C: A solution that has a greater osmotic pressure than blood is said to be hypertonic
    D: When red blood cells are immersed in a hypotonic solution they will shrink

14. **How many grams of sodium chloride should be added to 25 mL of a 1% w/v solution of tetracaine hydrochloride to make the solution isotonic? The freezing-point depression of 1% tetracaine hydrochloride is 0.109°C, the freezing-point depression of 1% NaCl is 0.576°C and the freezing point of blood serum is −0.52°C.**
    A: 0.884
    B: 0.273
    C: 1.092
    D: 0.178

15. **Indicate which of the following statements are correct.**
    A: The partition coefficient P is usually defined as the ratio of solubility in the aqueous phase to that in the non-aqueous phase
    B: The greater the value of log P, the higher the lipid solubility of the solute
    C: Ionised solutes will readily partition into the non-aqueous phase
    D: The partition coefficient of an amphoteric drug is at a maximum value at the isoelectric point

16. **Indicate which of the following statements are correct.**
    A: Drug molecules in solution will diffuse from a region of high chemical potential to one of low chemical potential
    B: The units of diffusion coefficient are $m\,s^{-1}$
    C: The diffusion coefficient decreases as the radius of the diffusing molecule increases
    D: The diffusion coefficient decreases when the viscosity of the solution is decreased
    E: The diffusion coefficient increases when the temperature is increased

CHAPTER 4

Drug stability

LEARNING OBJECTIVES

Upon completion of this chapter you should be able to:
- identify those classes of drugs that are particularly susceptible to chemical breakdown and outline some of the precautions that can be taken to minimise the loss of activity
- understand how reactions can be classified into various orders, and how to calculate the rate constant for a reaction under a given set of environmental conditions
- outline some of the factors that influence drug stability
- outline methods for accelerating drug breakdown using elevated temperatures and understand how to estimate drug stability at the required storage conditions from these measurements.

The chemical breakdown of drugs

The main ways in which drugs break down are as follows:

Hydrolysis
- Drugs containing ester, amide, lactam, imide or carbamate groups are susceptible to hydrolysis.
- Hydrolysis can be catalysed by hydrogen ions (specific acid catalysis) or hydroxyl ions (specific base catalysis).
- Solutions can be stabilised by formulating at the pH of maximum stability or, in some cases, by altering the dielectric constant by the addition of non-aqueous solvents.

Oxidation
- Oxidation involves the removal of an electropositive atom, radical or electron, or the addition of an electronegative atom or radical.
- Oxidative degradation can occur by autoxidation, in which a reaction is uncatalysed and proceeds quite slowly under the influence of molecular oxygen, or may involve chain processes consisting of three concurrent reactions: initiation, propagation and termination.
- Examples of drugs that are susceptible to oxidation include steroids and sterols, polyunsaturated fatty acids, phenothiazines, and drugs such as simvastatin and polyene antibiotics that contain conjugated double bonds.
- Various precautions should be taken during manufacture and storage to minimise oxidation:
  - the oxygen in pharmaceutical containers should be replaced with nitrogen or carbon dioxide

- contact of the drug with heavy-metal ions such as iron, cobalt or nickel, which catalyse oxidation, should be avoided
- storage should be at reduced temperatures
- antioxidants should be included in the formulation.

Key points

- Drugs may break down in solution and also in the solid state (for example, in tablet or powder form).
- It is often possible to predict which drugs are likely to decompose by looking for specific chemical groups in their structures.
- The most common causes of decomposition are hydrolysis and oxidation, but loss of therapeutic activity can also result from isomerisation, photochemical decomposition and polymerisation of drugs.
- It is possible to minimise breakdown by optimising the formulation and storing under carefully controlled conditions.

Isomerisation

- Isomerisation is the process of conversion of a drug into its optical or geometric isomers, which are often of lower therapeutic activity.
- Examples of drugs that undergo isomerisation include adrenaline (epinephrine: racemisation in acidic solution), tetracyclines (epimerisation in acid solution), cephalosporins (base-catalysed isomerisation) and vitamin A (*cis–trans* isomerisation).

Key points

- Reactions may be classified according to the order of reaction, which is the number of reacting species whose concentration determines the rate at which the reaction occurs.
- The most important orders of reaction are zero-order (breakdown rate is independent of the concentration of any of the reactants), first-order (reaction rate is determined by one concentration term) and second-order (rate is determined by the concentrations of two reacting species).
- The decomposition of many drugs can occur simultaneously by two or more pathways, which complicates the determination of rate constants.

Photochemical decomposition

- Examples of drugs that degrade when exposed to light include nifedipine, phenothiazines, hydrocortisone, prednisolone, riboflavin, ascorbic acid and folic acid.

- Photodecomposition may occur not only during storage, but also during use of the product. For example, sunlight is able to penetrate the skin to a depth sufficient to cause photodegradation of drugs circulating in the surface capillaries or in the eyes of patients receiving the drug. In the case of nifedipine, decomposition can occur during preparation of infusions; in some cases giving sets should be protected from light.
- Pharmaceutical products can be adequately protected from photo-induced decomposition by the use of coloured-glass containers (amber glass excludes light of wavelength <470 nm) and storage in the dark. Coating tablets with a polymer film containing ultraviolet absorbers has been suggested as an additional method for protection from light; drugs that are photosensitive may cause phototoxicity, photoallergy and photosensitivity (see **Chapter 11**).

Polymerisation

- Polymerisation is the process by which two or more identical drug molecules combine together to form a complex molecule.
- Examples of drugs that polymerise include amino-penicillins, such as ampicillin sodium in aqueous solution, and also formaldehyde. Polymers (or oligomers) of penicillins can be allergenic.

Kinetics of chemical decomposition in solution

Zero-order reactions:

- The decomposition proceeds at a constant rate and is independent of the concentrations of any of the reactants.
- The rate equation is:

$$dx/dt = k_0$$

- Integration of the rate equation gives:

$$x = k_0 t$$

- A plot of the amount decomposed (as ordinate) against time (as abscissa) is linear with a slope of k_0 (*Figure 4.1*).
- The units of k_0 are concentration time^{-1}.
- Many decomposition reactions in the solid phase or in suspensions apparently follow zero-order kinetics.

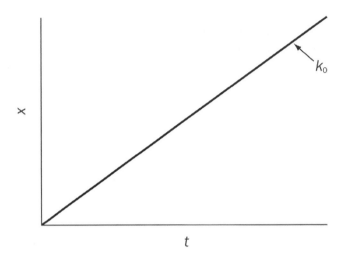

Figure 4.1: *Plot of the amount decomposed against time for a zero-order reaction.*

First-order reactions:
- The rate depends on the concentration of one reactant.
- The rate equation is:

$$dx/dt = k_1(a - x)$$

- Integration of the rate equation gives:

$$k_1 = \frac{2.303}{t} \log \frac{a}{a - x}$$

- Rearrangement into a linear equation gives:

$$t = \frac{2.303}{k_1} \log a - \frac{2.303}{k_1} \log (a - x)$$

- A plot of time (as ordinate) against the logarithm of the amount remaining (as abscissa) is linear with a slope $= -2.303/k_1$ (*Figure 4.2*).
- The units of k_1 are time^{-1}.
- If there are two reactants and one is in large excess, the reaction may still follow first-order kinetics because the change in concentration of the excess reactant is negligible. This type of reaction is a pseudo first-order reaction.
- The half-life of a first-order reaction is $t_{0.5} = 0.693/k_1$. The half-life is therefore independent of the initial concentration of reactants.

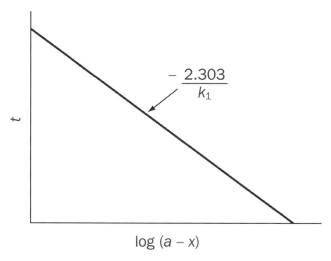

$$-\frac{2.303}{k_1}$$

$\log (a - x)$

Figure 4.2: *Plot of log amount of reactant remaining against time for a first-order reaction.*

Tips

The rate of decomposition of a drug A is the change of concentration of A over a time interval, t, i.e., $-d[A]/dt$ (note that this is negative because the drug concentration is decreasing). However, it is more usual to express the rate as dx/dt, where x is amount of drug which has reacted in time t.

We can show that $-d[A]/dt$ is equal to dx/dt as follows. If the initial concentration of drug A is a mol dm^{-3} and if we find experimentally that x mol dm^{-3} of the drug has reacted in time t, then the amount of drug remaining at a time t, i.e., $[A]$, is $(a - x)$ mol dm^{-3} and the rate of reaction is:

$-d[A]/dt = -d(a - x)/dt = dx/dt$

Notice that the term a is a constant and therefore disappears during differentiation.

So, when we say that a drug A decomposes by a first-order reaction it means that the rate is proportional to the concentration of A at any particular time, i.e., rate $\propto$ [A]. The rate of reaction is therefore given by $dx/dt = k[A]$, where the proportionality constant, k, is called the rate constant.

Second-order reactions:

- The rate depends on the concentrations of two reacting species, A and B.
- For the usual case where the initial concentrations of A and B are different, the rate equation is:

$$dx/dt = k_2(a - x)(b - x)$$

where a and b are the initial concentrations of reactants A and B, respectively.
- The integrated rate equation is:

$$k_2 = \frac{2.303}{t(a-b)} \log \frac{b(a-x)}{a(b-x)}$$

- Rearrangement into a linear equation gives:

$$t = \frac{2.303}{k_2(a-b)} \log \frac{b}{a} + \frac{2.303}{k_2(a-b)} \log \frac{(a-x)}{(b-x)}$$

- A plot of time (as ordinate) against the logarithm of $[(a - x)/(b - x)]$ (as abscissa) is linear with a slope $= 2.303/k_2(a - b)$ (*Figure 4.3*).
- The units of k_2 are concentration^{-1} time^{-1}.
- The half-life of a second-order reaction depends on the initial concentration of reactants and it is not possible to derive a simple expression to calculate it.

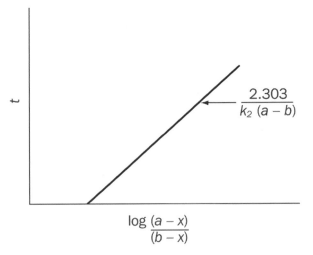

Figure 4.3: *Plot of log (amount of reactant A remaining/amount of reactant B remaining) against time for a second-order reaction.*

> **Tip**
>
> The half-life is the time taken for half the reactant to decompose. Therefore, to derive an expression for the half-life, substitute $t = t_{0.5}$, $x = a/2$, and $(a - x) = a - a/2 = a/2$ into the integrated-rate equation. This now becomes
>
> $$t_{0.5} = \frac{2.303}{k_1} \log \frac{a}{a/2}$$
>
> And hence
>
> $$t_{0.5} = \frac{2.303}{k_1} \log 2 = \frac{0.693}{k_1}$$

Complex reactions

These are reactions involving simultaneous breakdown by more than one route or by a sequence of reaction steps. Some examples include:

- Reversible reactions of the type

$$A \underset{k_r}{\overset{k_f}{\rightleftharpoons}} B$$

where k_f is the rate of the forward reaction and k_r is the rate of the reverse reaction. For these reactions the rate constants can be calculated from a plot of t (as ordinate) against
$\log[([A_o] - [A_{eq}])/([A] - [A_{eq}])]$, where $[A_o]$, $[A]$ and $[A_{eq}]$
represent the initial concentration, the concentration at time t and the equilibrium concentration of reactant A, respectively. The plot should be linear with a slope of $2.303/(k_f + k_r)$. k_f and k_r may be calculated separately if the equilibrium constant K is also determined, since
$K = k_f/k_r$.
- Parallel reactions in which the decomposition involves two or more pathways, the preference for each route depending on the conditions. Values of the rate constants k_A and k_B for each route may be evaluated separately by determining experimentally the overall rate constant, k_{exp}, and also the ratio R of the concentration of products formed by each reaction from $R = [A]/[B] = k_A/k_B$. It is then possible to calculate the rate constants from $k_A = k_{exp}(R/(R + 1))$ and $k_B = k_A/R$.
- Consecutive reactions in which drug A decomposes to an intermediate B which then decomposes to product C. Each of the decomposition steps has its own rate constant but there is no simple equation to calculate them.

Tip

Note that the rate equations used for plotting experimental data are linear equations of the form $y = mx + c$. It is important to remember this when plotting the data. For example, if you are fitting data to the equation

$$t = \frac{2.303}{k_1} \log a - \frac{2.303}{k_1} \log (a - x)$$

then $t = y$, $\log (a - x) = x$ and the gradient $m = -2.303/k_1$. If, for convenience, you plot t on the x-axis and $\log (a - x)$ on the y-axis, then the gradient will, of course, be $-k_1/2.303$.

Key points

The rate of decomposition is influenced by formulation factors such as the pH of the liquid preparation or the addition of electrolytes to control tonicity, and also by environmental factors such as temperature, light and oxygen. An understanding of the way in which these affect the rate of reaction often suggests a means of stabilising the product.

Factors influencing drug stability of liquid dosage forms

pH
- pH has a significant influence on the rate of decomposition of drugs that are hydrolysed in solution and it is usual to minimise this effect by formulating at the pH of maximum stability using buffers.
- The rate of reaction is, however, influenced not only by the catalytic effect of hydrogen and hydroxyl ions (specific acid–base catalysis), but also by the components of the buffer system (general acid–base catalysis). The effect of the buffer components can be large. For example, the hydrolysis rate of codeine in 0.05 M phosphate buffer at pH 7 is almost 20 times faster than in unbuffered solution at this pH.
- The general equation for these two effects is:

$$k_{obs} = k_0 + k_{H^+}[H^+] + k_{OH^-}[OH^-] + k_{HX}[HX] + k_{X^-}[X^-]$$

where k_{obs} is the experimentally determined hydrolytic rate constant, k_0 is the uncatalysed or solvent-catalysed rate constant, k_{H^+} and k_{OH^-} are the specific acid and base catalysis rate constants respectively, k_{HX} and k_{X^-} are the general acid and base catalysis rate constants respectively and [HX] and [X^-] denote the concentrations of protonated and unprotonated forms of the buffer.
- The ability of a buffer component to catalyse hydrolysis is related to its dissociation

constant, K, by the Brønsted catalysis law. The catalytic coefficient of a buffer component which is a weak acid is given by $k_A = aK_A{}^{\alpha}$; the catalytic coefficient of a weak base $k_B = bK_B{}^{\beta}$, where a, b, α, and β are constants, and α and β are positive and vary between 0 and 1.

- To remove the influence of the buffer, the reaction rate should be measured at a series of buffer concentrations at each pH and the data extrapolated back to zero buffer concentration. These extrapolated rate constants are plotted as a function of pH to give the required buffer-independent pH–rate profile (*Figure 4.4*)
- The rate constants for specific acid and base catalysis can be determined from the linear plots obtained when the corrected experimental rate constants, k_{obs}, are plotted against the hydrogen ion concentration [H^+] at low pH (gradient is k_{H^+}), and against the hydroxyl ion concentration at high pH (gradient is k_{OH^-}).
- Complex pH rate profiles are seen when the ionisation of the drug changes over the pH of measurement because of the differing susceptibility of the un-ionised and ionised forms of the drug to hydrolysis.
- The oxidative degradation of some drugs, for example prednisolone and morphine, in solution may be pH-dependent because of the effect of pH on the oxidation–reduction potential, E_0, of the drug.
- The photodegradation of several drugs, for example midazolam and ciprofloxacin, is also pH-dependent.

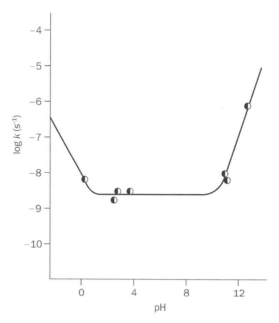

Figure 4.4: *A typical plot of log rate constant as a function of pH for a drug (codeine sulfate) which undergoes both acid and base catalysis. Modified from Powell MF. Enhanced stability of codeine sulfate: effect of pH, buffer and temperature on the degradation of codeine in aqueous solution. J Pharm Sci 1986;75:901–3 with permission.*

Temperature

- Increase in temperature usually causes a very pronounced increase in the hydrolysis rate of drugs in solution. This effect is used as the basis for drug stability testing.
- The equation which describes the effect of temperature on decomposition is the Arrhenius equation:

$$\log k = \log A - E_a/(2.303\ RT)$$

where E_a is the activation energy, A is the frequency factor, R is the gas constant $(8.314\ \text{J mol}^{-1}\ \text{K}^{-1})$ and T is the temperature in kelvins.

- The Arrhenius equation predicts that a plot of the log rate constant, k, against the reciprocal of the temperature should be linear with a gradient of $-E_a/2.303R$. Therefore, assuming that there is not a change in the order of reaction with temperature, we can measure rates of reaction at high temperatures (where the reaction occurs relatively rapidly) and extrapolate the Arrhenius plots to estimate the rate constant at room temperature (where reaction occurs at a very slow rate) (*Figure 4.5*). This method therefore provides a means of speeding up the measurements of drug stability during preformulation.
- If a drug formulation is particularly unstable at room temperature, for example injections of penicillin, insulin, oxytocin and vasopressin, it should be labelled with instructions to store in a cool place.

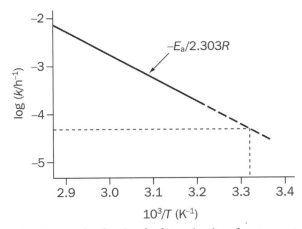

Figure 4.5: *A typical Arrhenius plot showing the determination of a rate constant at room temperature by extrapolation of data at high temperatures.*

Ionic strength

- The equation which describes the influence of electrolyte on the rate constant is the Brønsted–Bjerrum equation:

$$\log k = \log k_0 + 2Az_Az_B\sqrt{\mu}$$

where z_A and z_B are the charge numbers of the two interacting ions, A is a constant for a given solvent and temperature and μ is the ionic strength (see below).

- The Brønsted–Bjerrum equation predicts that a plot of log k against $\mu^{1/2}$ should be linear for a reaction in the presence of different concentrations of the same electrolyte with a gradient of $2Az_Az_B$ (*Figure 4.6*).
- The gradient will be positive (i.e. the reaction rate will be increased by electrolyte addition) when reaction is between ions of similar charge, for example, the acid-catalysed hydrolysis of a cationic drug ion.
- The gradient will be negative (i.e. the reaction rate will be decreased by electrolyte addition) when the reaction is between ions of opposite charge, for example, the base-catalysed hydrolysis of positively charged drug species.

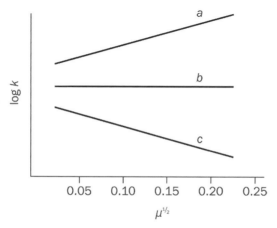

Figure 4.6: *The variation of rate constant, k, with square root of ionic strength, μ, for reaction between a: ions of similar charge, b: ion and uncharged molecule and c: ions of opposite charge.*

Tip

Ionic strength can be calculated from:

$$\mu = \tfrac{1}{2}\Sigma(mz^2)$$

$$= \tfrac{1}{2}(m_A z_A^2 + m_B z_B^2 + \ldots)$$

So, for example, if we have a monovalent drug ion of concentration $0.01 \, \text{mol kg}^{-1}$ in the presence of $0.001 \, \text{mol kg}^{-1}$ of Ca^{2+} ions, then the ionic strength of the solution will be $\mu = \tfrac{1}{2}[(0.01 \times 1^2) + (0.001 \times 2^2)] = 0.007 \, \text{mol kg}^{-1}$. Note that if the drug ion and the electrolyte ion are both monovalent, then the ionic strength will be equal to the total molality of the solution.

Solvent effects

- The equation that describes the effect of the dielectric constant, ε, on the rate of hydrolysis is:

$$\log k = \log k_{\varepsilon=\infty} - Kz_Az_B/\varepsilon$$

where K is a constant for a particular reaction at a given temperature, z_A and z_B are the charge numbers of the two interacting ions and $k_{\varepsilon=\infty}$ is the rate constant in a theoretical solvent of infinite dielectric constant.
- This equation predicts that a plot of $\log k$ against the reciprocal of the dielectric constant of the solvent should be linear with a gradient $-Kz_Az_B$. The intercept when $1/\varepsilon = 0$ (i.e. when $\varepsilon = \infty$) is equal to the logarithm of the rate constant, $k_{\varepsilon=\infty}$, in a theoretical solvent of infinite dielectric constant (*Figure 4.7*).
- The gradient will be negative when the charges on the drug ion and the interacting species are the same. This means that if we replace the water with a solvent of lower dielectric constant then we will achieve the desired effect of reducing the reaction rate (see Tips box on next page).
- The gradient will be positive if the drug ion and the interacting ion are of opposite signs and therefore the choice of a non-polar solvent will only result in an increase of decomposition.

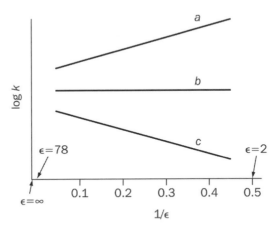

Figure 4.7: *The variation of rate constant with reciprocal of dielectric constant for reaction between a, ions of opposite charge, b, ion and uncharged molecule and c, ions of similar charge.*

> **Tips**
> - The dielectric constant (or relative permittivity) of a solvent is a measure of its polarity. Water has a high dielectric constant (approximately 78 at room temperature); other solvents have much lower values (for example, ε of ethanol is approximately 24).
> - Obviously, the particular solvent chosen to replace water in non-aqueous formulations must be non-toxic and alcohol–water or propylene glycol–water mixtures may be suitable for this purpose.

Oxygen
- The susceptibility of a drug to the presence of oxygen can be tested by comparing its stability in ampoules purged with oxygen to that when it is stored under nitrogen.
- Drugs which have a higher rate of decomposition when exposed to oxygen can be stabilised by replacing the oxygen in the storage container with nitrogen or carbon dioxide. These drugs should also be kept out of contact with heavy metals and should be stabilised with antioxidants.

Light
- The susceptibility of a drug to light can readily be tested by comparing its stability when exposed to light to that when stored in the dark.
- Photolabile drugs should be stored in containers of amber glass and, as an added precaution, should be kept in the dark.

Factors influencing drug stability of solid dosage forms

Moisture
- Water-soluble drugs in the solid dosage form will dissolve in any moisture layer which forms on the solid surface. The drug will now be in an aqueous environment and will be affected by many of the same factors as for liquid dosage forms.
- It is important to select packaging that will exclude moisture during storage.

Excipients
- Excipients such as starch and povidone have high water contents and affect stability by increasing the water content of the formulation.
- Chemical interactions between the excipients and the drug can sometimes occur and these lead to a decrease of stability. For example, stearate salts used as tablet lubricants can cause base-catalysed hydrolysis; polyoxyethlene glycols used as suppository bases can cause degradation of aspirin.

Temperature

- The effect of temperature on stability can sometimes be described by the Arrhenius equation (see below), but complications arise if the dosage form melts on temperature increase (e.g. suppositories) or if the drug or one of the excipients changes its polymorphic form.

Light and oxygen

- Solid dosage formulations containing photolabile drugs or drugs susceptible to oxidation should be stored in the same way as described for liquid dosage forms to protect from light and oxygen. Note also that moisture contains dissolved oxygen and hence the preparations should be stored in dry conditions.

Key points

- It is most important to be able to ensure that a particular formulation when packaged in a specific container will remain within its physical, chemical, microbiological, therapeutic and toxicological specifications on storage for a specified time period.
- In order to have such an assurance we need to conduct a rigorous stability testing programme on the product in the form that is finally to be marketed.
- To calculate the shelf-life it is necessary to know the rate constant at the storage temperature. However, the rate of breakdown of most pharmaceutical products is so slow that it would take many months to determine this at room temperature and it has become essential to devise a more rapid technique which can be used during product development to speed up the identification of the most suitable formulation.
- The method that is used for accelerated storage testing is based on the Arrhenius equation (see below).

Stability testing and calculation of shelf-life

The Arrhenius equation is used as the basis of a method for accelerating decomposition by raising the temperature of the preparations. This method provides a means for rapidly identifying the most suitable preparation during preformulation of the product. The main steps in the process are:

- Determination of the order of reaction by plotting stability data at several elevated temperatures according to the equations relating decomposition to time for each of the orders of reaction, until linear plots are obtained.
- Values of the rate constant k at each temperature are calculated from the gradient of these plots, and the logarithm of k is plotted against reciprocal temperature according to the Arrhenius equation

$$\log k = \log A - E_a/2.303RT$$

- A value of k can be interpolated from this plot at the required temperature.
- Alternatively, if only an approximate value of k is required at temperature T_1, then this may be estimated from measurements at a single higher temperature T_2 using

$$\log \left[\frac{k_2}{k_1} \right] = \frac{E_a(T_2 - T_1)}{2.303RT_2T_1}$$

where k_1 and k_2 are the rate constants at temperatures T_1 and T_2, respectively. A mid-range value of $E_a = 75\,\text{kJ mol}^{-1}$ may be used for these rough estimations.
- The shelf-life for the product can be calculated from the rate constant based on an acceptable degree of decomposition. For example, for decomposition which follows first-order kinetics, the time taken for 10% loss of activity is given by $t_{90} = 0.105/k_1$.

Tip

You can derive an expression for the time taken for 10% of the reactant to decompose by substituting $t = t_{0.9}$, $x = 0.1a$, $(a - x) = a - 0.1a = 0.9a$ into the integrated-rate equation for the relevant order of reaction. For example, substituting into the first-order rate equation gives

$$t_{0.9} = \frac{2.303}{k_1} \log \frac{a}{0.9a} = \frac{0.105}{k_1}$$

Memory maps

Drug stability in solid dosage forms

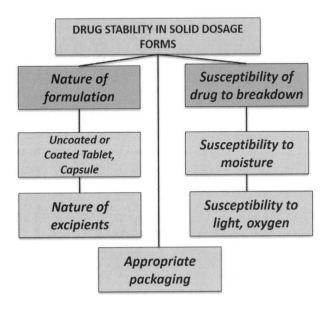

Factors affecting drug stability

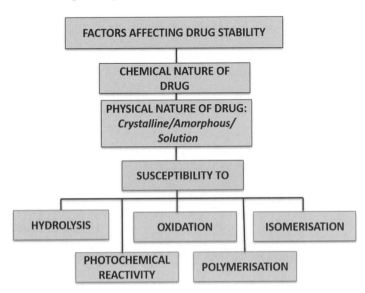

Questions

In questions 1–6 indicate which of the statements are true.

1. **In a zero-order reaction:**
   A: The rate of decomposition is independent of the concentration of the reactants
   B: The rate of decomposition is dependent on the concentration of one of the reactants
   C: A plot of the amount remaining (as ordinate) against time (as abscissa) is linear with a slope of $1/k$
   D: The units of k are (concentration^{-1} time^{-1})
   E: The half-life is $t_{0.5} = 0.693/k$

2. **In a second-order reaction:**
   A: The rate of reaction depends on the concentration of two reacting species
   B: A plot of time (as ordinate) against the logarithm of $[(a - x)/(b - x)]$ (as abscissa) is linear with a slope = $2.303/k_2(a - b)$
   C: The units of k are concentration $\times$ time^{-1}
   D: The half-life is independent of the concentration of the reactants

3. **In a study of the hydrolysis of a drug in aqueous solution a plot of logarithm of the amount of drug remaining (as ordinate) against time (as abscissa) is linear.**
   A: The reaction is zero-order
   B: The slope is $-2.303/k$
   C: The units of k are (concentration^{-1} time^{-1})
   D: The half-life is $t_{0.5} = 0.693/k$
   E: The half-life depends on the initial concentration of reactants

4. **The Arrhenius equation for effect of temperature on the hydrolysis of a drug in aqueous solution:**
   A: Predicts that the rate of reaction will decrease as temperature is increased
   B: Predicts that a plot of log k against temperature will be linear
   C: Predicts that a plot of log k against the reciprocal of temperature will be linear
   D: Predicts that there will be no change in the order of reaction when temperature is increased
   E: Is the basis of drug stability testing

5. **The Brønsted–Bjerrum equation:**
   A: Describes the influence of electrolyte on the rate constant
   B: Predicts that a plot of log k against ionic strength will be linear
   C: Predicts that a plot of log k against the reciprocal of ionic strength will be linear
   D: Predicts that the reaction rate will be increased by electrolyte addition when reaction is between ions of similar charge
   E: Predicts that the reaction rate will be decreased by electrolyte addition when the reaction is between ions of opposite charge

6. **The equation that describes the effect of dielectric constant on rate of reaction predicts that:**
   A: A plot of log k against the reciprocal of the dielectric constant of the solvent should be linear
   B: A plot of k against the reciprocal of the dielectric constant of the solvent should be linear
   C: Replacing the water with a solvent of lower dielectric constant will always reduce the reaction rate
   D: The rate of hydrolysis will increase when a less polar solvent is used if the drug ion and the interacting ion are of opposite charge
   E: The rate of hydrolysis will increase when a less polar solvent is used if the charges on the drug ion and the interacting species are the same

7. **Indicate which of the following statements relating to the effect of pH on drug stability are true.**
   A: The rate of acid-catalysed decomposition of a drug increases with pH
   B: The rate of base-catalysed decomposition of a drug increases with the concentration of hydroxyl ions.
   C: The effect of buffer components on decomposition is referred to as general acid–base catalysis
   D: A plot of the observed-rate constant (as ordinate) against pH (as abscissa) for an acid-catalysed reaction has a gradient equal to k_{H^+}

8. **What is the remaining concentration $(a - x)$ in mg mL^{-1} of a drug (initial concentration $a = 7$ mg mL^{-1}) after a time equivalent to 3 half-lives assuming that the decomposition follows first-order kinetics?**
   A: 2.33
   B: 3.5
   C: 1.75
   D: 0.875
   E: 1.167

9. **The time taken for 5% of a drug to decompose by first-order kinetics is:**
   A: $0.022/k_1$
   B: $0.051/k_1$
   C: $0.105/k_1$
   D: $k_1/0.051$
   E: $0.105\ k_1$

CHAPTER 5

Surfactants

LEARNING OBJECTIVES

Upon completion of this chapter you should be able to:
- understand why certain molecules have the ability to lower surface and interfacial tension and how the surface activity of a molecule is related to its molecular structure
- outline the properties of some surfactants that are commonly used in pharmacy
- outline the nature and properties of monolayers formed when insoluble surfactants are spread over the surface of a liquid
- outline some of the factors that influence adsorption onto solid surfaces and understand how experimental data from adsorption experiments may be analysed to gain information on the process of adsorption
- understand why micelles are formed, outline the structure of ionic and non-ionic micelles and outline some of the factors that influence micelle formation
- outline the properties of liquid crystals and surfactant vesicles
- outline the process of solubilisation of water-insoluble compounds by surfactant micelles and its applications in pharmacy.

Types of surfactant

Depending on their charge characteristics, surface-active molecules may be anionic, cationic, zwitterionic (ampholytic) or non-ionic.
- The most commonly encountered anionic surfactants have carboxylate, sulfate, sulfonate and phosphate polar groups in combination with counterions such as sodium and potassium (for water-solubility) or calcium and magnesium (for oil-solubility).
- In the most common cationic surfactants the charge is carried on a nitrogen atom as, for example, with amine and quaternary ammonium surfactants. The quaternary ammonium compounds retain this charge over the whole pH range, whereas the amine-based compounds only function as surfactants in the protonated state and therefore cannot be used at high pH.
- By far the most common non-ionic surfactants are those with one or more poly(oxyethylene) chains as their hydrophilic part.
- Zwitterionic and amphoteric surfactants possess polar head groups which on ionisation may impart both positive and negative charges.
  - The positive charge is almost always carried by an ammonium group and the negative charge is often a carboxylate.
  - If the ammonium group is quaternary the molecule will exist as a zwitterion over a wide pH range since the quaternary ammonium group will be permanently charged.

- — If not, the molecule will behave as a true amphoteric surfactant, that is, the molecule will change from net cationic to zwitterionic and finally to net anionic as the pH is increased; such surfactants will only therefore be zwitterionic over a certain range of pH which depends on the pK_a values of each charge group.
- — At the isoelectric point both charged groups will be fully ionised and the molecule will have properties similar to those of non-ionic surfactants. As the pH shifts away from the isoelectric point, the molecule will gradually assume the properties of either a cationic or anionic surfactant.
- — Common examples are N-alkyl derivatives of simple amino acids such as glycine (NH_2CH_2COOH), aminopropionic acid ($NH_2CH_2CH_2COOH$) and the alkyl betaines.

Key point

Surfactants have two distinct regions in their chemical structure, one of which is water-liking or hydrophilic and the other of which is water-hating or hydrophobic. These molecules are referred to as amphiphilic or amphipathic molecules or simply as surfactants or surface active agents.

Some typical surfactants

Examples of surfactants that are used in pharmaceutical formulation are as follows:

Anionic surfactants: Sodium Lauryl Sulfate BP
- is a mixture of sodium alkyl sulfates, the chief of which is sodium dodecyl sulfate, $C_{12}H_{25}SO_4^-Na^+$
- is very soluble in water at room temperature, and is used pharmaceutically as a preoperative skin cleaner, having bacteriostatic action against Gram-positive bacteria, and also in medicated shampoos
- is a component of emulsifying wax.

Cationic surfactants
- The quaternary ammonium and pyridinium cationic surfactants are important pharmaceutically because of their bactericidal activity against a wide range of Gram-positive and some Gram-negative organisms.
- They may be used on the skin, especially in the cleaning of wounds.
- Their aqueous solutions are used for cleaning contaminated utensils.

Non-ionic surfactants
- Polyoxyethylene alkyl ethers are glycol ethers of n-alcohols, also known as macrogol ethers, (macrogol being the nonproprietary name for polyethylene glycol). They tend to be mixtures of polymers of slightly varying molecular weights, and the numbers

used to describe their chain lengths are average values. A widely used example is Cetomacrogol 1000 BP (Macrogol Cetostearyl Ether), which is a water-soluble substance with the general structure $CH_3(CH_2)_m(OCH_2CH_2)_nOH$, where m may be 15 or 17 and the number of oxyethylene groups, n, is between 20 and 24. It is used in the form of Cetomacrogol Emulsifying Wax BP in the preparation of oil-in-water emulsions and also as a solubilising agent for volatile oils. Other macrogol ethers are commercially available as the Brij series.

- Polyoxyethylene castor oil derivatives are a series of non-ionic surfactants synthesised by reacting either castor oil or hydrogenated castor oil with varying amounts of ethylene oxide. The most widely used are the Cremophor series (BASF Corp). For example, Cremophor EL and Cremophor RH40 are used to solubilise the fat-soluble vitamins in aqueous solutions for oral and topical administration, Cremophor EL is also used as a solubilising agent in the preparation of intravenous anaesthetics.

- Polyglycolysed glycerides are produced by the partial pegylation of glycerides (fatty acid esters of glycerol) derived from fixed oils of vegetable origin - apricot kernel oil (mainly composed of oleic acid) in the case of Labrafil M-1944CS, corn oil (mainly linoleic acid) for Labrafil M-2125CS, coconut oil (mainly caprylic and capric acids) for Labrasol and palm kernel oil (mainly lauric and myristic acids) for Gelucire 44/14. The average polyoxyethylene chain lengths of these commercial products also vary. They are used mainly as micellar solubilising agents.

- Polyoxyethylene esters.
  - Widely used examples are Vitamin E TPGS and Sotulol HS-15. Vitamin E TPGS (D-α-tocopheryl polyethylene glycol 1000 succinate) is prepared by the esterification of the acid group of crystalline D-α-tocopheryl acid succinate by polyethylene glycol 1000. It is used as an emulsifier, micellar solubilising agent, an absorption enhancer and as a vehicle for lipid-based drug delivery formulations. It is also a water-soluble source of the water-insoluble oil Vitamin E (D-α-tocopherol).
  - Sotulol HS-15 (polyoxyethylene 660 hydroxystearate or macrogol 660) is a mixture of ~70% polyglycol mono- and di-esters of 12-hydroxystearic acid (lipophilic) and ~30% of free polyethylene glycol (hydrophilic). It is a water-soluble, micelle forming, solubilising agent used commercially in oral and parenteral formulations with lipophilic drugs and vitamins.

- Sorbitan esters are supplied commercially as Spans and are mixtures of the partial esters of sorbitol and its mono- and di-anhydrides with oleic acid. They are generally insoluble in water (low hydrophile–lipophile balance (HLB) value) and are used as water-in-oil emulsifiers and as wetting agents.

- Polysorbates are complex mixtures of partial esters of sorbitol and its mono-and di-anhydrides condensed with an approximate number of moles of ethylene oxide. They are supplied commercially as Tweens. The polysorbates are miscible with water, as reflected in their higher HLB values, and are used as emulsifying agents for oil-in-water emulsions.

- Poloxamers are synthetic block copolymers of hydrophilic poly(oxyethylene) and hydrophobic poly(oxypropylene) with the general formula $E_mP_nE_m$ where E = oxyethylene (OCH_2CH_2) and P = oxypropylene ($OCH_2CH(CH_3)$) and the subscripts m and n denote chain lengths. Properties such as viscosity, HLB and physical state (liquid, paste or solid) are dependent on the relative chain lengths of the hydrophilic and hydrophobic blocks. They are supplied commercially as Pluronics and are labelled using the Pluronic grid, for example as F127 or L62, where the letter indicates the physical state (F, P or L, denoting solid, paste or liquid, respectively). The last digit of this number is approximately one-tenth of the weight percentage of poly(oxyethylene); the first one (or two digits in a three-digit number) multiplied by 300 gives a rough estimate of the molecular weight of the hydrophobe. When polyoxyethylated surfactants are used in formulation it should be recognised that there can be batch to batch and brand to brand variations in PEG chain length as all are produced by polymerisation and have averaged PEG chain length.

- A wide variety of drugs, including the antihistamines and the tricyclic depressants, are surface-active.

> **Tip**
>
> HLB stands for hydrophile–lipophile balance. Compounds with a high HLB (greater than about 12) are predominantly hydrophilic and water-soluble. Those with very low HLB values are hydrophobic and water-insoluble.

Reduction of surface and interfacial tension

- When surfactants are dissolved in water they orientate at the surface so that the hydrophobic regions are removed from the aqueous environment, as shown in *Figure 5.1a*.
- The reason for the reduction in the surface tension when surfactant molecules adsorb at the water surface is that the surfactant molecules replace some of the water molecules in the surface and the forces of attraction between surfactant and water molecules are less than those between two water molecules, hence the contraction force is reduced.
- Surfactants will also adsorb at the interface between two immiscible liquids such as water and oil and will orientate themselves as shown in *Figure 5.1b*, with their hydrophilic group in the water and their hydrophobic group in the oil.
- The interfacial tension at this interface, which arises because of a similar imbalance of attractive forces as at the water surface, will be reduced by this adsorption.
- There is an equilibrium between surfactant molecules at the surface of the solution and those in the bulk of the solution which is expressed by the Gibbs equation:

$$\Gamma_2 = - \frac{1}{xRT} \frac{d\gamma}{2.303 \, d \log c}$$

where Γ_2 is the surface excess concentration, R is the gas constant ($8.314\,J\,mol^{-1}\,K^{-1}$), T is temperature in kelvins, c is the concentration in mol m^{-3} and x has a value of 1 for ionic surfactants in dilute solution.

- The area, A, occupied by a surfactant molecule at the solution–air interface can be calculated from $A = 1/N_A\Gamma_2$ where N_A is the Avogadro number (6.023×10^{23} molecules mol^{-1}) and dγ/d log c is the gradient of the plot of surface tension against log c measured at a concentration just below the critical micelle concentration (CMC).
- The surface activity of a particular surfactant depends on the balance between its hydrophilic and hydrophobic properties. For a homologous series of surfactants:
  - An increase in the length of the hydrocarbon chain (hydrophobic) increases the surface activity. This relationship between hydrocarbon chain length and surface activity is expressed by Traube's rule, which states that 'in dilute aqueous solutions of surfactants belonging to any one homologous series, the molar concentrations required to produce equal lowering of the surface tension of water decreases threefold for each additional CH$_2$ group in the hydrocarbon chain of the solute'.
  - An increase of the length of the ethylene oxide chain (hydrophilic) of a polyoxyethylated non-ionic surfactant results in a decrease of surface activity.

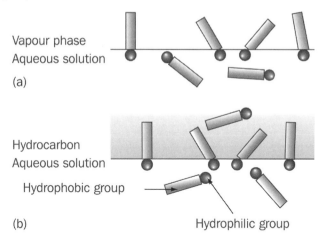

Figure 5.1: *Orientation of amphiphiles at (a) solution–vapour interface and (b) hydrocarbon–solution interface.*

Key points

- The molecules at the surface of water are not completely surrounded by other molecules as they are in the bulk of the water.
- As a result there is a net inward force of attraction exerted on a molecule at the surface from the molecules in the bulk solution, which results in a tendency for the surface to contract. This contraction is spontaneous and represents a minimum free energy state.
- We express the strength of contraction by the work required to increase the surface area by $1\,m^2$; this is referred to as the surface tension, γ.
- Units of surface and interfacial tension are $mN\,m^{-1}$.

Tip

- When substituting values into equations it is important to convert the values into the correct units. In the case of the Gibbs equation it is easy to forget to convert concentration into $mol\,m^{-3}$
  ($1\,mol\,L^{-1} = 1\,mol\,dm^{-3} = 10^3\,mol\,m^{-3}$).
- Remember when using Traube's rule that for every extra CH_2 group in the compound you need 3 times less of the compound to produce the same lowering of surface tension. So if you add 2 extra CH_2 groups you will require 9 times less of the compound (not 6 times less).
- Remember that an increase in surface activity means a decrease in surface tension. Compounds that are most effective in lowering the surface tension are those with a high surface activity.

Insoluble monolayers

- Insoluble amphiphilic compounds, for example surfactants with very long hydrocarbon chains, will also form films on water surfaces when the amphiphilic compound is dissolved in a volatile solvent and carefully injected onto the surface. Polymers and proteins may also form insoluble monolayers.
- The molecules are orientated at the surface in the same way as typical surfactants, i.e. with the hydrophobic group protruding into the air and the polar group acting as an anchor in the surface.
- The properties of the film can be studied using a Langmuir trough (*Figure 5.2*) as follows:
  - In use, the trough is filled completely so as to build up a meniscus above the level of the sides. The surface is swept clean with the movable barrier and any surface impurities are sucked away using a water pump.
  - The film-forming material is dissolved in a suitable volatile solvent and an accurately measured amount, usually about $0.01\,cm^3$, of this solution is carefully

distributed onto the surface. The solvent evaporates and leaves a uniformly spread film entirely contained in the well-defined surface area between the two barriers.
— The film is compressed by moving the movable barrier towards the fixed barrier in a series of steps. At each position of the two barriers the surface tension of the film-covered surface is measured directly using a Wilhelmy plate partially immersed in the subphase and attached to a sensitive electrobalance.
— The results are presented as plots of surface pressure π ($\pi = \gamma_o - \gamma_m$, where γ_o is the surface tension of the clean surface and γ_m is the surface tension of the film-covered surface) against area per molecule.
- There are three main types of insoluble monolayers (*Figure 5.3*):
  — Solid or condensed monolayers, in which the film pressure remains very low at high film areas and rises abruptly when the molecules become tightly packed on compression. The extrapolated limiting surface area is very close to the cross-sectional area of the molecule from molecular models.
  — Expanded monolayers, in which the π–A plots are quite steeply curved but extrapolation to a limiting surface area yields a value that is usually several times greater than the cross-sectional area from molecular models. Films of this type tend to be formed by molecules in which close packing into condensed films is prohibited by bulky side chains or by a *cis* configuration of the molecule.
  — Gaseous monolayers, in which there is only a gradual change in the surface pressure as the film is compressed. The molecules in this type of monolayer lie along the surface, often because they possess polar groups that are distributed about the molecule and anchor the molecules to the surface along its length. Monolayers of polymers and proteins are often of this type.
- Monolayers are useful models by which the properties of polymers used as packaging materials can be investigated. They may also be used as cell membrane models.

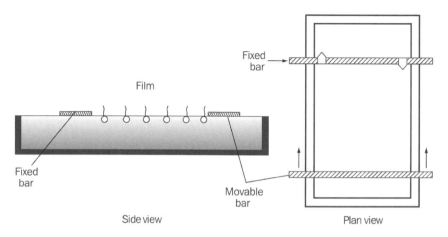

Figure 5.2: *Langmuir trough.*

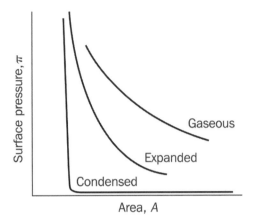

Figure 5.3: *Surface pressure, π, versus area per molecule, A, for the three main types of monolayer.*

Key point

The important difference between the film produced when surfactant molecules accumulate spontaneously at the surface of a surfactant solution and the film formed when insoluble amphiphilic compounds are injected onto a water surface is that in the former the surfactant molecules at the surface are in equilibrium with those in the bulk of the solution and continually move back and forward between the surface and the solution, whereas in insoluble monolayers all the molecules injected onto the surface stay at the surface.

Lung surfactant monolayers

- The lung surfactant membrane comprises a complex mixture of lipids and proteins that act to lower the surface tension of the alveolar air–water interface, thus facilitating the large surface area changes that occur during the successive compression–expansion cycles that accompany the breathing process.
- When formation of this membrane is incomplete, as may occur for example in prematurely born infants suffering from respiratory distress syndrome, breathing is laboured and there is insufficient transport of oxygen into the blood stream.
- Lung surfactant is a lipid–protein complex secreted as vesicles or other aggregates by type II pneumocytes into the thin aqueous layer that covers the alveoli; it spontaneously adsorbs from the aggregates to form a film at the air–water interface, which acts to moderate surface tension during breathing. Lung surfactant is a complex mixture of lipids and proteins consisting of 78–90% phospholipid, most of which is dipalmitoylphosphatidylcholine (DPPC), 5–10% protein and 4–10% neutral lipid, which is mainly cholesterol. The different components of lung surfactant

interact to determine the overall behaviour of the surfactant film.

- During inhalation phospholipid molecules are rapidly inserted into the expanding film to form a tightly packed rigid film with a surface tension of about $25\,mN\,m^{-1}$; this film is compressed during exhalation and as a result the surface tension is reduced to a low level (less than $5\,mN\,m^{-1}$). It is this very low surface tension that allows the lungs to inflate more easily during inhalation, so reducing the effort of breathing.
- Rigid monolayers formed by DPPC alone can provide the necessary low surface tension on compression of the alveolar interface that accompanies exhalation. However, pure DPPC is not able to spread rapidly enough to cover the greatly enlarged interface that is formed when the lungs expand during inhalation. The respreading of the film is greatly enhanced by the presence of the neutral lipids and the surfactant proteins.

Adsorption at the solid–liquid interface

- There are two general types of adsorption:
  1. Physical adsorption, in which the adsorbate is bound to the surface through the weak van der Waals forces.
  2. Chemical adsorption or chemisorption, which involves the stronger valence forces.
- Frequently both physical and chemical adsorption may be involved in a particular adsorption process.
- A simple experimental method of studying adsorption is to shake a known mass of the adsorbent material with a solution of known concentration at a fixed temperature until no further change in the concentration of the supernatant is observed, that is, until equilibrium conditions have been established.
- Adsorption data may be analysed using the Langmuir and Freundlich equations:
  - The Langmuir equation is:

$$x/m = abc/(1 + bc)$$

where x is the amount of solute adsorbed by a weight, m, of adsorbent, c is the concentration of solution at equilibrium, b is a constant related to the enthalpy of adsorption and a is related to the surface area of the solid. For practical usage the Langmuir equation is rearranged into a linear form as:

$$c/(x/m) = 1/ab + c/a$$

Values of a and b may then be determined from the intercept ($1/ab$) and slope ($1/a$) of plots of $c/(x/m)$ against concentration (*Figure 5.4*).
  - The Freundlich equation is:

$$x/m = ac^{1/n}$$

where a and n are constants, the form $1/n$ being used to emphasise that c is raised to a power less than unity. $1/n$ is a dimensionless parameter and is related to the intensity of drug adsorption. The linear form of this equation is:

$$\log (x/m) = \log a + (1/n) \log c$$

A plot of log (x/m) against log c should be linear, with an intercept of log a and slope of $1/n$ (*Figure 5.5*). It is generally assumed that, for systems that obey this equation, adsorption results in the formation of multilayers rather than a single monolayer.

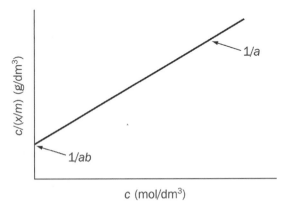

Figure 5.4: *A typical Langmuir plot.*

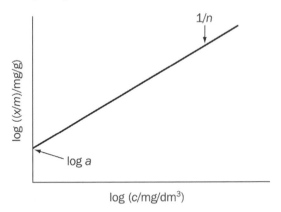

Figure 5.5: *A typical Freundlich plot.*

Key point

Note the difference between the term adsorption, which is used to describe the process of accumulation at an interface, and absorption, which means the penetration of one component throughout the body of a second.

Factors affecting adsorption

- Solubility of the adsorbate. In general, the extent of adsorption of a solute is inversely proportional to its solubility in the solvent from which adsorption occurs. This empirical rule is termed Lundelius' rule. For homologous series, adsorption from solution increases as the series is ascended and the molecules become more hydrophobic.
- pH. In general, for simple molecules adsorption increases as the ionisation of the drug is suppressed, the extent of adsorption reaching a maximum when the drug is completely un-ionised (*Figure 5.6*).
- Nature of the adsorbent. The most important property affecting adsorption is the surface area of the adsorbent; the extent of adsorption is proportional to the specific surface area. Thus, the more finely divided or the more porous the solid, the greater will be its adsorption capacity.
- Temperature. Since adsorption is generally an exothermic process, an increase in temperature normally leads to a decrease in the amount adsorbed.

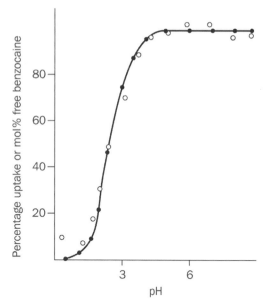

Figure 5.6: *The adsorption onto nylon of a typical weakly basic drug (O) and its percentage in un-ionised form (•) as a function of pH. Reproduced from Richards NE and Meakin BJ. The sorption of benzocaine from aqueous solution by nylon 6 powder.* J Pharm Pharmacol 1974;26:166–74 *with permission.*

Pharmaceutical applications and consequences of adsorption

- Adsorption of poisons/toxins. The 'universal antidote' for use in reducing the effects of poisoning by the oral route is composed of activated charcoal, magnesium oxide and tannic acid. Adsorbents are also used in dialysis to reduce toxic concentrations of drugs by passing blood through a haemodialysis membrane over charcoal and other adsorbents.
- Taste masking. Drugs such as diazepam may be adsorbed onto solid substrates to minimise taste problems, but care should be taken to ensure that desorption does not become a rate-limiting step in the absorption process.
- Haemoperfusion. Carbon haemoperfusion is an extracorporeal method of treating cases of severe drug overdoses and originally involved perfusion of the blood directly over charcoal granules. Activated charcoal granules are very effective in adsorbing many toxic materials, but they give off embolising particles and also lead to removal of blood platelets. These problems are removed by microencapsulation of activated charcoal granules by coating with biocompatible membranes such as acrylic hydrogels.
- Adsorption in drug formulation. Beneficial uses include adsorption of surfactants and polymers in the stabilisation of suspensions, and adsorption of surfactants onto poorly soluble solids to increase their dissolution rate through increased wetting. Problems may arise from the adsorption of medicaments by adsorbents such as antacids, which may be taken simultaneously by the patient, or which may be present in the same formulation; and from the adsorption of medicaments onto the container walls, which may affect the potency and possibly the stability of the product.

Micellisation

- Micelles are formed at the critical micelle concentration (CMC), which is detected as an inflection point when physicochemical properties such as surface tension are plotted as a function of concentration (*Figure 5.7*).
- The main reason for micelle formation is the attainment of a minimum free energy state. The main driving force for the formation of micelles is the increase of entropy that occurs when the hydrophobic regions of the surfactant are removed from water and the ordered structure of the water molecules around this region of the molecule is lost.
- Most micelles are spherical and contain between 60 and 100 surfactant molecules.
- The structure of the micelles formed by ionic surfactants (*Figure 5.8a*) consists of a:
  - hydrophobic core composed of the hydrocarbon chains of the surfactant molecule
  - Stern layer surrounding the core, which is a concentric shell of hydrophilic head groups with $(1 - a)N$ counterions, where a is the degree of ionisation and N is the aggregation number (number of molecules in the micelle). For most ionic micelles the degree of ionisation, a, is between 0.2 and 0.3; that is, 70–80% of the counterions may be considered to be bound to the micelles

- — Gouy-Chapman electrical double layer surrounding the Stern layer, which is a diffuse layer containing the aN counterions required to neutralise the charge on the kinetic micelle. The thickness of the double layer is dependent on the ionic strength of the solution and is greatly compressed in the presence of electrolyte.
- Micelles formed by non-ionic surfactants:
  - — are larger than their ionic counterparts and may sometimes be elongated into an ellipsoid or rod-like structure
  - — have a hydrophobic core formed from the hydrocarbon chains of the surfactant molecules surrounded by a shell (the palisade layer) composed of the oxyethylene chains of the surfactant (*Figure 5.8b*), which is heavily hydrated.
- Micelles formed in non-aqueous solution (reverse or inverted micelles) have a core composed of the hydrophilic groups surrounded by a shell of the hydrocarbon chains (Figure 5.8c).

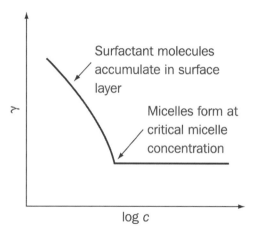

Figure 5.7: *Typical plot of the surface tension against logarithm of surfactant concentration, c, showing the critical micelle concentration.*

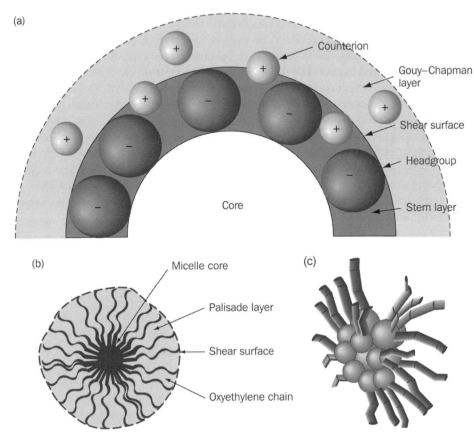

(a)

(b)

(c)

Figure 5.8: *(a) Partial cross-section of an anionic micelle showing charged layers; (b) cross-section of a non-ionic micelle; (c) diagrammatic representation of a reverse micelle, with the polar groups to the inside and the non-polar groups at the micelle surface.*

Key points

- Micelles are formed at the CMC.
- Micelles are dynamic structures and are continually formed and broken down in solution – they should not be thought of as solid spheres.
- The typical micelle diameter is about 2–3 nm and so they are not visible under a light microscope.
- There is an equilibrium between micelles and free surfactant molecules in solution.
- When the surfactant concentration is increased above the CMC, the number of micelles increases but the free surfactant concentration stays constant at the CMC value.

Tips

- Entropy is a thermodynamic property that is a measure of the randomness or disorder of a system.
- When a system becomes more chaotic its entropy increases, so the loss of water structure when micelles are formed will increase entropy.
- Entropy change, ΔS, is linked to free energy change, ΔG, by the equation $\Delta G = \Delta H - T\Delta S$.
- The enthalpy change, ΔH, when micelles are formed is very small and can be ignored, so you can see that an increase of entropy will lead to a decrease in free energy.
- Any change that leads to a free energy decrease will occur spontaneously because it leads to the formation of a more stable system. Micelle formation is therefore a spontaneous process.

Factors affecting the CMC and micellar size

Structure of the hydrophobic group

Increase in length of the hydrocarbon chain results in:

- a decrease in CMC, which for compounds with identical polar head groups is expressed by the linear equation:

$$\log [CMC] = A - Bm$$

where m is the number of carbon atoms in the chain and A and B are constants for a homologous series.
- corresponding increase in micellar size.

Nature of the hydrophilic group

- Non-ionic surfactants generally have very much lower CMC values and higher aggregation numbers than their ionic counterparts with similar hydrocarbon chains.
- An increase in the ethylene oxide chain length of a non-ionic surfactant makes the molecule more hydrophilic and as a consequence the CMC increases.

Type of counterion

- Micellar size increases for a particular cationic surfactant as the counterion is changed according to the series $Cl^- < Br^- < I^-$, and for a particular anionic surfactant according to $Na^+ < K^+ < Cs^+$.
- Ionic surfactants with organic counterions (e.g. maleates) have lower CMCs and higher aggregation numbers than those with inorganic counterions.

Addition of electrolytes

- Electrolyte addition to solutions of ionic surfactants decreases the CMC and increases the micellar size. This is because the electrolyte reduces the forces of repulsion between the charged head groups at the micelle surface, so allowing the micelle to grow.

- At high electrolyte concentration the micelles of ionic surfactants may become non-spherical.

Key points

- The properties of a surfactant are determined by the balance between the hydrophobic and hydrophilic parts of the molecule.
- If the hydrophobic chain length is increased then the whole molecule becomes more hydrophobic and micelles will form at lower solution concentrations, i.e. the CMC decreases.
- If the hydrophilic chain length is increased the molecule becomes more hydrophilic and the CMC will increase.

Effect of temperature

- Aqueous solutions of many non-ionic surfactants become turbid at a characteristic temperature called the cloud point.
- At temperatures up to the cloud point there is an increase in micellar size and a corresponding decrease in CMC.
- Temperature has a comparatively small effect on the micellar properties of ionic surfactants.

Formation of liquid crystals and vesicles

Lyotropic liquid crystals

- The liquid crystalline phases that occur on increasing the concentration of surfactant solutions are referred to as lyotropic liquid crystals; their structure is shown diagrammatically in *Figure 5.9*.
- Increase of concentration of a surfactant solution frequently causes a transition from the typical spherical micellar structure to a more elongated or rod-like micelle.
- Further increase in concentration may cause the orientation and close packing of the elongated micelles into hexagonal arrays; this is a liquid crystalline state termed the middle phase or hexagonal phase.
- With some surfactants, further increase of concentration results in the separation of a second liquid crystalline state – the neat phase or lamellar phase.
- In some surfactant systems another liquid crystalline state, the cubic phase, occurs between the middle and neat phases (*Figure 5.10*).
- Lyotropic liquid crystals are anisotropic, that is, their physical properties vary with direction of measurement.

- The middle phase, for example, will only flow in a direction parallel to the long axis of the arrays. It is rigid in the other two directions.
- The neat phase is more fluid and behaves as a solid only in the direction perpendicular to that of the layers.
- Plane-polarised light is rotated when travelling along any axis except the long axis in the middle phase and a direction perpendicular to the layers in the neat phase.

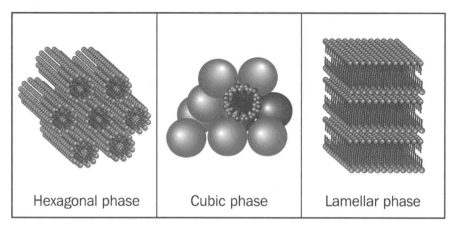

| Hexagonal phase | Cubic phase | Lamellar phase |

Figure 5.9: *Diagrammatic representation of forms of lyotropic liquid crystals.*

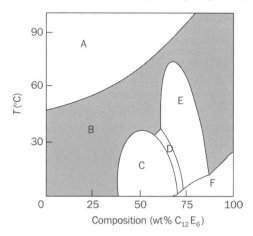

Figure 5.10: *Phase diagram of a typical non-ionic surfactant in water. A, two isotropic liquid phases; B, micellar solution; C, middle or hexagonal phase; D, cubic phase; E, neat or lamellar phase; F, solid phase. The boundary between phases A and B is the cloud point. Modified from Clunie JS, Goodman JF, Symons PC. Phase equilibria of dodecylhexaoxyethylene glycol monoether in water. Trans Farad Soc 1969;65:287–296.*

Key point

Because of their ability to rotate polarised light, liquid crystals are visible when placed between crossed polarisers, and this provides a useful means of detecting the liquid crystalline state.

Thermotropic liquid crystals

Thermotropic liquid crystals are produced when certain substances, for example the esters of cholesterol, are heated. The arrangement of the elongated molecules in thermotropic liquid crystals is generally recognisable as one of three principal types (*Figure 5.11*):

1. Nematic liquid crystals:
   - groups of molecules orientate spontaneously with their long axes parallel, but they are not ordered into layers
   - because the molecules have freedom of rotation about their long axis, the nematic liquid crystals are quite mobile and are readily orientated by electric or magnetic fields.
2. Smectic liquid crystals:
   - groups of molecules are arranged with their long axes parallel, and are also arranged into distinct layers
   - as a result of their two-dimensional order the smectic liquid crystals are viscous and are not orientated by magnetic fields.
3. Cholesteric (or chiral nematic) liquid crystals:
   - are formed by several cholesteryl esters
   - can be visualised as a stack of very thin two-dimensional nematic-like layers in which the elongated molecules lie parallel to each other in the plane of the layer
   - the orientation of the long axes in each layer is displaced from that in the adjacent layer and this displacement is cumulative through successive layers so that the overall displacement traces out a helical path through the layers
   - the helical path causes very pronounced rotation of polarised light, which can be as much as 50 rotations per millimeter
   - the pitch of the helix (the distance required for one complete rotation) is very sensitive to small changes in temperature and pressure and dramatic colour changes can result from variations in these properties
   - the cholesteric phase has a characteristic iridescent appearance when illuminated by white light due to circular dichroism.

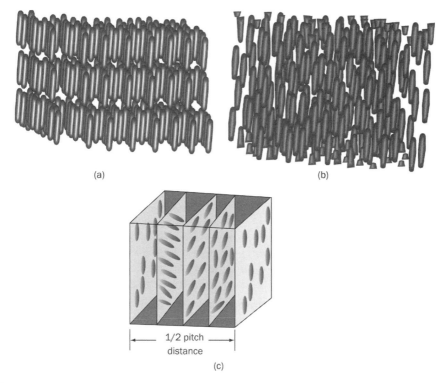

Figure 5.11: *Diagrammatic representation of forms of thermotropic liquid crystals: (a) smectic, (b) nematic and (c) cholesteric liquid crystals.*

Vesicles

Vesicles are formed by phospholipids and other surfactants having two hydrophobic chains. There are several types:

Liposomes

- Liposomes are formed by naturally occurring phospholipids such as lecithin (phosphatidyl choline).
- They can be multilamellar (composed of several bimolecular lipid lamellae separated by aqueous layers) or unilamellar (formed by sonication of solutions of multilamellar liposomes).
- They may be used as drug carriers; water-soluble drugs can be entrapped in liposomes by intercalation in the aqueous layers, whereas lipid-soluble drugs can be solubilised within the hydrocarbon interiors of the lipid bilayers (*Figure 5.12*).

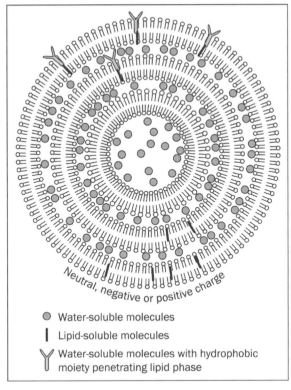

Figure 5.12: *Diagrammatic representation of a liposome in which three bilayers of polar phospholipids alternate with aqueous compartments. Water-soluble and lipid-soluble substances may be accommodated in the aqueous and lipid phases, respectively. Certain macromolecules can insert their hydrophobic regions into the lipid bilayers with the hydrophilic portions extending into water.*

Surfactant vesicles and niosomes

- Formed by surfactants having two alkyl chains.
- Sonication can produce single-compartment vesicles.
- Vesicles formed by ionic surfactants are useful as membrane models.
- Vesicles formed from non-ionic surfactants are called niosomes and have potential use in drug delivery.

Solubilisation

- The maximum amount of solubilisate that can be incorporated into a given system at a fixed concentration is termed the maximum additive concentration (MAC).
- Solubility data are expressed as solubility versus concentration curves or as three-component phase diagrams, which describe the effect of varying all three components of the system (solubilisate, solubiliser and solvent).

- The site of solubilisation within the micelle is closely related to the chemical nature of the solubilisate (*Figure 5.13*):
  - Non-polar solubilisates (aliphatic hydrocarbons, for example) are dissolved in the hydrocarbon core of ionic and non-ionic micelles (position 1 in *Figure 5.13*).
  - Water-insoluble compounds containing polar groups are orientated with the polar group at the core–surface interface of the micelle, and the hydrophobic group buried inside the hydrocarbon core of the micelle (positions 2 and 3 in *Figure 5.13*).
  - In addition to these sites, solubilisation in non-ionic polyoxyethylated surfactants can also occur in the polyoxyethylene shell (palisade layer) which surrounds the core (position 4 in *Figure 5.13*).

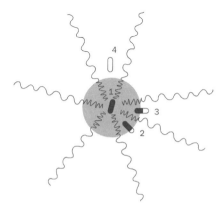

Figure 5.13: *Schematic representation of sites of solubilisation depending on the hydrophobicity of the solubilisate. Redrawn from Torchilin VP, J Control Release 2001;73:137–72.*

Key points

- Solubilisation is the process whereby water-insoluble substances are brought into solution by incorporation into micelles.
- There is a difference between this exact use of the term 'solubilisation' which is used in this chapter and its more general use to mean simply to dissolve in solution.

Factors affecting solubilisation capacity

Nature of the surfactant

- When the solubilisate is located within the core or deep within the micelle structure the solubilisation capacity increases with increase in alkyl chain length up to about C_{16}; further increase has little effect on solubilisation capacity.
- The effect of an increase in the ethylene oxide chain length of a polyoxyethylated non-ionic surfactant on its solubilising capacity is dependent on the location of the

solubilisate within the micelle and is complicated by corresponding changes in the micellar size. The aggregation number decreases with increase in the hydrophilic chain length so there are more micelles in a given concentration of surfactant and, although the number of molecules solubilised per micelle decreases, the total amount solubilised per mole of surfactant may actually increase.

Nature of the solubilisate
- For a simple homologous series of solubilisates a decrease in solubilisation occurs when the alkyl chain length is increased.
- A relationship between the lipophilicity of the solubilisate, expressed by the partition coefficient between octanol and water, and its extent of solubilisation has been noted for several surfactant systems.

Temperature
- With most systems the amount solubilised increases as temperature increases.
- This increase is particularly pronounced with some non-ionic surfactants where it is a consequence of an increase in the micellar size with temperature increase.
- In some cases, although the amount of drug that can be taken up by a surfactant solution increases with temperature increase, this may simply reflect an increase in the amount of drug dissolved in the aqueous phase rather than an increased solubilisation by the micelles.

Tips
- Remember that the micelle core is like a tiny reservoir of hydrocarbon and it is therefore not surprising that there is a close relationship between the distribution of a compound between octanol and water phases in a test tube and its distribution between micelles and water in a micellar solution.
- A very lipophilic solubilisate will mainly reside in the micelles rather than in the aqueous phase surrounding them. This compound will therefore have a high micelle/water partition coefficient and also a high octanol/water partition coefficient.
- On the other hand a hydrophilic compound will be partitioned mainly in the aqueous phase rather than the micelles and will have a low micelle/water and octanol/water partition coefficient.

Method of preparation of solubilised systems
The method of preparation of the solubilised system can have a significant influence on the solubilisation capacity.
- The simplest and most commonly used method of incorporation of the drug is the so-called 'shake flask' method, in which excess solid drug is equilibrated with the micellar solution and unsolubilised drug subsequently removed by filtration or centrifugation.

- Larger amounts of drug can often be solubilised by co-mixing the drug and surfactant at elevated temperature (typically about 60°C) and adding the resultant intimate mixture to water or buffer to form the solubilised micellar solution; this method is often referred to as 'melt loading'.
- In the dialysis method, drug and surfactant are dissolved in a water-miscible organic solvent followed by dialysis against water until the organic phase is replaced with water, leaving the solubilised solution.
- In the solvent evaporation method, the drug and surfactant are dissolved in volatile organic solvents which are allowed to evaporate at room temperature; the resultant dried drug/surfactant film is then pulverised and dispersed in water.
- In the cosolvent evaporation method, a micellar solution is formed by adding water slowly to a solution of drug and surfactant in a water-miscible organic solvent (cosolvent) and removing the organic solvent by evaporation.
- In the emulsion method, an oil-in-water emulsion is formed by mixing the organic solvent containing dissolved drug with an aqueous solution of the surfactant; the volatile solvent is then allowed to evaporate, leaving the solubilised micellar solution.

Pharmaceutical applications of solubilisation

- The solubilisation of phenolic compounds such as cresol, chlorocresol, chloroxylenol and thymol with soap to form clear solutions for use in disinfection.
- Solubilised solutions of iodine in non-ionic surfactant micelles (iodophors) for use in instrument sterilisation.
- Solubilisation of drugs (for example, steroids and water-insoluble vitamins), and essential oils by non-ionic surfactants (usually polysorbates or polyoxyethylene sorbitan esters of fatty acids).

Memory maps

Classification and properties of surfactants

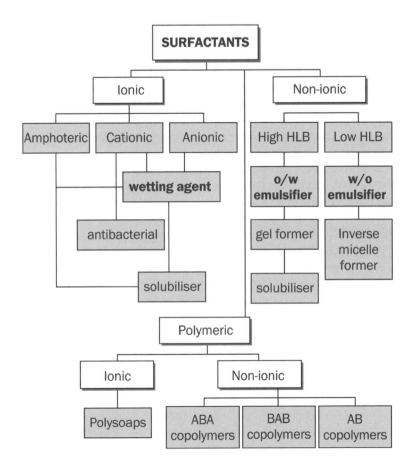

Properties of surfactants

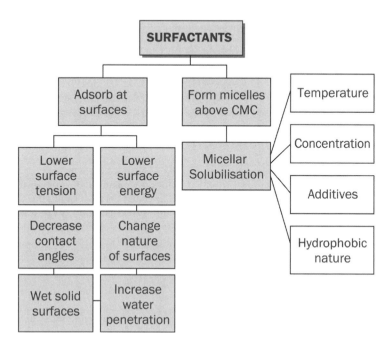

Factors affecting solubilisation in surfactant micelles

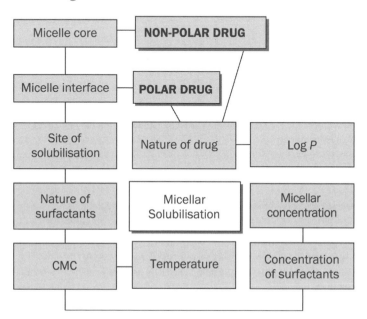

Questions

1. Using Traube's rule, calculate the concentration of a surfactant with a hydrocarbon chain length of 16 carbon atoms that would be required to achieve the same lowering of the surface tension of water as a 8×10^{-4} mol dm^{-3} solution of a surfactant in the same homologous series with a hydrocarbon chain length of 18 carbon atoms.
    A: 0.89×10^{-4} mol dm^{-3}
    B: 7.2×10^{-3} mol dm^{-3}
    C: 2.4×10^{-3} mol dm^{-3}
    D: 4.8×10^{-3} mol dm^{-3}
    E: 1.33×10^{-4} mol dm^{-3}

2. The slope of a plot of surface tension against logarithm of surfactant concentration for an aqueous surfactant solution measured at a concentration just below the CMC at a temperature of 30°C is -0.0115 N m^{-1}. Using the Gibbs equation, calculate the surface excess concentration in mol/m^2 given that $R = 8.314$ J mol^{-1} K^{-1}:
    A: 1.98×10^{-6} mol m^{-2}
    B: 2.00×10^{-5} mol m^{-2}
    C: 5.04×10^{5} mol m^{-2}
    D: 1.64×10^{-5} mol m^{-2}
    E: 4.56×10^{-6} mol m^{-2}

3. In relation to the surface tension at the air–water interface, indicate which of the following statements are true.
    A: Surface tension is due to spontaneous expansion of the surface
    B: Surface tension arises because of the downward pull of molecules in the water
    C: Surface tension represents a state of maximum free energy
    D: Surface tension has units of N m^{-1}
    E: Surface tension is lowered by surface-active agents

4. A surfactant has a structure $CH_3(CH_2)_{11}(OCH_2CH_2)_8OH$. Indicate which of the following statements are true.
    A: The surface activity of the surfactant will increase when the alkyl chain length is increased
    B: The CMC of the surfactant will increase when the alkyl chain length is increased
    C: The CMC of the surfactant will increase when the ethylene oxide chain length is decreased
    D: The hydrophobicity of the molecule will increase when the ethylene oxide chain length is increased
    E: Aqueous solutions of the surfactant will show a cloud point when heated

5. Indicate which of the following statements concerning the structure of micelles are correct.
    A: The core consists of the hydrophobic chains of the surfactant
    B: The Stern layer of ionic micelles contains the charged head groups
    C: In ionic micelles most of the counterions are contained in the Gouy–Chapman layer
    D: Micelles formed by non-ionic surfactants are generally much smaller than those formed by ionic surfactants with identical hydrophobic groups
    E: The Gouy–Chapman layer of an ionic micelle is compressed in the presence of electrolyte

6. **In relation to the adsorption of an ionisable drug molecule on to an uncharged solid surface from an aqueous solution, indicate which of the following statements are true.**
   A: The amount adsorbed usually increases as the ionisation of the drug decreases
   B: The amount adsorbed is not affected by change of pH
   C: The amount adsorbed usually decreases as the ionisation of the drug decreases
   D: The adsorptive capacity of the solid increases when its surface area is increased
   E: The adsorptive capacity of the solid is not affected by changes in its surface area

7. **In relation to insoluble monolayers formed on the surface of water, indicate which of the following statements are true.**
   A: Insoluble monolayers are formed by water-soluble surfactants
   B: The properties of insoluble monolayers are determined by an equilibrium between molecules in the monolayer and those in the bulk solution
   C: Polymers having several polar groups usually form gaseous films
   D: Molecules with bulky side chains usually form solid or condensed films
   E: The area occupied by a molecule in a gaseous film is greater than the cross-sectional area of the molecule

8. **In relation to liquid crystals, indicate which of the following statements are true.**
   A: Thermotropic liquid crystals are formed when concentrated surfactant solutions are heated
   B: In smectic liquid crystals the long axes of groups of molecules are parallel and organised in layers
   C: Variation of temperature and pressure of solutions of cholesteric liquid crystals can produce dramatic colour changes
   D: In the lamellar phase the surfactant molecules are arranged in bilayers
   E: The hexagonal phase is more fluid than the lamellar phase

9. **Indicate which one of the following statements is correct. The main reason why surfactants form micelles is because:**
   A: There is a decrease of entropy when surfactant molecules are transferred from water to a micelle
   B: There is an increase of entropy when surfactant molecules are transferred from water to a micelle
   C: There is a large decrease of enthalpy when micelles form
   D: There is a large increase of enthalpy when micelles form
   E: The free energy of the system increases when micelles form

10. **Indicate which one of the following statements is correct. In the solubilisation of poorly soluble drugs by aqueous surfactant solutions:**
    A: Non-polar drugs are usually solubilised in the palisade layer of a non-ionic micelle
    B: Polar drugs are usually solubilised in the micelle core
    C: Drugs with a high octanol/water partition coefficient will usually have a high micelle/water partition coefficient
    D: The solubilisation capacity of a non-ionic surfactant usually decreases with increase of temperature
    E: For a homologous series of solubilisates, an increase of solubilisation occurs when the alkyl chain length is increased

CHAPTER 6

Emulsions, suspensions and other dispersed systems

LEARNING OBJECTIVES

Upon completion of this chapter you should be able to:
- outline the variety of emulsions, suspensions and aerosols used in pharmacy
- understand what contributes to their physical stability
- outline the elements of colloid stability theory and understand how these assist in the design of formulations.

Colloid stability

- Water-insoluble drugs in fine dispersion form lyophobic dispersions. Because of their high surface energy they are thermodynamically unstable and have a tendency to aggregate.
- Emulsions and aerosols are thermodynamically unstable two-phase systems which only reach equilibrium when the globules have coalesced to form one macro-phase, when the surface area is at a minimum.
- Suspension particles achieve a lower surface area by flocculating or aggregating: they do not coalesce.
- In dispersions of fine particles in a liquid (or of particles in a gas) frequent encounters between the particles occur due to:
  - Brownian movement
  - creaming or sedimentation
  - convection.
- According to Stokes' law the rate of sedimentation (or creaming), v, of a spherical particle in a fluid medium, viscosity η, is given by:

$$v = \frac{2ga^2\,(\rho_1 - \rho_2)}{9\eta}$$

where the particle radius is a, ρ_1 is the density of the particles, ρ_2 is the density of the medium and g is the gravitational constant.

Key points

- Colloids can be broadly classified as:
  - lyophobic (solvent-hating) (= hydrophobic in aqueous systems)
  - lyophilic (solvent liking) (= hydrophilic in aqueous systems).
- Emulsions and suspensions are disperse systems – a liquid or solid phase dispersed in an external liquid phase.
  - The disperse phase is the phase that is subdivided.
  - The continuous phase is the phase in which the disperse phase is distributed.
- Emulsions and suspensions are intrinsically unstable systems that require stabilisers to ensure a useful lifetime.
- Emulsions exist in many forms:
  - oil-in-water
  - water-in-oil
  - oil_1-in-oil_2 (rare)
  - a variety of multiple emulsions such as water-in-oil-in-water systems and oil-in-water-in-oil systems.

Key points

- Pharmaceutical emulsions and suspensions are in the colloidal state, i.e. the disperse phase diameters range from nanometres to the visible (several micrometres). Microemulsions are formulated so that the disperse phase is in the nanometre size range.
- Suspensions may have an aqueous or oily continuous phase.
- Aerosols are dispersions of a liquid or solid in air.

DLVO theory of colloid stability

Forces of interaction between colloidal particles

- There are five possible forces between colloidal particles:
  1. van der Waals forces or electromagnetic forces (attraction)
  2. electrostatic forces (repulsion)
  3. Born forces – essentially short-range (repulsion)
  4. steric forces (repulsive) due to adsorbed molecules (particularly macromolecules) at the particle interface
  5. solvation forces (repulsive) due to reduction in the hydration of stabilising molecules on close approach.
- Consideration of the electrostatic repulsion and van der Waals forces of attraction by Deryagin, Landau, Verwey and Overbeek (DLVO) led to a theory of stability of hydrophobic suspensions.
- DLVO theory considers two spherical particles of radius a at a distance apart H (*Figure 6.1*).

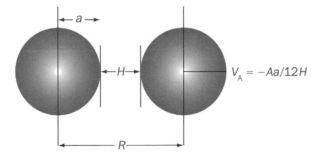

Figure 6.1: *Diagram of the interaction between two spheres of radius a at a distance of separation H with a centre-to-centre distance of R = H + 2a.*

In this theory:
- The combination of the electrostatic repulsive energy (V_R) with the attractive potential energy (V_A) gives the total potential energy of interaction:

$$V_{total} = V_A + V_R$$

- Attractive forces arise from van der Waals forces between particles of the same kind.
  - When the particles are large relative to the distance of separation, the attractive force (V_A) is written as:

$$V_A = - \frac{Aa}{12H}$$

  where A is the Hamaker constant.
- Repulsive forces arise from the electrical charge on particles, which is due either to ionisation of surface groups or to adsorption of ions:
  - A particle surface with a negative charge has a layer of positive ions attracted to its surface in the Stern layer, and a diffuse or electrical double layer which accumulates and contains both positive and negative ions (*Figure 6.2*).
  - Electrostatic forces arise from the interaction of these electrical double layers surrounding particles in suspension, leading to repulsion if the particles have both the same positive or negative surface charges.
  - The electrostatic repulsive force decays as an exponential function of the distance. It has a range of the order of the thickness of the electrical double layer, equal to the Debye–Hückel length, $1/\kappa$. An approximate equation for the repulsive interactions for small surface potentials and low values of κ is:

$$V_R = 2\pi\varepsilon\varepsilon_0 a\psi_\delta^2 \exp(-\kappa H)$$

where ε_0 is the permittivity of a vacuum, ε is the dielectric constant (or relative permittivity) of the dispersion medium and ψ_δ is the Stern potential, which can be approximated to the zeta potential (ζ) measured by microelectrophoresis.

- V_{total} plotted against the distance of separation, H, gives a potential energy curve (*Figure 6.3*) showing maximum and minimum energy states.

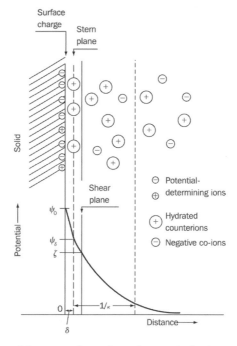

Figure 6.2: *Distribution of charges at the surface of a negatively charged solid.*

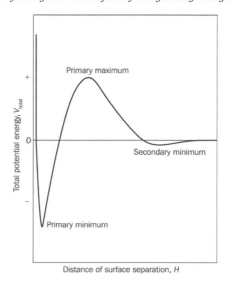

Figure 6.3: *Typical DLVO plot.*

Effect of electrolytes on stability

Figure 6.4 shows the effect of electrolyte on a typical DLVO plot. Changes in the plot arise because of compression of the double layer as the electrolyte concentration is increased, which increases κ, so decreasing $1/\kappa$.

- At low electrolyte concentrations the range of the double layer is high and V_R extends to large distances around the particles. Summation of V_R and V_A gives a total energy curve having a high primary maximum but no secondary minimum (see curve A in *Figure 6.4*).
- The decrease of the double layer when more electrolyte is added produces a more rapid decay in V_R and the result is a small primary maximum but, more importantly, a secondary minimum. This concentration of electrolyte would produce a stable suspension, since flocculation could occur in the secondary minimum. The small primary maximum would be sufficient to prevent coagulation in the primary minimum (see curve B in *Figure 6.4*).
- At high concentrations of added electrolyte, the range of V_R would be so small that the van der Waals attractive forces alone dictate the shape of the energy curve. The curve has no primary maximum or secondary minimum (see curve C in *Figure 6.4*).

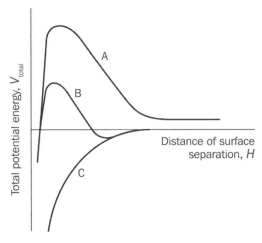

Figure 6.4: *The effect on the DLVO plot of A: low, B: medium and C: high concentrations of added electrolyte.*

Key points

- If the primary maximum is too small, two interacting particles may reach the primary minimum and the depth of this energy minimum means escape is improbable.
- When the primary maximum is sufficiently high, the two particles do not reach the stage of being in close contact.
- The depth of the secondary minimum is important in determining the stability of the system.
- If the secondary minimum is less than the thermal energy, kT (where k is the Boltzmann constant), the particles will always repel each other.

The magnitude of the effect of an electrolyte of a given concentration on V_R also depends on the valence of the ion of opposite charge to that of the particles (the counterion): the greater the valence of the added counterion, the greater its effect on V_R. These generalisations are known as the Schulze–Hardy rule. Notice that it does not matter which particular counterion of a given valence is added.

Repulsion between hydrated surfaces – steric stabilisation

The DLVO theory deals only with electrostatic repulsion whereas colloids can also be stabilised by the repulsive forces that arise from adsorption of macromolecules and surfactants to their surfaces. In aqueous media these adsorbed molecules will be hydrated. Stabilisation arises because of three effects:

1. Entropic effect:
   - Loss of freedom of movement of the chains of the adsorbed molecules.
   - The approach of two particles with adsorbed stabilising chains leads to a steric interaction when the chains interact.
   - The steric effect does not come into play until $H = 2\delta$, so the interaction increases suddenly with decreasing distance.
   - The loss of conformational freedom leads to a negative entropy change (ΔS). Each chain loses some of its conformational freedom and its contribution to the free energy of the system is increased, leading to the repulsion.
   - The steric effect depends on: (1) the chain length of the adsorbed molecule; (2) the interactions of the solvent with the chains; and (3) the number of chains per unit area of interacting surface.
2. Osmotic effect:
   - The 'osmotic effect' arises as the macromolecular chains on neighbouring particles crowd into each other's space, increasing the concentration of chains in the overlap region.
   - The repulsion which arises is due to the osmotic pressure of the solvent attempting to dilute out the concentrated region: this can only be achieved by the particles moving apart.

3. Enthalpic stabilisation:

— On close approach of the particles the hydrating water on the adsorbed molecules is released, which causes an increase in enthalpy leading to repulsion (*Figure 6.5*).

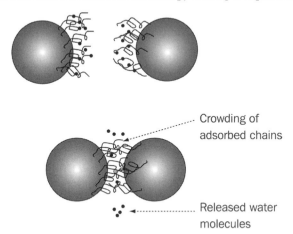

Crowding of adsorbed chains

Released water molecules

Figure 6.5: *Representation of enthalpic stabilisation of particles with adsorbed hydrophilic chains.*

Tips

In considering the reasons for the stabilising action of the adsorbed molecules the basic thermodynamic equation must be remembered:

$\Delta G = \Delta H - T\Delta S$

ΔG is the change in free energy of a process such as repulsion: effective repulsion of the particles is characterised by an increase of ΔG.

ΔH is the change in enthalpy: loss of water molecules leads to a positive change in enthalpy, hence an increase of free energy.

ΔS is the change in entropy: loss of freedom of movement of stabilising macromolecules leads to a negative entropy change, hence positive ΔG .

Disperse system flow

Colloidal systems, whether suspensions or emulsions, have flow and viscous properties which are important in a number of pharmaceutical processes. In this section we will examine the various types of flow, commencing with the simplest type of flow, Newtonian flow, which may be exhibited by dilute colloidal solutions, and then considering the various types of non-Newtonian flow, which are exhibited by the more complex colloidal systems.

Newtonian flow

- A diagrammatic representation of the flow of a liquid through a narrow tube is given in *Figure 6.6* which shows the movement of imaginary concentric annuli within the liquid over each other. The flow rate is highest in the centre of the tube and gradually decreases across the tube because of internal resistance to flow, reaching a minimum value at the tube walls.
- The gradient of velocity, u, in a direction, x, at right angles to the wall, i.e. du/dx, is the shear rate, D. The external force which is required to overcome the internal friction and to cause movement is called the shear force, F, or when it refers to unit surface area, A, is called the shear stress, τ.
- In a Newtonian liquid, the velocity gradient or shear rate is directly proportional to the shear stress, and the proportionality constant is the coefficient of viscosity, or more simply the viscosity, η, i.e. $\tau = \eta D$.
- The viscosity may be combined with the density, ρ, using the kinematic viscosity, $v = \eta/\rho$.
- In Newtonian flow, the viscosity is independent of the shear rate and this is characterised by linear plots of τ against D as shown in *Figure 6.7*. The gradient of these plots is η.
- The viscosity of a colloidal dispersion of spherical particles may be expressed using various terms as follows:
  - relative viscosity, $\eta_{rel} = \eta_*/\eta_0$
  - specific viscosity, $\eta_{sp} = \eta_{rel} - 1$
  - reduced viscosity $= \eta_{sp}/\varnothing$
  - intrinsic viscosity, $[\eta]$, is the value of $\eta_{sp}/\varnothing$ extrapolated to zero volume fraction where η_0 is the viscosity of the suspending fluid, and $\varnothing$ is particle volume fraction defined as the volume occupied by the particles divided by the total volume of the dispersion. η_* is the effective viscosity given by $\eta_* = \eta_0(1 + 2.5\varnothing)$ from which it is seen that the intrinsic viscosity in an ideal dispersion should equal 2.5; this is true only to spheres, asymmetric particles will produce coefficients greater than 2.5.

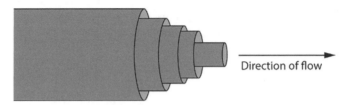

Direction of flow

Figure 6.6: *Diagrammatic representation of the flow of a liquid through a narrow tube as the movement of a series of concentric annuli.*

Tips

- Viscosity has SI units of N m^{-2} s but is usually given in centipoise, cP, where 1 cP = 1 mN m^{-2} s. This is a more convenient unit since water has a viscosity of 1 cP at 20°C.
- Kinematic viscosity has SI units of m^2 s^{-1} but is often given in centistokes, cSt, for example in describing the viscosity grade of several polymers. The two units are related by 1 cSt = 10^{-6} m^2 s^{-1}.

Non-Newtonian flow

When shear stress and shear rate are not linearly related the flow is described as non-Newtonian. There are several types of flow behaviour as follows:

Shear thinning (pseudoplastic flow)

- In shear thinning or pseudoplastic flow the apparent viscosity decreases with increasing shear rate. This type of flow is compared with Newtonian flow in *Figure 6.7a*. Since the apparent viscosity is derived by drawing tangents to this plot, it will generate the type of rheogram shown in *Figure 6.7b*.
- Shear thinning is particularly common to colloidal dispersions containing asymmetric particles such as methyl cellulose or tragacanth. These particles provide the greatest resistance to flow when they are randomly orientated at low velocity gradients. As the shear rate is gradually increased, they begin to align themselves with the flow lines and their resistance to flow is greatly reduced. The viscosity eventually becomes constant at high rates of shear when alignment is complete. This type of flow is also characteristic of systems in which particle aggregation occurs. Under shear, these aggregates break down releasing some of the solvent which they have immobilised, thus lowering the viscosity of the system.
- Pseudoplastic flow can be described by the Ostwald equation

$$\tau = KD^n$$

where K is a constant, often called the consistency index, and n is a number less than 1, referred to as the flow behaviour index. When $n = 1$ this equation represents Newtonian flow and K is the viscosity. From the logarithmic form of the equation, i.e,

$$\log \tau = \log K + n \log D$$

plots of log shear stress, τ, as a function of log shear rate, D, will be linear when the system exhibits shear thinning behaviour.

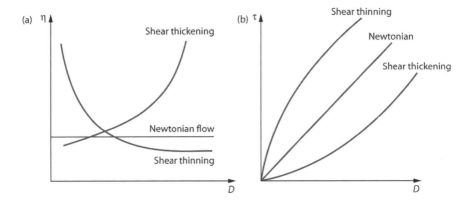

Figure 6.7: *Plots of (a) apparent viscosity η against shear rate D and (b) shear stress τ against shear rate D, comparing Newtonian and non-Newtonian flow characteristics.*

Shear thickening (dilatancy)

- In this type of flow the apparent viscosity increases with increasing shear rate (see *Figure 6.7a*). Dilatant systems obey the Ostwald equation with a value of $n > 1$.
- A well-known example of the dilatant effect is the drying out of wet sand when it is walked upon. As the shear rate is increased when the sand is compressed the dense packing is broken down to allow the particles to flow past each other. The resulting expansion leaves insufficient liquid to fill the voids and the system apparently 'dries out'. The dry footprint soon becomes wet again as the pressure is released. Similarly, starch paste stirs easily if you stir it slowly but soon thickens up and resists stirring if you try to stir it quickly.

Plastic flow

- This type of flow is similar to shear thinning except that the system does not flow noticeably until the shear stress exceeds a certain minimum value called the critical shear stress, τ_0.
- At high shear stresses the rheogram may become linear (see *Figure 6.8*) in which case we say that the system exhibits Bingham flow.
- Several characteristics describing the flow properties may be obtained from the rheogram:
  - the upper yield stress is the shear stress at the point where the plot becomes linear
  - extrapolation of the linear portion of the rheogram to zero shear rate gives the extrapolated yield stress
  - the shear stress at which flow is first observed (i.e. τ_0) is the lower yield stress.
- Some substances show a non-linear relationship between shear rate and shear stress after yielding and these are called Casson bodies.

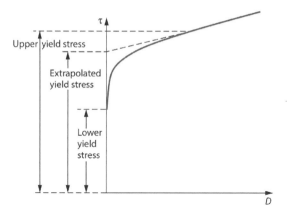

Figure 6.8: *A plot of shear stress τ against shear rate D for a colloidal dispersion exhibiting plastic flow properties.*

Thixotropy and rheopexy

- In a thixotropic system the apparent viscosity decreases as a continuous shear stress is applied at a constant rate of shear. If this system is allowed to stand for a while it regains its structure and its shear stress returns to its original value when shearing is recommenced at the same shear rate.
- A consequence of this time-dependent effect is that the rheogram exhibits a hysteresis loop, as seen in *Figure 6.9a*, when the shear rate is first increased and then decreased.
- Solutions of high molecular weight polymers are generally thixotropic because of chain entanglements, which are gradually reduced on shearing and then reform on standing due to Brownian motion.
- In a rheopectic system the apparent viscosity increases as continuous shear stress is applied at a constant rate of shear and then returns to its initial value after a regeneration period. This type of flow results in a hysteresis loop of the type shown in *Figure 6.9b*.

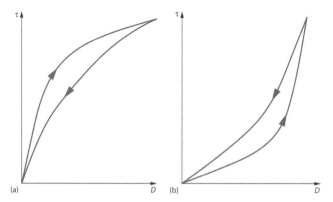

Figure 6.9: *Plots of shear stress τ against shear rate D for colloidal dispersions exhibiting (a) thixotropic and (b) rheopectic flow properties showing hysteresis loops resulting from time-dependent flow.*

Viscoelasticity

- Many dispersed systems exhibit the properties of both solids and liquids when a constant small shear stress is applied, i.e. they flow but they also show elasticity. When such dispersions are stressed they deform and the increase in deformation (strain) as a function of time is called creep. Creep compliance is the ratio of the strain to the applied constant stress.
- In the creep testing of a colloidal dispersion, the stress is applied for a given time and then removed and the recovery with time is studied.
- *Figure 6.10* shows a typical plot of creep compliance against time. As soon as a stress is applied there is an immediate strain which is represented by A–B. This is called the instantaneous elastic compliance, J_0, and is the region in which the bonds between the primary structural units in the system stretch elastically. The curvature in the region B–C gradually decreases and eventually the increase of creep compliance with time becomes linear over the region C–D. The region B–C represents the retarded elastic compliance, J_R, and C–D is the region of Newtonian compliance, J_N. When the stress at D is removed there is an instantaneous elastic recovery over the region D–E, followed by a retarded elastic recovery over the region E–F and then an eventual flattening of the curve beyond F. The vertical distance, F–G, to the time abscissa represents the non-recoverable strain per unit stress and this is related to the degree of structural alteration which has occurred during the test.

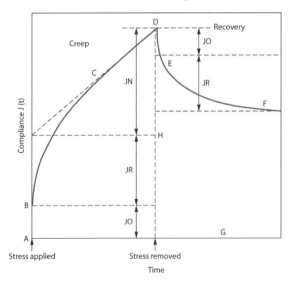

Figure 6.10: *Model plot of creep compliance against time. A–B is the region of instantaneous elastic modulus (compliance) in which the bonds between the primary structure units in the system stretch elastically. B–C is a time-dependent region. C–D is a region of Newtonian compliance; here some bonds rupture but do not reform in the period of the test. On removal of the stress the recovery curve is given by D–F. An instantaneous elastic recovery (D–E) of the same magnitude as A–B is followed by retarded elastic recovery to E–F. As bonds were irreversibly broken during the period of applied stress, this part of the structure is not recovered; hence F–G is equal to D–H.*

Key points

- In Newtonian flow, the viscosity is independent of the shear rate and this is characterised by linear plots of τ against D, the gradient of which is η. This type of flow is exhibited by dilute colloidal solutions.
- More complex colloidal dispersions exhibit non-Newtonian flow properties which may be:
  - shear thinning or pseudoplastic flow in which the apparent viscosity decreases with increasing shear rate
  - shear thickening or dilatant flow in which the apparent viscosity increases with increasing shear rate.
- Plastic flow which is similar to shear thinning except that the system does not flow noticeably until the shear stress exceeds a certain minimum value called the critical shear stress, τ_0.
- Thixotropic flow in which the apparent viscosity decreases when a continuous shear stress is applied at a constant rate of shear. If this system is allowed to stand for a while it regains its structure and its shear stress returns to its original value when shearing is recommenced at the same shear rate, giving a hysteresis loop in plots of τ against D.
- Rheopectic flow in which the apparent viscosity increases when a continuous shear stress is applied at a constant rate of shear and then returns to its initial value after a regeneration period, again producing a hysteresis loop in plots of τ against D.
- Viscoelastic systems exhibit the properties of both solids and liquids when a constant small shear stress is applied, i.e. they flow but they also show elasticity. They deform when stressed and the increase in deformation (strain) as a function of time is called creep. Creep compliance is the ratio of the strain to the applied constant stress.

Emulsions

Stability of oil-in-water and water-in-oil emulsions

- Adsorption of a surfactant at the oil–water interface lowers interfacial tension, hence it aids the dispersal of the oil into droplets of a small size and helps to maintain the particles in a dispersed state (*Figure 6.11*).
- Unless the interfacial tension is zero, there is a natural tendency for the oil droplets to coalesce to reduce the area of oil–water contact, but the presence of the surfactant monolayer at the surface of the droplet reduces the possibility of collisions leading to coalescence.
- Adsorption of charged surfactants will lead to an increase in zeta potential and will thus help to maintain stability by increasing V_R.
- Non-ionic surfactants such as the alkyl or aryl polyoxyethylene ethers or polyoxyethylene-polyoxypropylene-polyoxyethylene block copolymers are widely used in pharmaceutical emulsions. These adsorb onto the emulsion droplets and maintain

stability by creating a hydrated layer on the hydrophobic particle in oil-in-water emulsions.

- In water-in-oil emulsions the hydrocarbon chains of the adsorbed molecules protrude into the oily continuous phase. Stabilisation arises from steric repulsive forces.
- It is usually observed that mixtures of surfactants form more stable emulsions than do single surfactants, perhaps due to complex formation at the interface providing a more 'rigid' stabilising film.

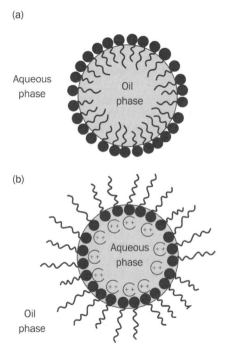

Figure 6.11: *Surfactant films at the oil–water interface for the stabilisation of (a) oil-in-water and (b) water-in oil emulsions.*

HLB system

- The hydrophile–lipophile balance (HLB) number is a measure of the balance between hydrophobic and hydrophilic portions of a surfactant.
- In selecting a surfactant for emulsion stabilisation it is essential that there is a degree of surfactant hydrophilicity to confer an enthalpic stabilising force and a degree of hydrophobicity to secure adsorption at the oil-in-water interface.
- The HLB of a surfactant is expressed using an arbitrary scale which for non-ionic surfactants ranges from 0 to 20.
  - At the higher end of the scale, the surfactants are hydrophilic and act as solubilising agents, detergents and oil-in-water emulsifiers.
  - Oil-soluble surfactants with a low HLB act as water-in-oil emulsifiers.

- HLB values can be calculated according to empirical but useful formulae:
  - For simple alkyl ethers in which the hydrophile consists only of ethylene oxide,

$$HLB = E/5$$

  where E is the weight percentage of ethylene oxide groups.
  - The HLB of polyhydric alcohol fatty acid esters such as glyceryl monostearate may be obtained from the equation:

$$HLB = 20\left(1 - \frac{S}{A}\right)$$

  where S is the saponification number of the ester and A is the acid number of the fatty acid (see below). The HLB of polysorbate 20 (Tween 20) calculated using this formula is 16.7, S being 45.5 and $A = 276$. The polysorbate (Tween) surfactants have HLB values in the range 9.6–16.7; the sorbitan ester (Span) surfactants have HLBs in the lower range of 1.8–8.6.
  - For those materials for which it is not possible to obtain saponification numbers, for example beeswax and lanolin derivatives, the HLB is calculated from:

$$HLB = (E + P)/5$$

  where P is the weight percentage of polyhydric alcohol groups (glycerol or sorbitol) in the molecule.
  - HLB values can also be calculated from group contributions using:

$$HLB = \sum(\text{hydrophilic group numbers}) + \sum(\text{lipophilic group numbers}) + 7$$

  - For a mixture of two surfactants containing fraction f of A and $(1 - f)$ of B it is assumed that the HLB is an algebraic mean of the two HLB numbers: $HLB_{mixture} = f\,HLB_A + (1 - f)HLB_B$
- The HLB system has several drawbacks:
  - The calculated HLB cannot take account of the effect of temperature or that of additives.
  - The presence of agents which salt-in or salt-out surfactants will, respectively, increase and decrease the effective (as opposed to the calculated) HLB values. Salting-out the surfactant (e.g. with NaCl) will make the molecules more hydrophobic (less hydrophilic).

> **Tip**
>
> Note that when calculating HLB from group contributions using
>
> HLB = $\sum$(hydrophilic group numbers) + $\sum$(lipophilic group numbers) + 7
>
> the lipophilic group contribution should be entered as a negative value. Some tables give these values as positive.

> **Tips**
>
> - The saponification number of the ester represents the number of milligrams of alkali (NaOH or KOH) required to hydrolyse 1 g of the ester. When the ester is an oil or fat the esterification leads to the formation of a soap, which is why the esterification reaction is called 'saponification'. As most of the mass of an oil or fat is in the fatty acids, it is a measure of the average molecular weight (or chain length) of all the fatty acids present.
> - The acid number is the number of milligrams of KOH required to neutralise 1 g of the fatty acid. The acid number is a measure of the number of carboxylic acid groups in the fatty acid.

Choice of emulsifier or emulsifier mixture

- The appropriate choice of emulsifier or emulsifier mixture can be made by preparing a series of emulsions with a range of surfactants of varying HLB.
- Mixtures of surfactants with high HLB and low HLB give more stable emulsions than do single surfactants.
- The solubility of surfactant components in both the disperse and the continuous phase maintains the stability of the surfactant film at the interface from the reservoir created in each phase.
- In the experimental determination of optimum HLB the system with the minimum creaming or separation of phases is deemed to have an optimal HLB. It is therefore possible to determine optimum HLB numbers required to produce stable emulsions of a variety of oils.
- At the optimum HLB the mean particle size of the emulsion is at a minimum, which explains the increased stability.
- The formation of a viscous network of surfactants in the continuous phase prevents the collision of droplets and this effect overrides the influence of the interfacial layer and barrier forces due to the presence of adsorbed layers.

Multiple emulsions

- Multiple emulsions are emulsions whose disperse phase contains droplets of another phase.

- They are made by emulsifying either a water-in-oil emulsion with a hydrophilic surfactant to produce a water-in-oil-in-water system, or an oil-in-water system with a low HLB surfactant to produce an oil-in-water-in-oil system. Other forms can also be made.
- Water-in-oil emulsions in which a water-soluble drug is dissolved in the aqueous phase may be injected by the subcutaneous or intramuscular routes to produce a delayed-action preparation. To escape, the drug has to diffuse through the oil to reach the tissue fluids, hence the delayed-release action.
- The main disadvantage of a water-in-oil emulsion is its high viscosity because of the oil continuous phase. Emulsifying a water-in-oil emulsion using surfactants which stabilise an oily disperse phase can produce multiple water-in-oil-in-water emulsions with an external aqueous phase and lower viscosity than the primary emulsion.
- Physical degradation of water-in-oil-in-water emulsions can arise by several routes:
  — coalescence of the internal water droplets
  — coalescence of the oil droplets surrounding them
  — rupture of the oil film separating the internal and external aqueous phases
  — osmotic flux of water to and from the internal droplets, possibly associated with inverse micellar species in the oil phase.

Microemulsions

- Microemulsions are homogeneous transparent systems of low viscosity which contain a high percentage of both oil and water and high concentrations (15–25%) of emulsifier mixture.
- Microemulsions form spontaneously when the components are mixed in the appropriate ratios and are thermodynamically stable.
- In their simplest form, microemulsions are small droplets (diameter 5–140 nm) of one liquid dispersed throughout another. The droplet size is therefore very much smaller than that of normal emulsions (which is why microemulsions are transparent) and the droplets are very much more uniform in size.
- They can be dispersions of oil droplets in water or water droplets in oil but more complex structures (bicontinuous structures) may exist when there are almost equal amounts of oil and water.
- An essential requirement for their formation and stability is the attainment of a very low interfacial tension,γ. Since microemulsions have a very large interface between oil and water (because of the small droplet size), they can only be thermodynamically stable if the interfacial tension is so low that the positive interfacial energy (given by γA, where A is the interfacial area) can be compensated by the negative free energy of mixing (ΔG_m).
- To achieve the very low interfacial tension required for their formation it is usually necessary to include a second amphiphile (the cosurfactant) such as a short-chain alcohol in the formulation. This cosurfactant is incorporated into the interfacial film around the droplets (*Figure 6.12*).

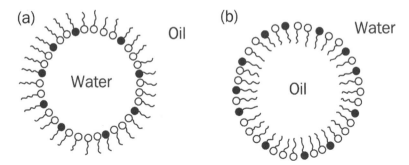

Figure 6.12: *Diagrammatic representation of the interfacial layers around microemulsion droplets in (a) water-in-oil and (b) oil-in-water microemulsions.*

Self-emulsifying drug delivery systems

- Utilisation of microemulsions and emulsions in therapy is aided by the development of self-emulsifying drug delivery systems (SEDDS) and the analogous self-microemulsifying delivery systems (SMEDDS), systems which disperse *in vivo* to form emulsions or microemulsions.

- Simple formulations comprising a solution of a lipophilic drug in an oil (for example a medium-chain-length triglyceride or vegetable oil) loaded into a gelatin capsule rely on the surfactants present in the gastrointestinal tract (bile salts and lecithin) to solubilise the lipophilic drug in a colloidal dispersion in the intestine from which the drug may be absorbed. The bioavailability of drugs from such formulations can vary considerably, mainly because the efficiency of solubilisation depends to a large extent on the bile salt concentration in the gastrointestinal tract, which can show a wide inter-patient variability. More reliable bioavailability is achieved from formulations in which suitable surfactants (and cosurfactants if required) are added to the oil/drug solution; on contact with water in the gastrointestinal tract these spontaneously form emulsions (SEDDS) or microemulsions (SMEDDS) depending on the formulation.

- The extent of absorption of poorly water-soluble drugs from oil-in-water dispersions is influenced by their droplet size; the smaller the droplet, the more rapid the breakdown of the triglycerides in which the drug is dissolved and hence the more rapidly the drug is released from the vehicle. As a consequence of their much smaller droplet size, SMEDDS formulations have the potential to achieve higher, less variable, bioavailability than SEDDS.

- An illustration of this is seen from the development of the Neoral formulation for the delivery of ciclosporin. This formulation incorporates the drug in a microemulsion preconcentrate (SMEDDS) that forms a microemulsion on dilution in aqueous fluids and shows improved bioavailability characteristics compared to the original formulation (Sandimmun) which was an emulsion preconcentrate (SEDDS).

Semi-solid emulsions (creams, ointments)

- Stable oil-in-water creams prepared with ionic or non-ionic emulsifying waxes are composed of (at least) four phases (*Figure 6.13*):
  1. A dispersed oil phase
  2. A crystalline gel phase
  3. A crystalline hydrate phase
  4. A bulk aqueous phase containing a dilute solution of surfactant.
- The interaction of the surfactant and fatty alcohol components of emulsifying mixtures which leads to high viscosity (body) is time-dependent, giving the name 'self-bodying' to these emulsions.
- The overall stability of a cream is dependent on the stability of the crystalline gel phase.
- The liquid crystalline phases form multilayers at the oil–water interface. These protect against coalescence by reducing the van der Waals forces of attraction and by retarding film thinning between approaching droplets; the viscosity of the liquid crystalline phases is often 100 times greater than that of phases without these structures.

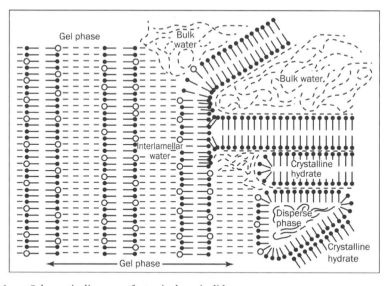

Figure 6.13: *Schematic diagram of a typical semisolid cream.*

Biopharmaceutical aspects of emulsions

- Traditionally, emulsions were used to administer oils such as castor oil and liquid paraffin in a palatable form. This is now a minor use.
- Emulsions are of interest as vehicles for drug delivery in which the drug is dissolved in

the disperse phase. For example, lipid oil-in-water emulsions are used as vehicles for lipophilic drugs (diazepam, propofol) for intravenous use.

- Griseofulvin and indoxole in emulsion formulations exhibit enhanced oral absorption.

Preservative availability in emulsified systems

- Microbial spoilage of emulsified products is avoided by the inclusion of appropriate amounts of a preservative in the formulation.
- Preservatives in emulsions may partition to the oily or micellar phases of complex systems and some are inactivated by surfactants, hence calculations must be made of the appropriate amounts.
- The presence of surfactant micelles alters the native partition coefficient of the preservative molecule because the micellar phase offers an alternative site for preservative molecules. Partitioning then occurs between the oil globule and the aqueous micellar phases, decreasing the amounts in the aqueous phase, where they are active.

Intravenous fat emulsions

- Cottonseed oil or soybean oil emulsions are used to supply a large amount of energy in a small volume of isotonic liquid; they supply the body with essential fatty acids and triglycerides.
- Fat emulsions for intravenous nutrition contain vegetable oil and phospholipid emulsifier.
- Several commercial fat emulsions are available, such as Intralipid, Lipiphysan, Lipofundin and Lipofundin S. They contain either cottonseed oil or soybean oil. Purified egg-yolk phospholipids are used as the emulsifiers in Intralipid.
- Isotonicity is obtained by the addition of sorbitol, xylitol or glycerol.
- Intralipid has also been used as the basis of an intravenous drug carrier, for example for diazepam (Diazemuls) and propofol (Diprivan).
- The addition of electrolyte or drugs to intravenous fat emulsions is generally contraindicated because of the risk of destabilising the emulsion.

The rheology of emulsions

- Most emulsions display both plastic and pseudoplastic flow behaviour rather than simple Newtonian flow (see before).
- The pourability, spreadability and 'syringeability' of an emulsion will, however, be directly determined by its rheological properties.
- The high viscosity of water-in-oil emulsions lead to problems with intramuscular administration of injectable formulations. Conversion to a multiple emulsion (water-in-oil-in-water) leads to a dramatic decrease in viscosity and consequent improved ease of injection.

Suspensions

Stability of suspensions

Flocculation of suspensions

- In deflocculated systems the particles are not associated; pressure on the individual particles can lead to close packing of the particles at the bottom of the container to such an extent that the secondary energy barriers are overcome and the particles are forced together in the primary minimum of the DLVO plot and become irreversibly bound together to form a cake.
- Caking of the suspension is usually prevented by including a flocculating agent in the formulation: it cannot be eliminated by reduction of particle size or by increasing the viscosity of the continuous phase.
- In flocculated systems (where the repulsive barriers have been reduced) particles form loosely bonded structures (flocs or flocculates) in the secondary minimum of the DLVO plot. The particles therefore settle as flocs and not as individual particles (*Figure 6.14*). Because of the random arrangement of the particles in the flocs, the sediment is not closely packed and caking does not readily occur. Clearance of the supernatant is, however, too rapid for an acceptable pharmaceutical formulation.
- The aim in the formulation of suspensions is, therefore, to achieve partial or controlled flocculation.
- Suspension stability may be assessed by measurement of:
  1. The ratio (R) of sedimentation layer volume (V_s) to total suspension volume (V_t). The height of the sedimented layer (h_∞) is usually measured against the height of the suspension (h_0) so that:

$$R = \frac{V_s}{V_t} \approx \frac{h_\infty}{h_0}$$

  2. The zeta potential of the suspension particles:
  - Most suspension particles dispersed in water have a charge acquired by specific adsorption of ions or by ionisation of ionisable surface groups. If the charge arises from ionisation, the charge on the particle will depend on the pH of the environment.
  - Repulsive forces arise because of the interaction of the electrical double layers on adjacent particles.
  - The magnitude of the charge can be determined by measurement of the electrophoretic mobility of the particles in an electrical field. The velocity of migration of the particles (μ_E) under unit-applied potential can be determined microscopically with a timing device and eye-piece graticule.
  - For non-conducting particles, the Henry equation is used to obtain ζ from μ_E. This equation can be written in the form:

$$\mu_E = \frac{\zeta\varepsilon}{4\pi\eta} f(\kappa a)$$

where $f(\kappa a)$ varies between 1, for small κa, and 1.5, for large κa; ε is the dielectric constant of the continuous phase and η is its viscosity. In systems with low values of κa the equation can be written in the form:

$$\mu_E = \frac{\zeta\varepsilon}{4\pi\eta}$$

— The zeta potential (ζ) is not the surface potential (ψ_o) as discussed earlier but is related to it. ζ can be used as a reliable guide to the magnitude of electric repulsive forces between particles. Changes in ζ on the addition of flocculating agents, surfactants and other additives can then be used to predict the stability of the system.

(a)   (b)

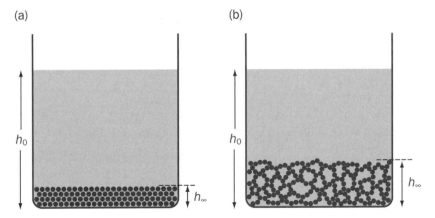

Figure 6.14: *Sedimentation of (a) deflocculated and (b) flocculated suspensions.*

Key points

- An acceptable suspension has the following characteristics:
  - suspended material should not settle too rapidly
  - particles that settle to the bottom of the container should not form a hard mass (cake) but should be easily redispersed on shaking.
- The suspension should not be too viscous to pour freely from a bottle or to flow through a needle.
- When a drug is suspended in a liquid, however, sedimentation, caking (leading to difficulty in resuspension), flocculation and particle growth (through dissolution and recrystallisation) can all occur.
- Formulation of pharmaceutical suspensions to minimise caking can be achieved by the production of flocculated systems.
- A flocculate or floc is a loose open structure or cluster of particles. A suspension consisting of particles in this state is termed flocculated; there are various states of flocculation and deflocculation.
- Flocculated systems clear rapidly and the preparation often appears unsightly, so a partially deflocculated formulation is more acceptable.

Controlled flocculation

- In suspensions of charged particles the flocculation may be controlled by the addition of electrolyte or ionic surfactants that reduce the zeta potential, and hence V_R, to give a satisfactory secondary minimum in which flocs may be formed. *Figure 6.15* shows the changes in a bismuth subnitrate suspension on addition of dibasic potassium phosphate as the flocculating agent.
- In the absence of charge on the particles flocculation may be controlled using non-ionic polymeric material including naturally occurring gums (e.g. tragacanth) and cellulose polymers (e.g. sodium carboxymethylcellulose). These polymers increase the viscosity of the aqueous vehicle, so hindering the movement of the particles, and also may form adsorbed layers on the particles which influence stability through steric stabilisation and, in some cases, bridging between particles.
- The ideal suspending agent for controlling flocculation should:
  - be readily and uniformly incorporated in the formulation
  - be readily dissolved or dispersed in water without resort to special techniques
  - ensure the formation of a loosely packed system which does not cake
  - not influence the dissolution rate or absorption rate of the drug
  - be inert, non-toxic and free from incompatibilities.

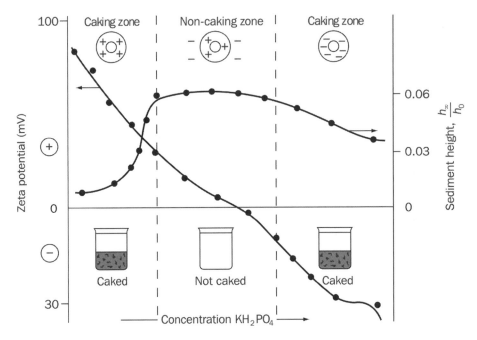

Figure 6.15: *Controlled flocculation of a bismuth subnitrate suspension using dibasic potassium phosphate (KH₂PO₄) as the flocculating agent.*

Non-aqueous suspensions

- Many pharmaceutical aerosols consist of solids dispersed in a non-aqueous propellant or propellant mixture.
- Low amounts of water adsorb at the particle surface and can lead to aggregation of the particles or to deposition on the walls of the container, which adversely affects the product.

Adhesion of suspension particles to containers

- When the walls of a container are wetted repeatedly an adhering layer of suspension particles may build up, and this subsequently dries to a hard and thick layer.
- Where the suspension is in constant contact with the container wall, immersional wetting occurs, in which particles are pressed up to the wall and may or may not adhere.
- Above the liquid line, spreading of the suspension during shaking or pouring may also lead to adhesion of the particles contained in the spreading liquid.
- Adhesion increases with increase in suspension concentration, and with the number of contacts the suspension makes with the surfaces.

Foams and defoamers

- Aqueous foams are formed from a three-dimensional network of surfactant films in air.
- Foams can be used as formulations for the delivery of enemas and topical drugs.
- Foams which develop in the production of liquids are troublesome, hence there is an interest in breaking foams and preventing foam formation. Small quantities of specific agents can reduce foam stability markedly. There are two types of such agent:
  1. Foam breakers, which are thought to act as small droplets forming in the foam lamellae.
  2. Foam preventives, which are thought to adsorb at the air–water interface in preference to the surfactants which stabilise the thin films.
- The most important action of an antifoam agent is to eliminate surface elasticity, the property that is responsible for the durability of foams. To do this the antifoam agent:
  — must displace any foam stabiliser
  — must therefore have a low interfacial tension in the pure state to allow it to spread when applied to the foam.
- Many foams can be made to collapse by applying drops of liquids such as ether, or long-chain alcohols such as octanol. Silcone fluids which have surface tensions as low as $20\,mN\,m^{-1}$ are effective and more versatile than soluble antifoams.

Memory maps

Types of colloidal systems

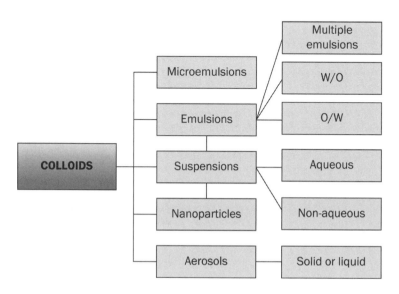

Stability of a hydrophobic colloidal system in an aqueous medium

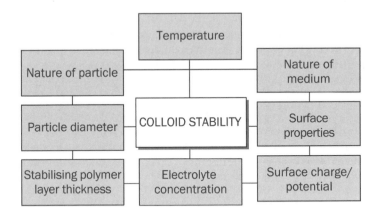

Questions

1. **According to Stokes' law, which of the following changes to a formulation of an oil-in-water emulsion would be expected to decrease the rate of creaming of the emulsion?**
   A: Decrease in the size of the oil droplets
   B: Increase in the viscosity of the continuous phase
   C: Increase in the difference in density between the oil and water phases

2. **Which of the following lead to attractive interaction between two particles?**
   A: Born forces
   B: Electrostatic forces
   C: van der Waals forces
   D: Steric forces
   E: Solvation forces

3. **Indicate which of the following statements are true. Two particles will repel each other when:**
   A: The primary maximum is very small
   B: The secondary minimum is less than the thermal energy
   C: The primary minimum is very deep

4. **Indicate which of the following statements are true. When electrolyte is added to a colloidal dispersion:**
   A: The double-layer thickness around the particles is increased
   B: Repulsion between particles is decreased
   C: van der Waals forces between particles are decreased
   D: The height of the primary maximum is decreased

5. **Indicate which of the following statements are true. Repulsion between hydrated surfaces:**
   A: Results from an increase in the freedom of movement of the chains of the adsorbed molecules
   B: Increases with increase of chain length of the adsorbed molecules
   C: Results from release of hydrated water molecules from the chains of the adsorbed molecules
   D: Increases with an increase of the number of chains per unit area of interacting surface

6. **Indicate which of the following statements are true. Stabilisation of oil-in-water emulsions by surfactants:**
   A: Arises because of a reduction of the oil–water interfacial tension
   B: Is a consequence of a decrease of the zeta potential of the oil droplets
   C: Is usually more effective when more than one surfactant is used
   D: Can only be achieved with ionic surfactants

7. **Indicate which of the following statements are true. Oil-soluble surfactants:**
   A: Have high HLB values
   B: Are hydrophilic
   C: Can be used as emulsifiers to produce water-in-oil emulsions
   D: Are efficient solubilising agents

8. **Which of the following properties are characteristic of microemulsions?**
   A: High surfactant content
   B: Droplet size greater than 1 μm
   C: Transparent systems
   D: Thermodynamically stable

9. **Which of the following properties are characteristic of deflocculated suspensions?**
   A: Close packing of the sediment to form a cake
   B: Slow sedimentation rate
   C: Formation of flocs
   D: Rapid clearance of supernatant

10. **A polysorbate has a molecular weight of 1300 Da, an ethylene oxide weight percentage of 68 and a sorbitol weight percentage of 14. The HLB of this surfactant is:**
    A: 15.0
    B: 13.6
    C: 16.4
    D: 2.8

11. **In relation to colloidal dispersions exhibiting Newtonian flow, indicate which of the following statements are true.**
    A: Shear rate is inversely proportional to shear stress
    B: Viscosity is independent of shear rate
    C: The gradient of plots of shear stress against shear rate is the reciprocal of the viscosity
    D: Kinematic viscosity is the viscosity of a dispersion divided by its density
    E: Viscosity has SI units of $N\ m^{-2}\ s$

12. **In relation to colloidal dispersions exhibiting non-Newtonian flow, indicate which of the following statements are true.**
    A: In pseudoplastic flow the apparent viscosity decreases with increasing shear rate
    B: In systems exhibiting dilatancy the apparent viscosity increases with increasing shear rate
    C: Systems exhibiting plastic flow do not flow until the shear stress exceeds a certain minimum value
    D: In thixotropic systems the apparent viscosity increases when a continuous shear stress is applied at a constant rate
    E: In rheopectic systems the apparent viscosity decreases when a continuous shear stress is applied at a constant rate

CHAPTER 7

Polymers

LEARNING OBJECTIVES

Upon completion of this chapter you should be able to:
- outline the variety of structures formed by polymers and the properties of polymers in solution
- outline the gelation of polymers and the characteristic properties of polymer gels
- outline the structure and properties of some typical polymers used in pharmacy and medicine
- outline some of the many applications of polymers in the fabrication of drug delivery devices.

Polymer structure

Polymers consist of a large number of monomer units linked together in a long chain:
- For example, polyethylene is composed of repeating ethylene monomers:

$$CH_2{=}CH_2 \rightarrow -CH_2-CH_2-CH_2-CH_2-$$

Polymers such as polyethylene in which all the monomer units are identical are referred to as homopolymers: other examples include polystyrene, poly(vinyl alcohol), polyacrylamide and polyvinylpyrrolidone.
- There are usually between about 100 and 10 000 monomer units in a chain.
- Homopolymers exist with much smaller chains including dimers (2 monomer units), trimers (3 units) and tetramers (4 units). These small chains are called oligomers.

Side chains or substituents (R) may be attached to the repeating monomer units, as for example in vinyl polymers of the type $-H_2C-CH(R)-$. These may have:
- all the R groups on the same side of the polymer backbone (isotactic)
- a regular alternation of the R groups above and below the backbone (syndiotactic)
- a random arrangement of R groups above and below the backbone (atactic)
  (*Figure 7.1*).

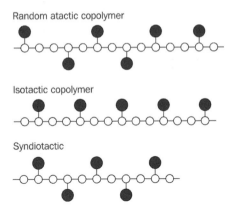

Figure 7.1: *Representation of isotactic, syndiotactic and atactic polymers showing the position of the substituent group* ● *in relation to the polymer backbone -o-o-o-o-.*

Polymers formed from more than one type of monomer are referred to as copolymers. There are several different types of copolymer (*Figure 7.2*).
- The different monomers can be arranged in a linear chain in either a random manner or in an alternating pattern along the chain.
- The linear polymer chains may be constructed from blocks of each monomer and are then referred to as block copolymers. These may be:
  - Diblock copolymers in which there is a block composed of monomer A chains attached to a block of monomer B chains (AB diblocks).
  - Triblock copolymers which are composed of either a block of A chains attached to a block of B chains attached to a block of A chains (ABA triblocks) or alternatively arranged as BAB triblocks. Well-known examples of ABA triblock copolymers are poloxamers in which the A chains are polyoxyethylene and the B chains are polyoxypropylene i.e.

$$HO(CH_2CH_2O)_x(CH(CH_3)CH_2O)_y(CH_2CH_2O)_x H$$

  x and *y* denote the numbers of monomer units in each of the blocks.
- The chains may be composed of a backbone of repeat units of one monomer on to which is grafted chains of the second monomer in a comb-like manner. These copolymers are called graft copolymers.

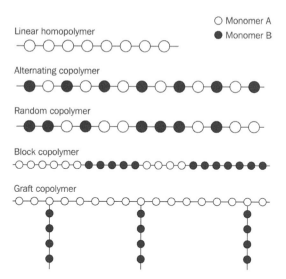

Figure 7.2: *Varieties of copolymer structure attainable through the polymerisation of two different monomers represented by • and o.*

Polymer chains can be either linear (forming random coils in solution) or branched. There may be cross-linking between chains to form three-dimensional networks. Highly branched and spherical or quasi-spherical polymers (dendrimers) built around a central core can be synthesised with a range of sizes depending on the generation of the dendrimer (see **Chapter 13**). Polymers do not form perfect crystals but have crystalline regions surrounded by amorphous regions (*Figure 7.3*).

- The melting point of polymers is not as well defined as in low-molecular-weight crystalline solids because of the presence of the poorly structured regions which melt over a range of temperatures.
- As well as the melting point the polymer may also exhibit a glass transition temperature, T_g. Below T_g the chains are 'frozen' in position and the polymer is glassy and brittle; above T_g the chains are mobile and the polymer is tougher and more flexible.

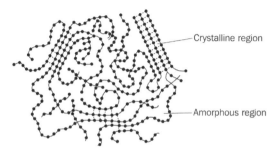

Figure 7.3: *Diagrammatic representation of a solid polymer showing regions of crystallinity and regions which are amorphous.*

Key points

- Polymers are substances of high molecular weight made up of repeating monomer units.
- Polymer molecules may be linear or branched, and separate linear or branched chains may be joined by cross-links. Extensive cross-linking leads to a three-dimensional and often insoluble polymer network.
- Polymers in which all the monomeric units are identical are referred to as homopolymers; those formed from more than one type of monomer are called copolymers.

Solution properties of polymers

Polydispersity

Nearly all synthetic polymers and naturally occurring macromolecules possess a range of molecular weights. The exceptions to this are proteins and natural polypeptides. The molecular weight is thus an average molecular weight and depending on the experimental method used to measure it may be:

- a number average molecular weight, M_n, (determined by chemical analysis or osmotic pressure measurement) which, in a mixture containing n_1, n_2, n_3... moles of polymer with molecular weights M_1, M_2, M_3..., respectively, is defined by:

$$M_n = \frac{n_1 M_1 + n_2 M_2 + n_3 M_3 + \ldots\ldots}{n_1 + n_2 + n_3 + \ldots\ldots} = \frac{\sum n_i M_i}{\sum n_i}$$

- a weight average molecular weight, M_w (determined by light scattering methods):

$$M_w = \frac{m_1 M_1 + m_2 M_2 + m_3 M_3 + \ldots\ldots}{m_1 + m_2 + m_3 + \ldots\ldots} = \frac{\sum n_i M_i^2}{\sum n_i M_i}$$

where m_2, m_3... are the masses of each species.

The weight average molecular weight, M_w, is biased towards large molecules and in a polydisperse polymer is always greater than M_n. The ratio M_w/M_n expresses the degree of polydispersity.

Tip

Remember that the mass, m_i, of a particular species is obtained by multiplying the molecular weight of each species by the number of molecules of that weight; that is, $m_i = n_i M_i$. Thus the molecular weight appears as the square in the numerator of the equation for the weight average molecular weight.

Viscosity

- Assuming that the polymer solution exhibits Newtonian flow properties (see **Chapter 6**), the viscosity can be expressed by:
  - The relative viscosity, η_{rel}, defined as the ratio of the viscosity of the solution, η, to the viscosity of the pure solvent, η_0, i.e,
    $\eta_{rel} = \eta/\eta_0$.
  - The specific viscosity, η_{sp}, of the solution defined by $\eta_{sp} = \eta_{rel} - 1$.
  - The intrinsic viscosity, $[\eta]$, obtained by extrapolation of plots of the ratio η_{sp}/c (called the reduced viscosity) against concentration c to zero concentration.
- If the polymer forms spherical particles in dilute solution then
  $\eta_{rel} = 1 + 2.5\Phi$ where Φ is the volume fraction (volume of the particles divided by the total volume of the solution).
  - Therefore, a plot of η_{sp}/Φ against Φ should have an intercept of 2.5.
  - Departure of the limiting value from this theoretical value may result from either hydration of the particles, or particle asymmetry, or both.
- A change in shape due to changes in polymer–solvent interactions (*Figure 7.4*) and the binding of small molecules with the polymer may lead to significant changes in solution viscosity:
  - In 'good' solvents linear macromolecules will be expanded as the polar groups will be solvated.
  - In 'poor' solvents the intramolecular attraction between the segments is greater than the segment–solvent affinity and the molecule will tend to coil up.
- The viscosity of ionised polymers is complicated by charge interactions which vary with polymer concentration and additive concentration, especially of added salts.
  - Flexible, charged macromolecules will vary in shape with the degree of ionisation.
  - At maximum ionisation they are stretched out due to mutual charge repulsion and the viscosity increases.
  - On addition of small counterions the effective charge is reduced and the molecules contract; the viscosity falls as a result.
- The intrinsic viscosity of solutions of linear high-molecular-weight polymers is proportional to the molecular weight M of the polymer as given by the Staudinger equation:

$$[\eta] = KM^a$$

where a is a constant in the range 0–2 (for most high polymers a has a value between 0.6 and 0.8) and K is a constant for a given polymer–solvent system.

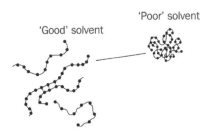

Figure 7.4: *Representation of the conformation of a polymer in 'good' and 'poor' solvents.*

Key points

- There is usually a range of sizes of the polymer chains in a solution, i.e. polymer solutions are polydisperse, as polymerisation reactions produce a range of molecular weight material.
- As a consequence of polydispersity the measured molecular weight varies depending on the experimental method used – some techniques such as light scattering are more influenced by the larger molecules than others such as osmometry.
- The viscosity of a polymer solution depends not only on its concentration but also on polymer–solvent interactions, charge interactions and the binding of small molecules to the chains.

Properties of polymer gels

Gels can be divided into two groups, depending on the nature of the bonds between the chains of the network:

- Gels of type I are irreversible systems with a three-dimensional network formed by covalent bonds between the macromolecules. They include swollen networks that have been formed by polymerisation of a monomer in the presence of a cross-linking agent:
    - Examples include poly(hydroxyethyl methacrylate) (poly[HEMA]) which may be cross-linked with, for example, ethylene glycol dimethacrylate (EGDMA).
    - These polymers swell in water but cannot dissolve as the cross-links are stable.
    - This expansion on contact with water has been put to many uses, such as in the fabrication of expanding implants from cross-linked hydrophilic polymers which imbibe body fluids and swell to a predetermined volume.
    - Hydrophilic contact lenses (such as Soflens) are made from cross-linked poly[HEMA]s.
- Type II gels are heat-reversible, being held together by intermolecular bonds such as hydrogen bonds:
    - The temperature at which gelation occurs is called the gel point and gelation

can be induced either by cooling (e.g. poly(vinyl alcohol)) or heating (e.g. water-soluble methylcelluloses) to this temperature depending on the type of temperature variation of solubility.

— The gel point can be influenced by the presence of additives which can induce gel formation by acting as bridge molecules (for example, with borax and poly(vinyl alcohol)) or by the addition of solvents such as glycerol.

— Because of their gelling properties poly(vinyl alcohol)s are used for application of drugs to the skin; on application the gel dries rapidly leaving a plastic film with the drug in intimate contact with the skin.

— Solutions of some poly(oxyethylene)-poly(oxypropylene)-poly(oxyethylene) block copolymers form reversible gels by the close packing of their micelles when concentrated solutions are warmed.

- Swollen gels may exhibit syneresis, which is the separation of solvent phase from the gel. This may be explained as follows:

— During gel formation the polymer network is stretched as the gel swells by taking in the solvent.

— At equilibrium the contracting force of the polymer network is balanced by the swelling forces determined by the osmotic pressure.

— If the osmotic pressure decreases, for example on cooling or by changing the ionisation of the polymer molecules, water may be squeezed out of the gel and the gel appears to 'weep'.

— Syneresis may often be decreased by the addition of electrolyte, glucose and sucrose or by increasing the polymer concentration.

Key points

- A gel is a polymer–solvent system containing a three-dimensional network which can be formed by swelling of solid polymer or by reduction in the solubility of the polymer in the solution.
- When gels are formed from solutions, each system is characterised by a critical concentration of gelation below which a gel is not formed.
- Gelation is characterised by a large increase in viscosity above the gel point, the appearance of a rubber-like elasticity and a yield point stress at higher polymer concentrations.
- Gels can be irreversible or reversible systems depending on the nature of the bonds between the chains of the network.

Polymers and macromolecules in solution may:

- form complexes, as for example between high-molecular-weight polyacids and polyethylene glycols, polyvinylpyrrolidone and poly(acrylic acid)s, and hyaluronic acid and the proteoglycans in the intracellular matrix in cartilage.
- bind ions present in solution to form gels, as for example when Ca^{2+} ions are bound by alginate molecules.

- adsorb at interfaces, for example:
  - insulin in solution will adsorb onto the surface of glass and poly(vinyl chloride) infusion containers, and plastic tubing used in giving sets, so reducing its concentration in solution
  - gelatin, acacia, poly(vinyl alcohol) will adsorb at the interface between oil and water in emulsions or on the surface of dispersed suspension particles and so stabilise these colloidal dispersions.
- imbibe large quantities of water. This is utilised:
  - in the manufacture of paper and sanitary towels, nappies and surgical dressings
  - in the treatment of constipation and in appetite suppression.

Tips
- Note that di- and triblock copolymers in which the A block is poly(oxyethylene) and the B block is poly(oxypropylene) are amphiphilic because poly(oxyethylene) is hydrophilic and poly(oxypropylene) is hydrophobic.
- These polymers are surface active and may form micelles in aqueous solution.
- At high solution concentrations the micelles pack so closely that the solution becomes immobile, i.e. gelation occurs.
- Gelation may also occur when concentrated solutions are warmed because the solubility of poly(oxyethylene) decreases as temperature increases, i.e. it becomes more hydrophobic. Therefore more micelles form at the higher temperature and gelation occurs as they pack closely together.

Some water-soluble polymers used in pharmacy and medicine

Important examples
- Carboxypolymethylene (Carbomer, Carbopol):
  - is a high-molecular-weight polymer of acrylic acid, containing a high proportion of carboxyl groups
  - is used as a suspending agent in pharmaceutical preparations, as a binding agent in tablets, and in the formulation of prolonged-action tablets.
- Cellulose derivatives:
  - Methylcellulose is a methyl ether of cellulose containing about 29% of methoxyl groups. It is slowly soluble in water. Low-viscosity grades are used as emulsifiers for liquid paraffin and other mineral oils. High-viscosity grades are used as thickening agents for medicated jellies and as dispersing and thickening agents in suspensions.
  - Hydroxypropylmethylcellulose (hypromellose) is a mixed ether of cellulose containing 27–30% of $-OCH_3$ groups and 4–7.5% of $-OC_3H_6OH$ groups. It forms

a viscous colloidal solution and is used in ophthalmic solutions to prolong the action of medicated eye drops and is employed as an artificial tear fluid.

- Natural gums and mucilages:
  - Gum arabic (acacia) is a very soluble polyelectrolyte whose solutions are highly viscous due to the branched structure of the macromolecular chains. It is used in pharmacy as an emulsifier.
  - Gum tragacanth partially dissolves in water to give highly viscous solutions. It is one of the most widely used natural emulsifiers and thickeners and is an effective suspending agent.
  - Alginates are block copolymer polysaccharides derived from seaweed consisting of β-D-mannuronic acid and α-L-guluronic acid residues joined by 1,4 glycosidic linkages. They form very viscous solutions and gel on addition of acid or calcium salts. They are used chiefly as stabilisers and thickening agents.
  - Pectin is a purified carbohydrate product from extracts of the rind of citrus fruits and consists of partially methoxylated polygalacturonic acid. It readily gels in the presence of calcium or other polyvalent cations.
  - Chitosan is a polymer obtained by the deacetylation of the polysaccharide chitin. The degree of deacetylation has a significant effect on the solubility and rheological properties of the polymer. Chitosan will form films, gels and matrices, making it useful for solid dosage forms such as granules or microparticles.
  - Dextran is a branched-chain polymer of anhydroglucose, linked through α-1,6 glucosidic linkages. Partially hydrolysed dextrans are used as plasma substitutes or 'expanders'.
  - Polyvinylpyrrolidone is a homopolymer of N-vinylpyrrolidone used as a suspending and dispersing agent, a tablet-binding and granulating agent, and as a vehicle for drugs such as penicillin, cortisone, procaine and insulin to delay their absorption and prolong their action. It forms hard films which are utilised in film-coating processes.
  - Macrogols (polyoxyethylene glycols) are liquid over the molecular weight range 200–700 Da and are used as solvents for drugs such as hydrocortisone. Higher-molecular-weight members of the series are semisolid and waxy and may be used as suppository bases. Polyoxyethylene glycols (PEGs) play an important role in the stability of polymeric nanoparticles *in vivo* and *in vitro* when they are applied covalently or by adsorption to the nanoparticle surface, achieving as discussed in **Chapter 13**, enthalpic stabilisation. Pegfilgrastim is a PEGylated form of recombinant human granulocyte colony-stimulating factor used to stimulate bone marrow to enhance production of neutrophils during chemotherapy. The parent filgrastim has a short half-life of some 3–4 h while the PEGylated drug has a human half-life of between 15 to 80 h.

Key points

- Water-soluble (hydrophilic) polymers are widely used in pharmacy, for example as suspending agents, emulsifiers, binding agents in tablets, thickeners of liquid dosage forms and in film coating of tablets.
- Water-insoluble (hydrophobic) polymers are mainly used in packaging material and tubing, and in the fabrication of membranes and films.
- Important properties of hydrophobic polymers which affect their suitability for use in pharmacy are their permeability to drugs and gases and their tendency to adsorb drugs.

Properties

Bioadhesivity

- Bioadhesivity arises from interactions between polymer chains and the macromolecules on mucosal surfaces – for maximum adhesion there should be maximum interaction (*Figure 7.5*).
- The charge on the molecules will be important – for two anionic polymers maximum interaction will occur when they are not charged.

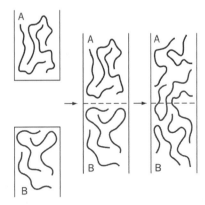

Figure 7.5: *Schematic representation of two phases, adhesive (A) and mucus (B), which adhere due to chain adsorption and consecutive chain entanglement during mucoadhesion. Reproduced from Peppas NA, Mikos AG (1990) In: Gurney R, Junginger H (eds) Bioadhesion. Stuttgart: Wiss Verlagsgesellschaft.*

Note: Adhesion between polymeric tablet coatings and human tissue can also be an unwanted problem leading, as discussed in **Chapter 11**, to issues such as oesophageal adhesion.

Crystallinity

Defects in polymer crystals allow preparation of microcrystals, e.g. microcrystalline cellulose (Avicel) by disruption of larger crystals.

> **Tip**
>
> Refer to **Chapter 6** to see the mechanism of stabilisation of suspensions and emulsions by polymers.

Water-insoluble polymers

Water-insoluble polymers play an important role in pharmacy and are used in the fabrication of membranes, containers and tubing. Important properties include:

- Degree of crystallinity – affects rigidity, fluidity, resistance to diffusion of small molecules and degradation.
- Permeability to drugs:
    - Diffusion of solutes in a non-porous solid polymer is governed by Fick's first law, which for polymer membranes of thickness l becomes:

$$J = \frac{DK\Delta c}{l}$$

    where J is the flux, Δc represents the difference in solution concentration of drug at the two faces of membrane, D is the diffusion coefficient of the drug in the membrane and K is the distribution coefficient of the permeant (drug) towards the polymer.
    - Permeability within a given polymer is a function of the degree of crystallinity, which itself is a function of polymer molecular weight.
    - Permeation of drug molecules through a solid polymer is a function of the solubility of the drug in the polymer and will be reduced by the presence of inorganic fillers in which the drug is insoluble.
    - The permeability of a polymer film is affected by the method of preparation of the film.
    - Drug flux through dense (non-porous) polymer membranes is by diffusion; flux through porous membranes will be by diffusion and by transport in solvent through pores in the film.
- Permeability to gases – this is important when polymers are used as packaging materials:
    - Permeability depends on the polarity of the polymer – more polar films tend to be more ordered and less porous, hence less oxygen-permeable. The less polar films are more porous, permitting the permeation of oxygen but not necessarily of the larger water molecules.

- — Water permeability can be controlled by altering the hydrophilic/hydrophobic balance of the polymer.
- Affinity of drugs for plastics:
  - — Steroids are adsorbed from solutions passing through polyethylene tubing.
  - — Glyceryl trinitrate has a high affinity for lipophilic plastics and migrates from tablets in contact with plastic liners in packages, causing a reduction of the active content of some stored tablets to zero.
- Ion-exchange properties:
  - — Synthetic organic polymers comprising a hydrocarbon cross-linked network to which ionisable groups are attached have the ability to exchange ions attracted to their ionised groups with ions of the same charge present in solution. They are used in the form of beads as ion-exchange resins.
  - — The resins may be either cation exchangers, in which the resin ionisable group is acidic, for example, sulfonic, carboxylic or phenolic groups, or anion exchangers, in which the ionisable group is basic, either amine or quaternary ammonium groups.
  - — Cation-exchange resins effect changes in the electrolyte balance of the plasma by exchanging cations with those in the gut lumen. In the ammonium form, cation-exchange resins are used in the treatment of retention oedema and for the control of sodium retention in pregnancy. These resins are also used (in their calcium and sodium forms) to treat hyperkalaemia.
  - — Anion-exchange resins such as polyamine methylene resin and polyaminostyrene have been used as antacids.
  - — Ion-exchange resins are used in the removal of ionised impurities from water and in the prolongation of drug action by forming complexes with drugs.
- Silicones are water-insoluble polymers with a structure containing alternate atoms of Si and O. Examples include:
  - — Dimeticones – a range of fluid polymers with a wide spectrum of viscosities. Commonly used as barrier substances, silicone lotions and creams acting as water-repellent applications protecting the skin against water-soluble irritants.
    - » Dimeticone 200 has been used as a lubricant for artificial eyes and to replace the degenerative vitreous fluid in cases of retinal detachment. It can also act as a simple lubricant in joints.
    - » Activated dimeticone (activated polymethylsiloxane) is a mixture of liquid dimeticones containing finely divided silica to enhance the defoaming properties of the silicone.

Application of polymers in drug delivery

Film coating

Polymer solutions allowed to evaporate produce polymeric films which can act as protective layers for tablets or granules containing sensitive drug substances or as a rate-controlling barrier to drug release.

- Film coats have been divided into two types: those that dissolve rapidly and those that behave as dialysis membranes, allowing slow diffusion of solute or some delayed diffusion by acting as gel layers.
- Materials that have been used as film formers include shellac, zein, cellulose acetate phthalate, glyceryl stearates, paraffins, and a range of anionic and cationic polymers such as the Eudragit polymers (see also **Chapter 2**).

Key point

Control of the rate of release of a drug when administered by oral or parenteral routes can be achieved by the use of polymers that function as a barrier to drug movement.

Matrices

Methods of drug delivery from matrices include the use of:

- A non-eroding matrix: the mechanism of sustained release is:
    - the passage of drug through pores in the matrix if this is made of water-insoluble polymer (hydrophobic matrices)
    - the entry of water into the polymer matrix followed by swelling and gelation and then diffusion of drug through the viscous gel when water-soluble matrices (hydrophilic matrices) are used.
- A reservoir system – drug contained in the reservoir releases by leaching or slow diffusion through the wall of the retaining polymer membrane.
- An eroding matrix – drug is released when the polymer matrix in which the drug is dissolved or dispersed erodes by either bulk erosion or surface erosion (*Figure 7.6*).

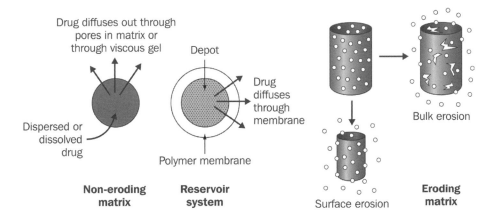

Figure 7.6: *Matrix systems for drug delivery.*

Microcapsules and microspheres

- In microcapsules drug is encapsulated as small particles or as a solution in a polymer film or coat, whereas microspheres are solid polymeric spheres which entrap drug. Equivalent structures with particle diameters ranging from 50 to ~200 nm are referred to as nanocapsules and nanoparticles (see **Chapter 13**).
- Microcapsules can be prepared by three main processes:
  1. Coacervation – the liquid or solid to be encapsulated is dispersed in a solution of a macromolecule (such as gelatin, gum arabic, carboxymethylcellulose or poly(vinyl alcohol)) in which it is immiscible. A suitable non-solvent (such as ethanol and isopropranol) is added which is miscible with the continuous phase but a poor solvent for the polymer and causes the polymer to form a coacervate (polymer-rich) layer around the disperse phase. This coating layer may then be treated to give a rigid coat of capsule wall.
  2. Interfacial polymerisation – reactions between oil-soluble monomers and water-soluble monomers at the oil–water interface of water-in-oil or oil-in-water dispersions can lead to interfacial polymerisation resulting in the formation of polymeric microcapsules, the size of which is determined by the size of the emulsion droplets. Alternatively, reactive monomer can be dispersed in one of the phases and induced to polymerise at the interface, or to polymerise in the bulk disperse phase and to precipitate at the interface due to its insolubility in the continuous phase. One monomer which has been used to prepare both microspheres and nanospheres is cyanoacrylate which when dissolved in the non-aqueous phase polymerises in contact with the aqueous phase and forms a poly(cyanoacrylate) membrane at the surface. Cyanoacrylates are also used as tissue adhesives in surgery.
  3. Physical methods – the spray drying process involves dispersion of the core material in a solution of coating substance and spraying the mixture into an environment which causes the solvent to evaporate. The process of pan coating has been applied in the formation of sustained-release beads by application of waxes such as glyceryl monostearate in organic solution to granules of drug. It can only be used for particles greater than 600 μm in diameter. Details of the use of spray drying and pan coating in the preparation of tablets and capsules are given in **Chapter 2**.
- Microspheres and nanoparticles can be prepared by modification of the coacervation process:
  - For example, gelatin nanoparticles have been prepared by desolvation (for example, with sodium sulfate) of a gelatin solution containing drug bound to the gelatin, in a process which terminates the desolvation just before coacervation begins.
  - In this manner colloidal particles rather than the larger coacervate droplets are obtained.
  - Hardening of the gelatin particles is achieved by glutaraldehyde which cross-links with gelatin.

Methods of preparing nanoparticulate systems for drug delivery are discussed in **Chapter 13**.

Rate-limiting membranes and devices

Rate-limiting membranes are utilised to control the movement of drugs from a reservoir.

- Drug release rate is controlled by choice of polymer, membrane thickness and porosity.
- Examples include the Progestasert device designed to release progesterone into the uterine cavity, the Ocusert device for delivery to the eye and the Transiderm therapeutic system for transdermal medication.

Osmotic pumps

A variety of devices have been described:

- In the oral osmotic pump (Oros) (*Figure 7.7*):
  - The drug is mixed with a water-soluble core material.
  - This core is surrounded by a water-insoluble semipermeable polymer membrane in which is drilled a small orifice.
  - Water molecules can diffuse into the core through the outer membrane to form a concentrated solution inside.
  - An osmotic gradient is set up across the semipermeable membrane with the result that drug is pushed out of the orifice.
  - For example, the osmotic tablet of nifedipine consists of a semipermeable cellulose acetate coating, a swellable hydrogel layer of polyoxyethylene glycol and hydroxypropylmethylcellulose, and a drug chamber containing nifedipine in hydroxypropylmethylcellulose and polyoxyethylene glycol.

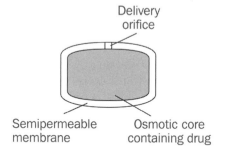

Figure 7.7: *Diagrammatic representation of the Oros osmotic pump.*

Transdermal delivery systems

- There are two groups of transdermal delivery systems (*Figure 7.8*):
  - Membrane systems generally consist of a reservoir, a rate-controlling membrane and an adhesive layer. Diffusion of the active principle from the reservoir through the controlling membrane governs release rate. The active principle is usually present in suspended form; liquids and gels are used as dispersion media. Examples of membrane systems include Transiderm Nitro, in which the rate-controlling membrane is composed of a polyethylene/vinyl acetate copolymer

having a thin adhesive layer and the reservoir contains nitroglycerin dispersed in the form of a lactose suspension in silicone oil.

— In matrix systems the active principle is dispersed in a matrix which consists of either a gel or an adhesive film. Examples of matrix systems include the Nitro-Dur system which consists of a hydrogel matrix (composed of water, glycerin, poly(vinyl alcohol) and polyvinylpyrrolidone) in which a nitroglycerin/lactose triturate is homogeneously dispersed.

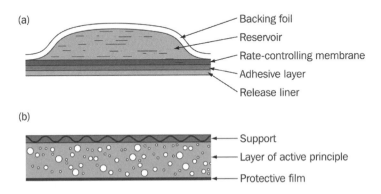

Figure 7.8: *Structures of commercial transdermal (a) membrane-controlled and (b) matrix systems.*

Polymer fibres

- Polymer fibres are formed by a process of electrospinning in which a high voltage is applied to the tip of a syringe needle containing polymer solution (see *Figure 7.9*). This causes the liquid droplets emerging from the needle to stretch and at a critical point to emerge as a stream of liquid (known as Taylor cone formation).
- As the jet travels out of the needle, tensile forces brought about by surface charge repulsion lead to a bending motion and the polymer chains in the jet orient to form microfibres or nanofibres depending on the polymer, its viscosity, surface tension and the capillary diameter; the polymer is then deposited and collected on an earthed plate.
- These techniques allow the formation of fibres with a variety of internal structures and dimensions, having potential for drug delivery or as materials for wound dressings, and transdermal delivery systems.

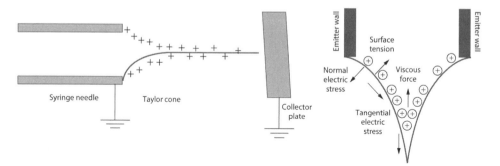

Figure 7.9: *Left: The formation of a Taylor cone, showing the effect of the application of a high voltage to a needle tip, causing surface charges to accumulate on the liquid, leading to the deformation of the spherical drop into a cone. Increase in the voltage beyond this level causes the formation of a liquid jet. Right: The forces acting on the system which shape the nature of the jet include surface tension, viscous forces and normal and tangential electrical stresses.*

Polymers in wound dressings

Wound dressings involve synthetic or natural polymers and macromolecules and rely for some of their benefits on physical phenomena such as capillarity and wicking. They can generally be classified in groups depending on their nature and properties, e.g.:

- Hydrocolloids: Hydrocolloids are composed of gel-forming substances such as gelatin or NaCMC (sodium carboxymethylcellulose). Hydrofiber is a NaCMC dressing with a high cohesive dry and wet tensile strength which absorbs up to 25 times its weight in fluid. NaCMC is spun into fibres (see also alginates, below) and is produced in ribbon and sheet formats.

- Alginates: Sodium alginates are soluble, but binding to calcium results in hydrated poorly soluble systems in the form of gels, beads, films and fibres. Calcium alginate fibres are made by extruding sodium alginate solutions through spinnerets into calcium-containing solutions where the fibres precipitate. This approach can be used to prepare zinc alginate and silver alginate fibres.

- Polymer foams: Polyurethane is most commonly used to prepare foam dressings. Synthaderm is a 'synthetic skin' of a modified polyurethane foam, hydrophilic on one side (placed in contact with the wound) and hydrophobic on the other. Lyofoam is a soft, hydrophobic, polyurethane foam sheet 8 mm thick. The side of the dressing that is to be placed in contact with the skin or wound has been heat-treated to collapse the cells of the foam, and thus enable it to absorb liquid by capillarity.

- Hydrogels: Hydrogel dressings are most commonly able to conform to the shape of a wound. A secondary, non-absorbent dressing is needed. These dressings are generally used to donate liquid to dry sloughy wounds and facilitate debridement of necrotic tissue; some also have the ability to absorb very small amounts of exudate. Hydrogel sheets have a fixed structure and limited fluid-handling capacity.

- Antimicrobial-releasing dressings: Dressings containing antimicrobials such as polihexanide (polyhexamethylene biguanide) or dialkylcarbamoyl chloride are available for use on infected wounds. Cadexomer is a dextrin derivative which forms a complex with iodine, cadexomer–iodine, which releases free iodine (acts as an antiseptic on the wound surface) when it is exposed to wound exudate.

Memory maps

Properties of polymers

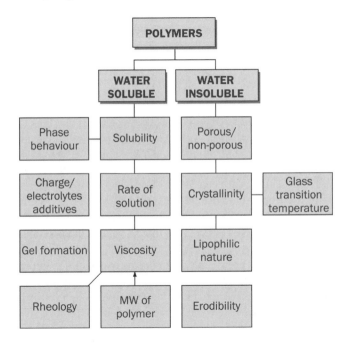

Release of drug from polymer matrices

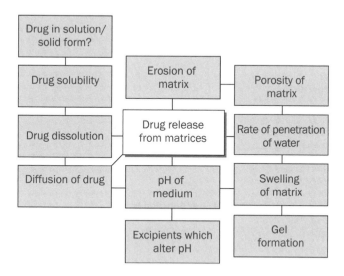

Properties of soluble polymers

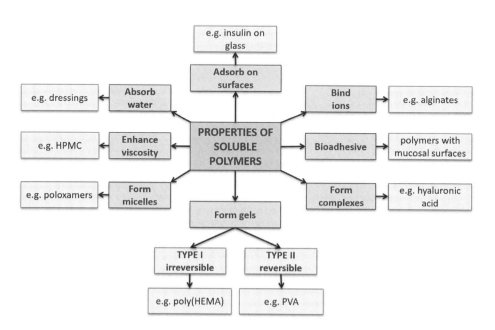

Questions

In questions 1–8 indicate the statements which are true.

1. **Polymers with regular alternation of the side chains on the polymer backbone are referred to as:**
    A: Isotactic
    B: Atactic
    C: Syndiotactic

2. **The copolymer $HO(CH_2CH_2O)_x (CH(CH_3)CH_2O)_y(CH_2CH_2O)_xH$ is an example of a:**
    A: Graft copolymer
    B: Diblock copolymer
    C: Homopolymer
    D: Triblock copolymer
    E: Poloxamer

3. **The intrinsic viscosity of a polymer solution is:**
    A: Relative viscosity −1
    B: The ratio of the viscosity of the solution to the viscosity of pure solvent
    C: Proportional to the molecular weight of the polymer
    D: Obtained by extrapolation of plots of reduced viscosity against concentration to infinite dilution
    E: Of an approximate value of 2.5 for spherical, non-hydrated particles

4. **Type I lyophilic gels are:**
    A: Held together by weak intermolecular bonds such as hydrogen bonds
    B: Heat reversible
    C: Formed by aqueous solutions of high molecular weight block copolymers
    D: Formed by covalent bonding of macromolecular chains
    E: Formed when poly(vinyl alcohol) solutions are cooled below the gel point

5. **Cross-linked poly[HEMA] gels:**
    A: Are type II gels
    B: Can swell in water but cannot dissolve
    C: Are heat reversible
    D: May exhibit syneresis
    E: May be used to form hydrophilic contact lenses

6. **The diffusion of small molecules through films formed from water-insoluble polymers:**
    A: Is not affected by the degree of crystallinity of the polymer
    B: Is a function of the polymer molecular weight
    C: Is not affected by the solubility of the molecule in the polymer
    D: Is governed by Fick's first law
    E: Is affected by the method of preparation of the polymer film

7. **Drug release from a non-eroding hydrophilic matrix involves:**
   A: Swelling and gelation of the matrix
   B: Coacervation
   C: Diffusion of drug through a gel layer
   D: Diffusion of drug through a semipermeable membrane
   E: Passage of drug through pores in the matrix

8. **Typical microcapsules:**
   A: May be prepared by interfacial polymerisation
   B: Release drugs by an osmotic gradient across a gel layer
   C: Have diameters of about 50 nm
   D: May be prepared by a coacervation process
   E: Release drug through a small orifice

CHAPTER 8

Drug absorption and delivery

LEARNING OBJECTIVES

Upon completion of this chapter you should be able to:
- outline the structure and function of biological membranes and the factors influencing the transport of drugs through them
- summarise the special features of a number of routes for drug administration either for systemic or local action, including:
  - oral route and oral absorption
  - buccal and sublingual absorption
  - intramuscular (i.m.) and subcutaneous (s.c.) injection
  - transdermal delivery
  - delivery to the eye and ear
  - vaginal absorption
  - lung and respiratory tract (inhalation therapy)
  - nasal and rectal routes
  - intrathecal drug administration, and the use of devices such as microneedles, implantable pumps and arterial stents.

The delivery and absorption of proteins and monoclonal antibodies are discussed in **Chapter 12**.

Biological membranes and drug transport

Drug absorption is controlled by the nature of the biological membrane involved, its degree of internal bonding and rigidity, its surface charge and by the physicochemical properties of the drug, as well as by the delivery system. Note that cellular efflux mechanisms centred on P-glycoproteins exist. Some drugs are ejected from cells by these 'pumps' so that these drugs have a lower apparent absorption than predicted on physicochemical grounds.

Biological membranes

Membrane structure
- *Figure 8.1* shows a diagram of the fluid mosaic model of a biological membrane.
- The fluid mosaic model illustrates the protein–lipid complexes which form either hydrophilic or hydrophobic 'gates' to allow transport of molecules with different characteristics.

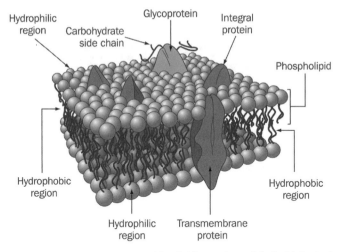

Figure 8.1: *Diagrammatic representation of the fluid mosaic model of a biological membrane.*

Cholesterol

- Cholesterol is a major component of most mammalian biological membranes.
- Its shape allows it to fit closely in bilayers with the hydrocarbon chains of unsaturated fatty acids.
- It complexes with phospholipids and reduces the permeability of phospholipid membranes to water, cations, glycerol and glucose.
- Its removal (e.g. by surfactants) causes the membrane to lose its structural integrity and to become highly permeable.

Key points

- Absorption generally requires the passage of the drug in a molecular form across one or more barrier membranes and tissues.
- The majority of conventional (non-biological) drugs are administered as solid or semisolid dosage forms.
- Tablets or capsules will disintegrate, and the drug will then be released for subsequent absorption.
- Many tablets contain granules or drug particles which must deaggregate to facilitate the solution process.
- If the drug has the appropriate physicochemical properties, it will pass by passive diffusion from a region of high concentration to a region of low concentration across the membrane.
- Soluble drugs can, of course, also be administered as solutions in appropriate solvents.

Key points

- The main function of biological membranes is to contain the aqueous contents of cells and separate them from an aqueous exterior phase.
- Membranes are lipoidal in nature.
- To allow nutrients to pass into the cell and waste products to move out, biological membranes are selectively permeable.
- There are specialised transport systems to assist the passage of water-soluble materials and ions through their lipid interior.
- Some drugs are absorbed byway of transport systems and do not necessarily obey the pH partition hypothesis.
- Lipid-soluble agents can pass by passive diffusion through the membrane.
- Biological membranes are composed of bilayers of phospholipids and cholesterol or other related structures.
- Embodied in the matrix of lipid molecules are proteins, generally hydrophobic in nature.
- Membranes have a hydrophilic, negatively charged exterior and a hydrophobic interior.

Lipophilicity and absorption

If the percentage absorption versus log P is plotted a parabolic relationship is obtained, with the optimum value designated as log P_0 (*Figure 8.2*). The optimal partition coefficient differs for different absorbing membranes.

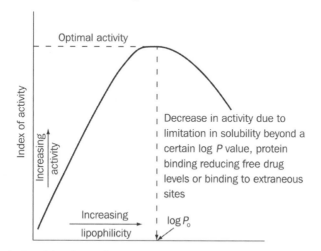

Figure 8.2: *Typical activity–log P plot.*

Drugs with high log *P* values

Drugs with high log *P* values are protein-bound, have low aqueous solubility and bind to extraneous sites. They have a lower bioavailability than anticipated from their log *P*, giving rise to the parabolic curve shown in *Figure 8.2*.

Drugs with low log *P* values

May be too hydrophilic to have any affinity for the barrier cell membranes and hence may be poorly absorbed.

Molecular weight and drug absorption

- The larger drug molecules are, the poorer will be their absorption.
- Lipinski devised a 'rule of five' defining drug-like properties. The rule is that good oral absorption is more likely when:
  - the drug molecule has fewer than 5 hydrogen bond donors (−OH groups or −NH groups)
  - the molecular weight of the drug is less than 500
  - the log *P* of the drug is less than 5
  - there are fewer than 10 H-bond acceptors.

  but note:
  - compounds that are substrates for transporters are exceptions to the rule
  - proteins and agents such as monoclonal antibodies because of their large size and physical properties present specific problems in relation to absorption, which are discussed in **Chapter 12**.

Permeability and the pH-partition hypothesis

Assumption

- Only drugs in their un-ionised form (more lipid-soluble) pass through membranes.
- As most drugs are weak electrolytes it is to be expected that the un-ionised form (U) of either acids or bases, the lipid-soluble species, will diffuse across the membrane, while the ionised forms (I) will be rejected. Hence, it is important to be able to calculate their ionisation, as below.

Calculation of percentage ionisation

- For weakly acidic drugs (such as aspirin and indometacin) the ratio of ionised to un-ionised species is given by the equations:

$$\text{pH} - \text{p}K_a = \log \frac{[\text{ionised form}]}{[\text{unionised form}]} = \log \frac{[\text{I}]}{[\text{U}]}$$

- For weakly basic drugs the equation takes the form:

$$\text{pH} - \text{p}K_a = \log \frac{[\text{unionised form}]}{[\text{ionised form}]} = \log \frac{[\text{U}]}{[\text{I}]}$$

Tips

The following example illustrates the calculation of the percentage ionisation from the equations before. The amount of drug in the un-ionised form of acetylsalicylic acid ($pK_a = 3.5$) at pH 4 is:

$4 - 3.5 = \log([I]/[U])$

Therefore $[I]/[U] = 3.162$

Percentage un-ionised

$= ([U] \times 100)/([U] + [I])$

$= 100/\{1 + ([I]/[U])\}$

$= 100/(1 + 3.162)$

$= (100/4.162) = 24.03\%$

- In choosing the correct equation you need to be able to distinguish between weakly acidic and basic drugs. You can usually tell the type of drug salt from the drug name. For example:
  - The sodium of sodium salicylate means that it is the salt of the strong base sodium hydroxide and the weak acid salicylic acid, i.e. sodium (or potassium) in the drug name implies the salt of a strong base.
  - The hydrochloride of ephedrine hydrochloride means that it is the salt of a strong acid (hydrochloric acid) and a weak base (ephedrine), i.e. hydrochloride (or bromide, nitrate, sulfate, etc.) in the drug name implies the salt of a strong acid.

Discrepancies between expected and observed absorption

- Absorption is often much greater than one would expect, although the trend is usually as predicted. For example, the absorption of acetylsalicylic acid is 41% at pH 4 (although only 24% is in un-ionised form) and 27% at pH 5 (only 3.1% is in un-ionised form).
- Two possible explanations exist:
  1. Absorption and ionisation are both dynamic processes so that even small amounts of un-ionised drug can be absorbed and are then quickly replenished and absorbed.
  2. The bulk pH is not the actual pH at the membrane. A local pH exists at the membrane surface which differs from the bulk pH. This local pH is lower than the bulk because of the attraction of hydrogen ions by the negative groups of the membrane components (see below).

Problems in the quantitative application of the pH-partition hypothesis

There are several reasons why the pH-partition hypothesis cannot be applied quantitatively in practical situations:

Variability in pH conditions

- Although the normally quoted range of stomach pH is 1–3, studies using pH-sensitive radiotelemetric capsules have shown a greater spread of values, ranging up to pH 7.
- The scope for variation in the small intestine is less, although in some pathological states the pH of the duodenum may be quite low due to hypersecretion of acid in the stomach.

pH at membrane surfaces

- pH at the membrane surface is lower than that of the bulk pH, hence the appropriate pH has to be inserted into equations, the solubility of drug will change in the vicinity of the membrane.
- The secretion of acidic and basic substances in many parts of the gut wall is also a complicating factor.

Convective water flow

- The movement of water molecules into and out of the GI tract, due to differences in osmotic pressure between blood and the contents of the lumen, and differences in hydrostatic pressure between the lumen and perivascular tissue, affects the rate of absorption of small molecules.
- Absorption of water-soluble drugs will be increased if water flows from the lumen to the serosal blood side across the mucosa, provided that drug and water are using the same route.
- Water movement is greatest within the jejunum.

Unstirred water layers

- A layer of relatively unstirred water lies adjacent to all biological membranes.
- During absorption drug molecules must diffuse across this layer, which is an additional barrier.

Effect of the drug

The drug must be in its molecular form before diffusional absorption processes take place.

- Basic drugs are therefore expected to be more soluble than acidic drugs in the stomach.
- Although the basic form of a drug as its hydrochloride salt should be soluble to some extent in this medium, this is not always so. The free bases of chlortetracycline and methacycline are more soluble than their hydrochloride salts in the stomach.

Other complicating factors

- The very high surface area of the small intestine also upsets the calculation of absorption based on considerations of theoretical absorption across identical areas of absorbing surface.
- Co-administration of drugs such as famotidine and nizatidine can raise stomach pH from below 2 to near neutrality.
- The drugs which may not be absorbed as expected include those which are:
  - unstable in the gastrointestinal tract (for example, erythromycin)

— metabolised on their passage through the gut wall
— hydrolysed in the stomach to active forms (e.g. prodrugs)
— bound to mucin to form complexes with bile salts; and those
— in the charged form, which interact with other ions to form absorbable species with a high lipid solubility – ion-pair formation.

Key points

- The nature of the formulation often has a large effect on drug absorption from some sites.
- The important features are always the interplay between:
  - drug
  - vehicle (formulation)
  - the route of administration.
- The same drug may be absorbed from different sites, often in quite different amounts. For example: cocaine with a P of 28 requires a sublingual/s.c. dosage ratio of 2 to obtain equal effects, atropine with a P of 7 requires eight times the s.c. dose sublingually, and for codeine (P ~2) over 15 times the s.c. dose is required when it is given sublingually.

Routes of administration

The oral route and oral absorption

Drug absorption from the gastrointestinal tract

Factors affecting absorption from oral dosage forms (in addition to the properties of the drug) include:

- the extent and rate of dissolution of the drug
- the rate of gastric emptying
- the site of absorption
- in some cases, and deliberately, the nature of the formulation (see Formulation effects).

Key points

- The functions of the gastrointestinal tract are the digestion and absorption of foods and nutrients and it is not easy to separate these from drug delivery.
- The natural processes in the gut can influence the absorption of drugs.
- The pH of the gut contents and the presence of enzymes, foods, bile salts, fat and the microbial flora can influence drug absorption.
- The complexity of the absorbing surfaces means that a simple physicochemical approach to drug absorption remains an approach to the problem and not the complete picture, as described before.

Structure of the gastrointestinal tract (*Figure 8.3*)

The stomach
- The stomach is not an organ designed for absorption.
- Its volume varies with the content of food (it may contain a few millilitres or a litre or more of fluid).
- Hydrochloric acid is liberated from the parietal cells (at a concentration of 0.58%).
- The gastric glands produce around 1000–1500 cm^3 of gastric juice per day.

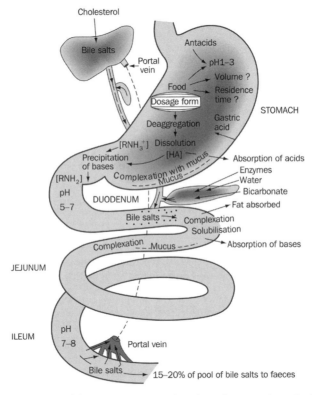

Figure 8.3: *Representation of the processes occurring along the gastrointestinal tract.*

The small intestine
- The small intestine is the main site of absorption.
- The small intestine is divided anatomically into three sections, duodenum, jejunum and ileum, with no clear transition between them.
- All three are involved in the digestion and absorption of foodstuffs; absorbed material is removed by the blood and the lymph.
- The absorbing area is enlarged by surface folds in the intestinal lining which are macroscopically apparent: the surface of these folds possesses villi (*Figure 8.4*).
- The human small intestine has a calculated active surface area of approximately 100 m^2.

- The surface area of the small intestine of the rat is estimated to be 700 cm², a difference of 1440-fold.
- Differences in the absorptive areas and volumes of gut contents in different animals are important when comparing experimental results on drug absorption in various species.

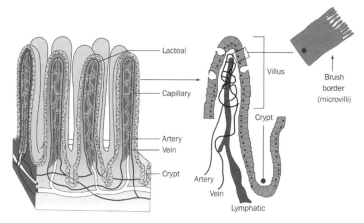

Figure 8.4: *Representation of the epithelium of the small intestine showing intestinal villi and microvilli.*

The large intestine
- The large intestine is primarily concerned with the absorption of water and the secretion of mucus to aid the intestinal contents to slide down the intestinal 'tube'.
- Villi are completely absent from the large intestine.

Carrier-mediated and specialised transport
There is the possibility of absorption of drugs by way of:
- tight junctions (the paracellular route)
- carrier-mediated uptake mechanisms
- endocytosis (*Figure 8.5*).

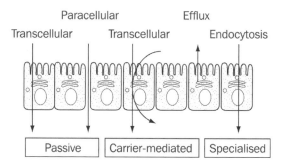

Figure 8.5: *Gastrointestinal membrane transport.*

Bile salts and fat absorption pathways
- Fat is absorbed by special mechanisms in the gut.
- Bile salts secreted into the jejunum are efficient emulsifiers and disperse fat globules, so increasing the surface area for absorption.
- Lipase activity is enhanced at the resulting large surface area.
- Medium-chain triglycerides are thought to be directly absorbed.
- Long-chain triglycerides are hydrolysed.
- Monoglycerides and fatty acids produced form mixed micelles with the bile salts and are either absorbed directly in the micelle or, more probably, brought to the microvillous surface by the micelle and transferred directly to the mucosal cells.
- There have been suggestions that lipid-soluble drugs may be absorbed by fat absorption pathways.
- The administration of drugs in an oily vehicle can significantly enhance absorption, e.g. of griseofulvin and ciclosporin.

Tips
Remember that:
- Bile salts are amphiphilic compounds and can form micelles or aggregates in solution in the gastrointestinal tract.
- Monoglycerides and fatty acids are also amphiphilic and so will be incorporated into the bile salt micelles, resulting in mixed micelle formation.

Gastric emptying, motility and volume of contents
- The volume of the gastric contents will determine the concentration of a drug which finds itself in the stomach.
- The time the drug or dosage form resides in the stomach will determine many aspects of absorption from solid dose forms:
  - If the drug is absorbed in the intestine, stomach emptying rates will determine the delay before absorption begins.
  - If a drug is labile in acid conditions, longer residence times in the stomach will lead to greater breakdown.
  - If the dosage form is non-disintegrating then retention in the stomach can influence the pattern of absorption.
- The stomach empties liquids faster than solids.
- Gastric emptying is a simple exponential or square-root function of the volume of a test meal – a pattern that holds for meals of variable viscosity.
- Acids have been found to slow gastric emptying, but acids with relatively high molecular weights (for example, citric acid) are less effective than those, like hydrochloric acid, with very low molecular weights.
- When considering the effect of an antacid, therefore, the effect of volume change and pH change and the effect on gastric emptying must be considered.

- Food affects not only transit but also pH in the gastrointestinal tract.
- Natural triglycerides inhibit gastric motility.

Key point

The formulation of a drug may influence drug absorption through an indirect physiological effect, e.g. whether it is solid or liquid, acidic or alkaline, aqueous or oily, may influence gastric emptying.

Buccal and sublingual absorption

- The absorption of drugs through the oral mucosa provides a route for systemic administration.
- This route avoids exposure of drug to the gastrointestinal tract.
- Drugs bypass the liver (and so avoid metabolism there) and have direct access to the systemic circulation.
- Drugs such as glyceryl trinitrate have traditionally been administered in this way. This drug exerts its pharmacological action 1–2 minutes after sublingual administration.
- Mucosal adhesive systems are used for administration of buprenorphine through the gingiva (gums).

Mechanisms of absorption

- The oral mucosa functions primarily as a barrier and it is not highly permeable. It comprises:
  - a mucous layer over the epithelium
  - a keratinised layer in certain regions of the oral cavity
  - an epithelial layer
  - a basement membrane
  - connective tissue
  - a submucosal region.
- Most drugs are absorbed by simple diffusion.
- There is a linear relationship between percentage absorption through the buccal epithelium and log P of a homologous drug series.
- Buccal absorption of basic drugs increases and that of acidic drugs decreases, with increasing pH of their solutions.
- Nicotine in a gum vehicle is absorbed through the buccal mucosa.
- The buccal route has the advantages of the sublingual route
  - the buccal mucosa is similar to sublingual mucosal tissue
  - but a sustained-release tablet can be held in the cheek pouch for several hours if necessary.
- A log P of 1.6–3.3 is optimal for drugs to be used by the sublingual route.

Intravenous injection and infusion

- For rapid systemic effects and for fluid replacement, the intravenous (i.v.) route is commonplace.
- Normally, solutions are administered, although lipid emulsions of carefully controlled size are employed in intravenous feeding.
- Suspensions are less commonly used because of the risk of embolism but suspensions in the nanometre size range (with all particles less than 1 µm in diameter) may be employed.
- Solutions can precipitate when they reach the blood so that rate of administration is often important.
- Vehicles of mixed solvents are prone to precipitation as the solvency changes on dilution in blood.
- Drugs administered in admixture in i.v. therapy via giving sets can be incompatible (see **Chapter 10**).
- Intra-arterial injections can be used when venous access is difficult, as with paediatric patients.
- Implantable infusion pumps can be implanted under the skin to deliver drugs at predetermined rates into the venous or arterial circulation. These can be used for the long-term administration of agents such as heparin.

Intramuscular and subcutaneous injection

- Not all drugs are efficiently or uniformly released from i.m. or s.c. sites.
- The s.c. region has a good supply of capillaries, although there are few lymph vessels in muscle proper.
- Drugs can diffuse through the tissue and pass across the capillary walls and thus enter the circulation via the capillary supply.
- Molecular size of soluble drugs is important: mannitol rapidly diffuses from the site of injection, insulin (molecular weight ~6000 Da) less rapidly and dextran (molecular weight 70 000 Da) disperses more slowly. Insulin is generally given by s.c. injection.
- Hydrophobic drugs may bind to muscle protein, leading to a reduction in free drug and perhaps to prolongation of action:
  - Dicloxacillin is 95% bound to protein; ampicillin is bound to the extent of 20%, hence as a consequence dicloxacillin is absorbed more slowly from muscle than is ampicillin.

Site of injection

- The regions into which the injection is administered are composed of both aqueous and lipid components (*Figure 8.6*).
- Muscle tissue is more acidic than normal physiological fluids.
- The pH of the tissue will determine whether or not drugs will dissolve in the tissue fluids or precipitate from formulations.
- The deliberate reduction of the solubility of a drug achieves prolonged action by both the i.m. and s.c. routes.

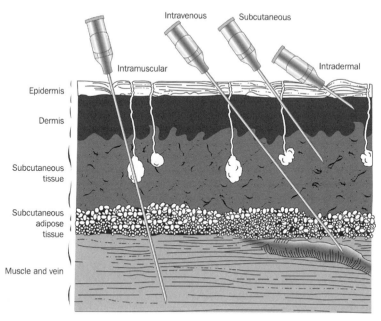

Figure 8.6: *Routes of parenteral medication. Modified from Quackenbusch DS (1969) In: Martin EW (ed.)* Techniques of Medication. *Philadelphia, PA: Lippincott.*

Vehicles
- Many i.m. injections are formulated in water-miscible solvents such as polyethylene glycol 300 or 400, or propylene glycol or ethanol mixtures.
- Dilution by the tissue fluids may cause the drug to precipitate.
- Three main types of formulation are used:
  1. Aqueous solutions, which are rapidly removed.
  2. Aqueous suspensions of less soluble drugs.
  3. Oily solutions from which drugs (e.g. fluphenazine decanoate) can diffuse slowly for prolonged action.

Blood flow
- Different rates of blood flow in different muscles mean that the site of i.m. injection can be crucial.
- Resting blood flow in the deltoid region is significantly greater than in the *gluteus maximus* muscle; flow in the *vastus lateralis* is intermediate.

Formulation effects
- Crystalline suspensions of fluspirilene, certain steroids and procaine benzylpenicillin can be prepared in different size ranges to produce different pharmacokinetic profiles following i.m. or s.c. injection.

- Variability in response to a drug, or differences in response to a formulation from different manufacturers, can be the result of the nature of the formulation.
- The depth of the injection is significant. If, in addition, the blood supply to the region is limited, there will be an additional restriction to rapid removal.

Insulin
- Insulin presents a classic example of how pharmacokinetics can be controlled by manipulation of the properties of the drug molecule and its formulation.
- Modification of the crystallinity of insulin allows control over solubility and duration of activity.
- Long-acting insulins are mainly protamine insulin and zinc insulins.
- Protamine insulins are salt-like compounds formed between the acid (insulin) polypeptide and the protamine polypeptide (primarily of arginine). They are used in the form of neutral suspensions of protamine insulin crystals (isophane insulin).
- Prolonged-acting insulins have been designed to have intermediate durations of action.
- Variable insulin activity may result from the mixing of protamine-zinc-insulin and soluble insulin prior to administration.
- As a general rule, insulin formulations of different pH should not be mixed.

Transdermal delivery
The barrier layer of the skin is the *stratum corneum*, which behaves like a passive diffusion barrier (*Figure 8.7*).

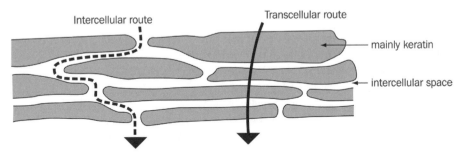

Figure 8.7: *Simplified model of the stratum corneum, illustrating possible pathways of drug permeation. Reproduced from Moghimi HR et al. A lamellar matrix model for stratum corneum intercellular lipids. II. Effect of geometry of the stratum corneum on permeation of model drugs 5-fluorouracil and oestradiol. Int J Pharm 1996;131:117.*

The vehicle in which the drug is applied influences the rate and extent of absorption, but formulations can change rapidly once they have been spread on the skin, with absorption of some excipients and evaporative loss of water.

Routes of skin penetration
- Solute molecules may penetrate the skin not only through the *stratum corneum* but also by way of the hair follicles or through the sweat ducts.

- Only in the case of molecules that move very slowly through the *stratum corneum* may absorption by these other routes predominate.
- The major pathway of transport for water-soluble molecules is transcellular, involving passage through cells and cell walls.
- The pathway for lipid-soluble molecules is presumably the endogenous lipid pathway within the *stratum corneum*; the bulk of this is intercellular.
- Passage through damaged skin is increased over normal skin. For example, skin with a disrupted epidermal layer will allow up to 80% of hydrocortisone to pass into the dermis compared to 1% through intact skin.
- The physicochemical factors that control drug penetration include:
  - the hydration of the *stratum corneum* (occluded skin may absorb up to 5–6 times its dry weight of water – see Tip below)
  - temperature
  - pH
  - drug concentration
  - the molecular characteristics of the penetrant
  - the vehicle.

Tip

Occlusive dressings are those that have low permeability to water vapour. When these are left on the skin they prevent water loss from the skin surface and therefore increase the hydration of the *stratum corneum* .

Influence of drug

- The diffusion coefficient of the drug in the skin will be determined by factors such as molecular size, shape and charge.
- The effective partition coefficient will be determined not only by the properties of the drug but also by the vehicle as this represents the donor phase, the skin being the receptor phase.
- The peak activity in a drug series coincides with an optimal partition coefficient – one that favours neither lipid nor aqueous phase. Examples include:
  - Triamcinolone is 5 times more active systemically than hydrocortisone, but has only one-tenth of its topical activity.
  - Triamcinolone acetonide has a topical activity 1000 times that of the parent steroid because of its favourable lipid solubility.
  - Betamethasone is 30 times as active as hydrocortisone systemically but has only four times the topical potency.
  - Of 23 esters of betamethasone, the 17-valerate ester possesses the highest topical activity. The vasoconstrictor potency of betamethasone 17-valerate is 360 (fluocinolone acetonide = 100), its 17-acetate 114, the 17-propionate 190, and the 17-octanoate 10.
- Clearly, not all drugs are suitable for transdermal delivery.

Formulations

- Many are washable oil-in-water systems.
- Simple aqueous lotions are also used as they have a cooling effect on the skin.
- Ointments are used for the application of insoluble or oil-soluble medicaments and leave a greasy film on the skin, inhibiting loss of moisture and encouraging the hydration of the keratin layer.
- Aqueous creams combine the characteristics of lotions and ointments.
- Ointments are generally composed of single-phase hydrophobic bases, such as pharmaceutical grades of soft paraffin or microcrystalline paraffin wax.
- 'Absorption' bases have a capacity to facilitate absorption by the skin but the term also alludes to their ability to take up considerable amounts of water to form water-in-oil emulsions.

Drug release from vehicles

- In emulsions the relative affinity of drug for the external and internal phases is an important factor.
- A drug dissolved in an internal aqueous phase of a water-in-oil emulsion must be able to diffuse through the oily layer.
- Three cases can be considered: (1) solutions; (2) suspensions; and (3) emulsion systems.

Solutions

- Release rate is proportional to the square root of the diffusion coefficient and hence release is slower from a viscous vehicle.

Suspensions

- Release rate is proportional to the square root of the total solubility of the drug in the vehicle and hence for a drug in suspension to have any action it must have a degree of solubility in the base used.

Emulsion systems

- Release rate is proportional to the diffusion coefficient of the drug in the continuous phase and inversely proportional to the partition coefficient between the phases.

Patches and devices

The ease with which some drugs can pass through the skin barrier into the circulating blood means that the transdermal route of medication is a possible alternative to the oral route. Theoretically there are several advantages:

- For drugs that are normally taken orally, administration through the skin can eliminate the vagaries that influence gastrointestinal absorption, such as pH changes and variations in food intake and intestinal transit time.
- A drug may be introduced into the systemic circulation without initially entering the portal circulation and passing through the liver.
- Constant and continuous administration of drugs may be achieved by a simple application to the skin surface.

- Continuous administration of drugs percutaneously at a controlled rate should permit elimination of pulse entry into the systemic circulation, an effect that is often associated with side-effects.
- Absorption of medication can be rapidly terminated whenever therapy must be interrupted.

Patches

There are currently four basic forms of patch systems (*Figure 8.8*):
1. matrix
2. reservoir
3. multilaminate
4. drug-in-adhesive.

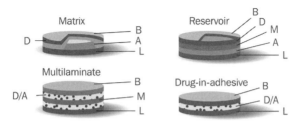

Matrix   Reservoir

Multilaminate   Drug-in-adhesive

B - Backing   D - Drug   M - Membrane   A - Adhesive   L - Liner

Figure 8.8: *The four main types of transdermal patch. Courtesy of 3M.*

Microneedles

- Microneedles comprise arrays of needles less than 1000 μm which create small pores in the skin without the pain produced by larger needles. *Figure 8.9* shows the four main types of microneedle and the manner of drug dispersion.
- Solid and coated systems are made from metals while dissolving systems are fabricated from biocompatible and water-soluble materials.

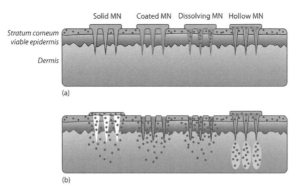

Figure 8.9: *Different types of microneedles for transdermal delivery: solid, coated, dissolving and hollow systems. From Ita K. Dissolving microneedles for transdermal drug delivery: Advances and challenges.* Biomed Pharmacother 2017;93:1116–1127. © 2017 Elsevier Masson SAS. All rights reserved.

Iontophoresis

- Iontophoresis is the process by which the migration of ionic drugs into tissues is enhanced by the use of an electrical current.
- Enhancement of permeability results from several possible sources:
  - ion–electric field interaction (electrorepulsion)
  - convective flow (electro-osmosis)
  - current-induced increases in skin permeability.

Ultrasound and transdermal penetration

- Therapeutic ultrasound first expands and then collapses air bubbles in the *stratum corneum* (the process of cavitation).
- Cavitation tends to liquefy the solid fats and allows molecules such as insulin to pass through the skin.
- The permeability of the skin increases as the frequency of ultrasound decreases.

Jet injectors

- The systems are based on the high-velocity ejection of particles through an orifice.
- Drug delivery is then due to either or both of skin 'failure' and convective flow through the skin.

The eye

- A wide range of drug types are placed in the eye, including antimicrobials, antihistamines, decongestants, mydriatics, miotics and cycloplegic agents.
- Drugs are usually applied to the eye in the form of drops or ointments for local action.
- The absorbing surface is the cornea.
- Drug absorbed by the conjuctiva enters the systemic circulation.
- The eye has two barrier systems:
  1. a blood–aqueous barrier.
  2. a blood–vitreous barrier.

Tears

- Tears contain electrolytes – sodium, potassium and some calcium ions, chloride and other counterions, and glucose.
- Macromolecular components include some albumin, globulins and lysozyme.
- Lipids form a monolayer over the tear fluid surface.
- Drugs or excipients may interact with components of the tear fluid, so that tear coverage of the eye is disrupted.
- Dry-eye syndrome (xerophthalmia) may arise because of premature break-up of the tear layer, resulting in dry spots on the corneal surface.

Absorption of drugs applied to the eye

The cornea is the main barrier to absorption and comprises an epithelium, a stroma and an endothelium:

- The endothelium and the epithelium have a high lipid content and are penetrated by drugs in their un-ionised lipid-soluble forms.
- The stroma lying between the two other structures has a high water content. Thus drugs which have to negotiate the corneal barrier successfully must be both lipid-soluble and water-soluble to some extent.

Aqueous humour
- Both water-soluble and lipid-soluble drugs can enter the aqueous humour.
- The pH-partition hypothesis thus accounts only imperfectly for different rates of entry into the aqueous humour.

Key points

- As tears have some buffering capacity, the pH-partition hypothesis for drug absorption has to be applied with some circumspection.
- However, in agreement with the pH-partition hypothesis, raising the pH from 5 to 8 results in a two- to threefold increase in the amount of pilocarpine reaching the anterior chamber.

Influence of formulation
- Some ingredients of eye medications may increase the permeability of the cornea.
- Surface-active agents are known to interact with membranes to increase permeability:
  - Benzalkonium chloride (bacteriostat and bactericide) has surfactant properties and may well have some effect on corneal permeability.
  - Chlorhexidine acetate and cetrimide, both of which are surface-active, are also used.

Eye drops
- Are usually formulated to be isotonic with tear fluid.
- The rate of drainage of drops decreases as their viscosity increases and this can contribute to an increased concentration of the drug in the precorneal film and aqueous humour:
  - Hydrophilic polymeric vehicles, such as poly(vinyl alcohol) and hydroxypropylmethylcellulose are used to adjust viscosity.
- Most of the dose applied to the eye in the form of drops reaches the systemic circulation and typically less than 5% acts on ocular tissues.

Prodrugs
A prodrug of adrenaline (epinephrine), the dipivoyl derivative of adrenaline, is absorbed to a greater extent and is then hydrolysed to the active parent molecule in the aqueous humour.

Reservoir systems
- Soft lenses can be used as drug reservoirs leaching drug over 24 h.
- The Ocusert device releases controlled amounts of pilocarpine over a period of 7 days.

The ear
- Medications are administered to the ear only for local treatment.
- Drops and other vehicles administered to the ear will occupy the external auditory meatus, which is separated from the middle ear by the tympanic membrane.
- The acidic environment of the ear skin surface (around pH 6), sometimes referred to as the acid mantle of the ear, is thought to be a defence against invading microorganisms.

Absorption from the vagina
- The vagina cannot be considered to be a route for the systemic administration of drugs, although oestrogens for systemic delivery have been applied intravaginally.
- Certain drugs, however, are absorbed when applied to the vaginal epithelium. Steroids, prostaglandins, iodine and some antibiotics and antifungals such as econazole and miconazole are appreciably absorbed.
- The pH in the vagina decreases after puberty, varying between pH 4 and 5 depending on the point in the menstrual cycle and also on the location within the vagina, the pH being higher near the cervix.
- There is little fluid in the vagina.
- The absorbing surface is under constant change, therefore absorption is variable.
- Mucus may retard absorption.
- Lymph vessels drain the vagina, and vaginal capillaries are found in close proximity to the basal epithelial layer.

Formulations
- Conventional vaginal delivery systems include vaginal tablets, foams, gels, suspensions and pessaries.
- Vaginal rings have been developed to deliver contraceptive steroids. These commonly comprise an inert silicone elastomer ring covered with an elastomer layer containing the drug.
- Hydrogel-based vaginal pessaries to deliver prostaglandin E_2 and bleomycin have been developed.
- Tablets often contain excipients which increase viscosity and are bioadhesive, e.g. hydroxypropyl cellulose, sodium carboxymethylcellulose and poly(acrylic acid) (such as Carbopol 934).
- Micropatches in the size range 10–100 μm in diameter prepared from starch, gelatin, albumin, collagen or dextrose will gel on contact with vaginal mucosal surfaces and adhere.

Inhalation therapy

- The respiratory system provides a route of medication administration.
- The contact area of its surfaces extends to more than $30\,m^2$.
- There are 2000 km of capillaries in the lungs.
- The route has been widely used in attempts to avoid systemic side-effects, such as adrenal suppression, but evidence suggests that inhaled steroids are absorbed systemically to a significant extent.
- The respiratory tract epithelium has permeability characteristics similar to those of the classical biological membrane, so lipid-soluble compounds are absorbed more rapidly than lipid-insoluble molecules.
- Compared to the gastrointestinal mucosa, the pulmonary epithelium possesses a relatively high permeability to water-soluble molecules, which is an advantage with drugs such as sodium cromoglicate.
- The efficiency of inhalation therapy is often low because of the difficulty in targeting particles to the sites of maximal absorption.
- Only about 8% of the inhaled dose of sodium cromoglicate administered from a dry-powder device reaches the alveoli.

Tips

Difference between physical diameter and aerodynamic diameter:
- The aerodynamic diameter of a particle, d_a, is related to the particle diameter (d) and density (ρ) by the equation:

$$d_a = \rho^{0.5}d$$

- To overcome problems of powder flow and agglomeration, porous particles (i.e. particles with a low density) have been developed. A particle of 10 µm diameter with a density of $0.1\,g\,cm^{-3}$ has an aerodynamic diameter ~3 µm (i.e. $(0.1)^{0.5} \times 10$).

Physical factors affecting deposition of aerosols

- Deposition of particles in the various regions of the respiratory tract is dependent on particle size (*Figure 8.10*).
- The major processes that influence deposition of drug particles in the respiratory tract are:
  - interception
  - impaction
  - gravitational settling
  - electrostatic attractions
  - Brownian diffusion.
- Very fine particles (<0.5 µm) are deposited on the walls of the smallest airways by diffusion, the result of bombardment of the particles by gas molecules.

- Particle size, or particle size distribution, is obviously important in several of these processes and will be affected by the nature of the aerosol-producing device and by the formulation.
- Particles of hygroscopic materials are removed from the air stream more effectively than are non-hygroscopic particles, because of their growth through uptake of water from the moist air in the respiratory tract.

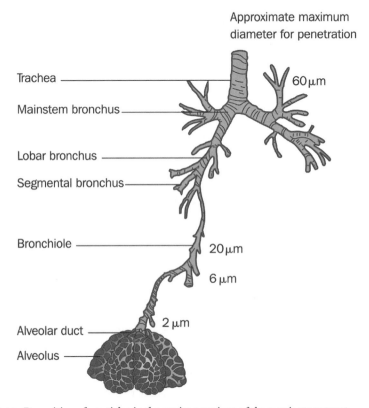

Approximate maximum
diameter for penetration

Trachea — 60 μm

Mainstem bronchus —

Lobar bronchus —

Segmental bronchus —

Bronchiole — 20 μm

6 μm

2 μm

Alveolar duct —

Alveolus —

Figure 8.10: *Deposition of particles in the various regions of the respiratory tract.*

Delivery devices

Pressurised aerosols

- Single-phase and two-phase systems are utilised.
- In two-phase systems the propellant forms a separate liquid phase, whereas in the single-phase form the liquid propellant is the liquid phase containing the drug in solution or in suspension in the liquefied propellant gas.
- Spacers are chambers which are attached to aerosols which control the impact of the particles emitted from the aerosol device (see *Figure 8.11*). Large particles are deposited in the chamber before inhalation and thus the inhaled aerosol contains higher levels

of the smaller particles. Such spacers are valuable for use by children. Without the spacer a large percentage of drug deposits in the mouth and throat.

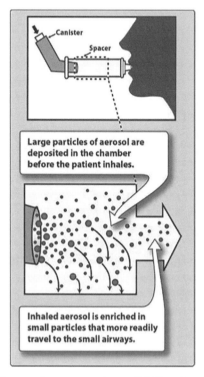

Figure 8.11: *The effect of the use of a spacer on the availability of small particles released from the aerosol. The inhaled fraction has a higher ratio of small particles hence absorption and effect is improved by this change in dynamics.*

Nebulisers

- Modern nebulisers for domestic and hospital use generate aerosols continuously for chronic therapy of respiratory disorders.
- The particle size distribution varies with the design and sometimes mode of use.

The nasal route

Three main classes of medicinal agents are applied by the nasal route:

1. Drugs for the alleviation of nasal symptoms.
2. Drugs that are inactivated in the gastrointestinal tract following oral administration.
3. Where the route is an alternative to injection, such as for peptides and proteins.

- Delivery of peptides and proteins such as insulin, luteinising hormone-releasing hormone analogues such as nafarelin, vasopressin, thyrotropin-releasing hormone analogues and adrenocorticotrophic hormone is feasible.

- Factors such as droplet or particle size which affect deposition in the respiratory tract are involved if administration is by aerosol (*Figure 8.12*).
- The physiological condition of the nose, its vascularity and mucus flow rate are therefore of importance.
- Formulation factors which can affect activity include:
  - the volume
  - concentration
  - viscosity
  - pH
  - tonicity of the applied medicament.
- As with all routes, absorption decreases with the increasing molecular weight of the active.

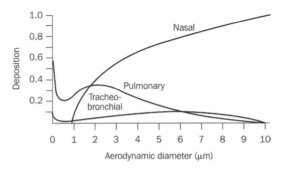

Figure 8.12: *Regional deposition of inhaled particles as a function of aerodynamic diameter. Reproduced from Muir DCF (ed.).* Clinical Aspects of Inhaled Particles *Heinemann Medical, London, 1972.*

Rectal absorption of drugs

- Drugs administered by the rectal route in suppositories are placed in intimate contact with the rectal mucosa, which behaves as a normal lipoidal barrier.
- The pH in the rectal cavity lies between 7.2 and 7.4, but the rectal fluids have little buffering capacity.
- As with topical medication, the formulation of the suppository can have marked effects on the activity of the drug.
- Factors such as retention of the suppository for a sufficient duration of time in the rectal cavity also influence the outcome of therapy; the size and shape of the suppository and its melting point may also determine bioavailability.
- Modern suppository vehicles include polyoxyethylene glycols of molecular weight 1000–6000 Da and semisynthetic vegetable fats.
- The appropriate bases must be carefully selected for each substance. The important features of excipient materials are melting point, speed of crystallisation and emulsifying capacity.
- If the medicament dissolves in the base it is likely that the melting point of the base will be lowered, so that a base with a melting point higher than 36–37°C has to be chosen.

- If the drug substance has a high density it is preferable that the base crystallises rapidly during production of the suppositories to prevent settling of the drug.

The rectal cavity
- The rectum is the terminal 15–19 cm of the large intestine.
- The mucous membrane of the rectal ampulla, with which suppositories come into contact, is made up of a layer of cylindrical epithelial cells without villi.
- The main artery to the rectum is the superior rectal (haemorrhoidal) artery.
- Veins of the inferior part of the submucous plexus become the rectal veins, which drain to the internal pudendal veins.
- Drug absorption takes place through this venous network. Superior haemorrhoidal veins connect with the portal vein and thus transport drugs absorbed in the upper part of the rectal cavity to the liver; the inferior veins enter into the inferior *vena cava* and thus bypass the liver.

Fate of drug
- The particular venous route the drug takes is affected by the extent to which the suppository migrates in its original or molten form further up the gastrointestinal tract, and this may be variable.
- The rectal route does not necessarily, or even reproducibly, avoid the liver.

Absorption from formulations
- The rate-limiting step in drug absorption from suppositories made from a fatty base is the partitioning of the dissolved drug from the molten base, not the rate of solution of the drug in the body fluids.
- Absorption from the rectum depends on the concentration of drug in absorbable form in the rectal cavity and, if the base is not emulsified, on the contact area between molten excipient and rectal mucosa.
- Water-soluble active substances will be insoluble in fatty bases, while the less water-soluble material will tend to be soluble in the base, and will thus diffuse from the base more slowly.
- Water-soluble drugs are better absorbed from a fatty excipient than from a water-soluble one.
- Addition of surfactants may increase the ability of the molten mass to spread and tends to increase the extent of absorption.
- Hygroscopicity of some hydrophilic bases such as the polyoxyethylene glycols results in the abstraction of water from the rectal mucosa, causing stinging and discomfort, and probably affects the passage of drugs across the rectal mucosa.

Incompatibility between base and drug
Various incompatibilities exist:
- Phenolic substances complex with glycols, probably by hydrogen bonding between the phenolic hydroxy group and the glycol ether oxygens.

- Polyoxyethylene glycol bases are incompatible with tannic acid, ichthammol, aspirin, benzocaine, vioform and sulfonamides.
- Glycerogelatin bases are prepared by heating together glycerin, gelatin and water:
  — Use of untreated gelatin renders the base incompatible with acidic and basic drugs.
  — Two types of treated gelatin are employed with different characteristics to avoid incompatibilities:
    » Type A is acidic and cationic, with an isoelectric point between pH 7 and 9.
    » Type B is less acidic and anionic, with an isoelectric point between pH 4.7 and 5.

Intrathecal drug administration

- Administration of drugs in solution by intrathecal catheter provides an opportunity to deliver drugs to the brain and spinal cord (*Figure 8.13*).
- Relatively hydrophilic drugs such as methotrexate (log P = −0.5), which do not cross the blood–brain barrier in significant amounts, have been infused intrathecally to treat meningeal leukaemia, and baclofen (log P = −1.0) to treat spinal cord spasticity.
- High lumbar cerebrospinal fluid concentrations are achieved.
- The spinal cerebrospinal fluid has a small volume (70 cm³) and a relatively slow clearance (20–40 cm³ h⁻¹) of hydrophilic drugs.
- The cerebrospinal fluid pharmacokinetics of three drugs, morphine (log P = 0.15), clonidine (log P = 0.85) and baclofen (log P = −1.0), were found to be similar, leading to the suggestion that bulk flow mechanisms may be the dominant factor in determining distribution.

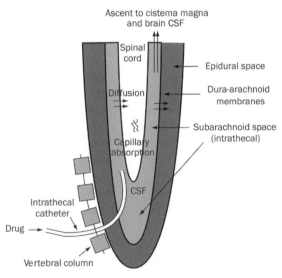

Figure 8.13: *Anatomical structures and absorption routes for a drug administered via an intrathecal catheter. CSF, cerebrospinal fluid. Reproduced from Kroin JS. Intrathecal Drug Administration. Clin Pharmacokinet 1992;22:319–26.*

Brain implants

- To overcome the blood brain barrier to drug access, direct implantation of devices loaded with anticancer agents have been used. The only licensed product is Gliadel™ containing the anticancer drug carmustine for the treatment of brain tumours. Implanted Gliadel wafers are shown in *Figure 8.14*.
- Drug release is dictated by the nature of the polymer and its erosion but the extent of diffusion in brain tissue is the main limitation on the distribution of the active. After 1 week one drug, human nerve growth factor, diffused only 2 mm from its implant.
- Development of implantable systems with activated release mechanisms is underway.

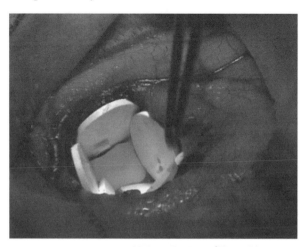

Nature Reviews | Drug Discovery

Figure 8.14: *Implants of the polyanhydride-based Gliadel wafers containing carmustine (BCNU); drug release is controlled both by diffusion of the drug and erosion of the polymer matrix. Reproduced with permission from Lesniak MS, Brem H. Targeted therapy for brain tumours.* Nature Rev Drug Discov 2004;3:499–508.

Coronary artery stents

- Stents comprise a mesh which can be inserted into an artery on a balloon carrier to maintain vessel potency. See *Figure 8.15*.
- Cardiovascular stents are employed to enlarge diseased arteries. Coated stents contain a drug within the polymer coating on the wire mesh, forming a reservoir for controlled drug release.
- Drug diffusion coefficients in arterial tissues vary considerably, for example rapamycin has a diffusion coefficient of circa 2×10^{-4} mm^2/s; that of Paclitaxel is 2.6×10^{-6} mm^2/s.

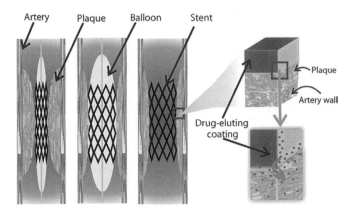

Figure 8.15: *The placement of a drug-eluting stent in a diseased coronary artery. Drug is released from the polymer coating to diffuse into the artery wall. Simulating this in vitro is difficult. From Vo T et al. Modelling chemistry and biology after implantation of a drug-eluting stent. Part I: Drug transport.* American Institute of Mathematical Sciences 2017;14(2):491–509.

Key points

- Each route has its own special characteristics. The nature of the absorption barrier in each is discussed on the basis of differences in liquid volume, pH, blood flow and drainage.
- The optimal lipophilicity of absorbing membranes depends on the nature of the membrane.
- Some barriers (as in the eye and skin) are complex, having the characteristics of typical lipid barriers, interspersed with more aqueous hurdles.
- In some cases (e.g. i.m. injections) the nature of the surrounding tissue, whether fatty or aqueous, is the key to the process of transferring drug into the blood.
- The overriding importance of lipophilicity is clear when drug is absorbed in molecular form, although water-soluble drugs can gain access, e.g. in the lung due to the very large surface area of contact between the absorbing membrane and the blood.
- When drug is delivered as a suspension (as in an aerosol) the paramount importance of particle size in first getting the drug to the site of action is clear; once it has reached that site (the alveoli), its rate of solution and its lipophilicity are again important.

Memory maps

Passive drug absorption: influence of drug and other factors

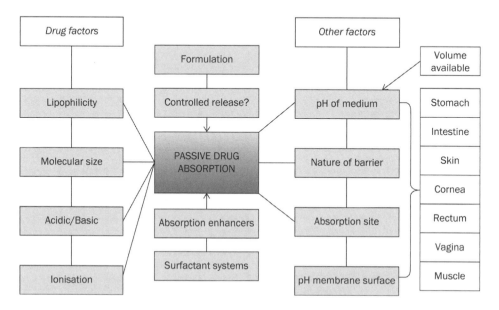

Oral dosage forms: factors affecting absorption

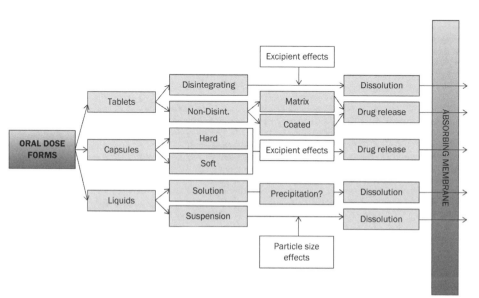

Controlled release formulations: routes and systems

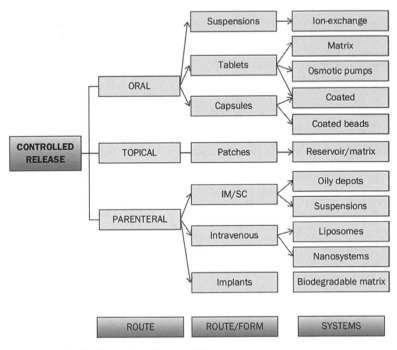

See also **Chapter 7** for the discussion of some of these systems.

Drug particle size: consequences in different delivery situations

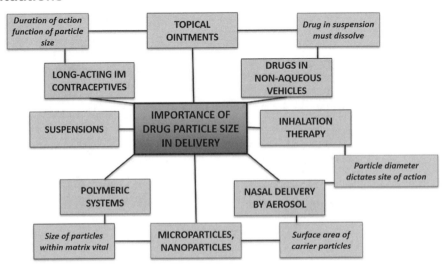

Questions

1. In relation to the absorption of drugs across membranes, indicate which of the following statements are correct.
    - **A:** The percentage absorption increases linearly with increase in log P
    - **B:** The percentage absorption decreases linearly with increase in log P
    - **C:** There is an optimum log P for absorption
    - **D:** Drugs with a high log P are strongly protein-bound

2. Good oral absorption is favoured when:
    - **A:** The molecular weight of the drug is high
    - **B:** Log P is less than 5
    - **C:** There are more than 5 hydrogen bond donors
    - **D:** There are fewer than 10 hydrogen bond acceptors

3. Indicate which of the following statements is correct. According to the pH-partition hypothesis:
    - **A:** Only ionised drugs pass through membranes
    - **B:** Weakly acidic drugs are absorbed well when the pH is below their pK_a
    - **C:** Weakly basic drugs are absorbed well when the pH is below their pK_a
    - **D:** Drug absorption is not usually affected by ionisation of the drug molecule

4. In relation to absorption from the gastrointestinal tract, which of the following statements are correct?
    - **A:** The stomach is the main site of absorption in the gastrointestinal tract
    - **B:** The absorbing area of the large intestine is enlarged by the presence of villi
    - **C:** The stomach volume varies with the content of food
    - **D:** Bile salts are secreted into the jejunum
    - **E:** The stomach empties solids faster than liquids
    - **F:** Natural triglycerides inhibit gastric motility
    - **G:** The large intestine is mainly concerned with the absorption of water

5. In relation to buccal and sublingual absorption, which of the following statements are correct?
    - **A:** Drugs absorbed by these routes bypass the liver
    - **B:** Absorption through the buccal epithelium is not affected by the partition coefficient of the drug
    - **C:** Buccal absorption of basic drugs increases with increasing pH of their solutions
    - **D:** Buccal absorption of acidic drugs increases with increasing pH of their solutions
    - **E:** There is an optimum log P for sublingual absorption

6. In relation to absorption of drugs from i.m. and s.c. injections, which of the following statements are correct?
    - **A:** Dispersion of soluble drugs from the injection site is more rapid the lower the molecular weight of the drug
    - **B:** Binding to muscle protein increases the rate of absorption
    - **C:** Hydrophilic drugs bind strongly to muscle protein
    - **D:** Muscle tissue is more acidic than normal physiological fluids
    - **E:** Oily vehicles may be used to provide diffusion over a prolonged period

7. **In relation to transdermal delivery of drugs, which of the following statements are correct?**
    A: The main barrier of the skin is the *stratum corneum*
    B: Solute molecules may penetrate the skin through sweat ducts
    C: The major absorption pathway for lipid-soluble molecules is the transcellular route
    D: Passage of drugs through damaged skin is more rapid than through normal skin
    E: There is an optimal partition coefficient for absorption

8. **In relation to the absorption of drugs from the eye, which of the following statements are correct?**
    A: The absorbing surface is the cornea
    B: Eye drops are usually formulated to be isotonic with tears
    C: Ionised drugs are more readily absorbed than un-ionised drugs
    D: The rate of drainage of eye drops decreases as their viscosity decreases
    E: Most of a drug applied in the form of eye drops acts on ocular tissues

9. **In relation to inhalation therapy, which of the following statements are correct?**
    A: The pulmonary epithelium has a relatively high permeability to water-soluble molecules compared to the gastrointestinal mucosa
    B: Particles of hygroscopic materials are less readily removed from the air stream than non-hygroscopic particles
    C: Lipid-soluble molecules are less readily absorbed than lipid-insoluble molecules
    D: Only very fine particles are able to reach the alveoli

10. **In relation to rectal absorption of drugs, which of the following statements are correct?**
    A: The melting point of the suppository base is usually increased when a drug is dissolved in it
    B: Administration of drugs rectally ensures that the liver is bypassed
    C: The rate-limiting step in drug absorption from suppositories is the rate of solution of the drug in the body fluids
    D: Water-soluble drugs are more readily absorbed from a fatty excipient than from a water-soluble one
    E: Addition of surfactants to the suppository may increase the extent of absorption

CHAPTER 9

Paediatric and geriatric medicines

LEARNING OBJECTIVES

Upon completion of this chapter you should be able to:
- give an overview of pharmaceutical aspects of formulations for use in paediatric and geriatric practice
- understand the need for special formulations for individual cases
- understand the general needs of the population at the different ends of the age spectrum, i.e. 'age-specific' medicine
- outline systems devised to facilitate safe dosing in contrasting age groups.

Introduction

- Personalised medicine is often construed as driven by a patient's disease-related genetic information.
- However, to achieve more precision requires personalised medications, not only the proper drug but perhaps special dose forms, as summarised in *Figure 9.1* on the next page.
- The emphasis on early and late life in this chapter simply highlights the need for all patients to be assessed more closely and their medication (drug and dose form) to be patient-specific, especially age-specific.
- Advances in pharmaceutical sciences (e.g. 3D printing) are key to aid this goal.

Key points

- Age is one factor in drug dosing and administration.
- Adaptable dosage forms designed for individuals or groups are preferable to those prepared from standard forms such as tablets.
- Using sustained release formulations other than in their licensed form can lead to unpredictable reactions.

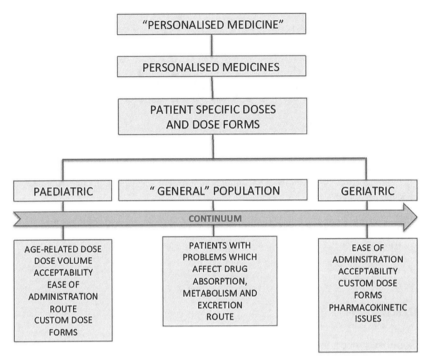

Figure 9.1: *Factors in the choice of medicines for children, the general population and the elderly.*

Key points

- Childhood covers more than a decade of life and involves large changes in metabolism, weight, height, gastric pH, gastric emptying, sensitivity to drugs and excipients, and many other parameters.
- Old age can span decades.
- Formulations for children prepared from existing adult products are not ideal.
- Medication for the elderly, often demands specialised formulations.

The drivers of formulation development are summarised in *Figure 9.2.*

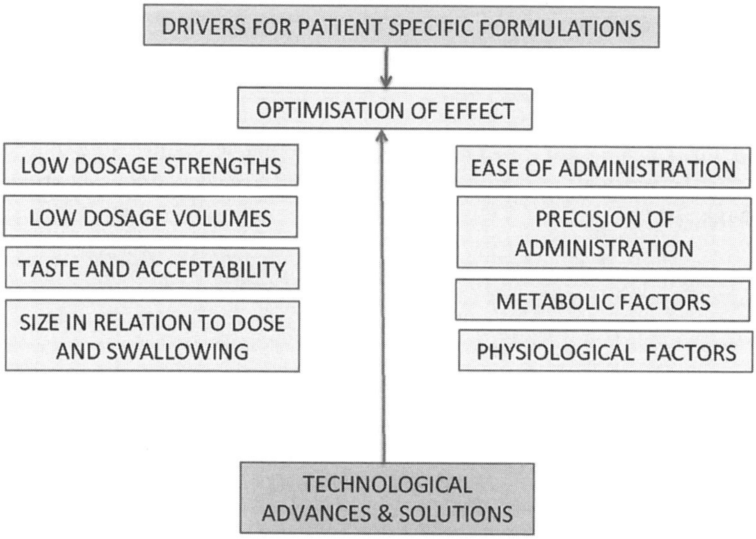

Figure 9.2: *The matrix of drivers for special formulations and means of administration.*

Paediatric medication

Children are not a homogeneous group, ranging from
- pre-term newborn infants (premature) (average weight <3.4 kg),
- full-term infants (neonates) (0–27 days),
- infants and toddlers (28 days to 23 months) (3.4–12.4 kg),
- children (2 to 11 years) (12.4–39 kg), to
- adolescents (12 to 16/18 years) (average 39–72 kg for males and 60 kg for females).

There are age-related developmental changes in the pharmacokinetics and pharmacodynamics of drugs. Changes occur in gastric acidity, drug clearance, and receptor expression. Many of these changes are relevant to drug absorption. Some 60 years ago it was shown that there was a 6 fold greater absorption of penicillin in neonates than in children. Why?
- Neonatal stomachs are achlorhydric soon after birth, enabling acid-labile drugs like penicillin to survive the passage through the stomach.
- The rate of gastric emptying falls as infants get older. It is faster in the neonate than in adults, but slower in infants and children than in adults. Because the liver takes up a relatively large percentage of body volume in infants, drug clearance rates often exceed those in adults.

> **Key point**
>
> Extrapolation of data on the absorption or the behaviour of dose forms in adults to children's medication is hazardous.

Figure 9.3 illustrates the variety of approaches to paediatric dosing using solutions, powder, granules or dividing solid dose forms, except those whose coating provides sustained release.

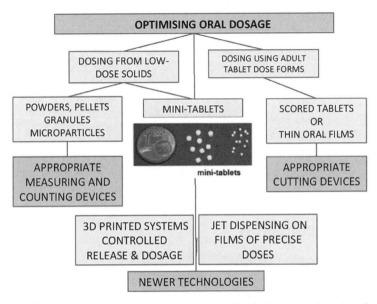

Figure 9.3: *A diagram of the approaches to dosing for individual patients, based on the diagram by Wening K and Breitkreuz J.* Int J Pharm *2011;404:1–9.*

Appropriateness of paediatric medication

Appropriateness involves the characteristics of both the child and the characteristics of the medicinal product such as:

- palatability
- ease of swallowing
- complexity of any required modification prior to administration
- required dose
- dosing frequency and duration of treatment
- mode of administration and suitability of any administration device.

These factors also apply to medicines designed for the elderly.

Extemporaneous formulations

> **Key points**
>
> - Extemporaneous formulations may be necessary where no proprietary medication form is available.
> - Conventional pharmaceutical controls must be applied to both the drug (source and purity) and to the final dose form (stability, release rate).
> - If tablets are crushed to provide drug for extemporaneous formulations, the process must be standardised as far as possible and the particle size distribution must be evaluated, as minimal quality procedures.
> - Sustained release tablet formulations should not normally be subdivided.

Figure 9.4 illustrates some of the basic approaches used when converting existing formulations of tablets, capsules and injections into alternative forms.

- It may be that the contents of an injection can be incorporated directly into a suitable vehicle.
- The contents of soft-gelatin capsules may be amenable to emulsification depending on their nature.
- In all cases key parameters should be determined: stability, particle size distribution of granules and powders, purity of drug substance.

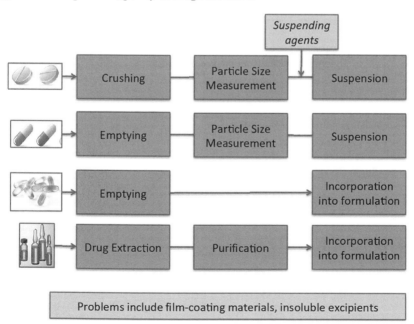

Figure 9.4: *Stratagems applied when there is a need to convert tablets, capsules, soft gelatin capsules and injections into patient-appropriate medicines.*

Developing paediatric medicines: liquid or solid oral forms?

- Liquid formulations are often favoured because of the ease of administration and acceptability to the child.
- Taste masking is more of an issue with liquid formulations, but solid-dose forms can be difficult to swallow.
- Liquid formulations suffer somewhat from variability of measurement of dose, although oral injectors can reduce this frequent domestic error. The teaspoon is far from a standard measure, delivering in use between 2.5 and 9 mL.

Excipients

There are some restrictions in the range of excipients that can be used in paediatric formulations.

- As neonates do not metabolise alcohol efficiently, ethanol should be used with caution.
- Glycerin is often a suitable alternative.

Doses in paediatric medication

- In the case of insulin, it has been suggested that for the lowest dose, insulin should be given diluted for greater accuracy of dose measurement. Insulin pens accurately deliver 5U doses but have shown no advantage over syringes in terms of accuracy.
- For other proteins, questions of their solution viscosity might dictate choice of dosing method (see **Chapter 12**).

Key point

Low doses can cause difficulties, not least in the reliable measurement of small volumes.

Tablets designed for division

- The use of mini-tablets, 1–3 mm in diameter, to aid swallowing has been investigated in children aged from 2 to 6 years.
- Such products also avoid, as we have discussed, the need for subdivision of adult dose forms.
- Recent developments have also led to new tablets designed for division as shown in *Figure 9.5*.

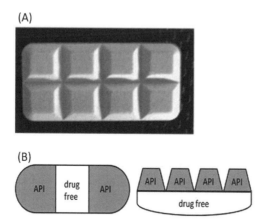

Figure 9.5: *(A) A design of rectangular divisible tablets; (B) systems which provide drug free regions to aid the accurate breaking of the tablet. Reproduced from Kayitare E et al. Development of fixed dose combination tablets containing zidovudine and lamivudine for paediatric applications.* Int J Pharm 2009;370:41–46.

Other routes of administration

Oral mucosal delivery
- Delivery to the oral mucosa is discussed in **Chapter 8**. It has some advantages in infants.
- Oral transmucosal fentanyl citrate is used as an anesthetic premedication in children undergoing surgery or painful diagnostic or therapeutic procedures within a monitored care setting. Rapid drug absorption can be achieved.

Sublingual delivery
- The advantages of sublingual and buccal administration have also been discussed in **Chapter 8**.
- There can be occasions when these routes are appropriate, such as for comatose babies who cannot swallow.

Subcutaneous injection
- The skin of children is thinner and their subcutaneous (s.c.) tissue thickness is lower compared to adults, hence shorter syringe needles (e.g. 4 mm) are employed to avoid unwanted results of injection into muscular tissue.
- Insulin injections should be given into the s.c. tissue and optimally avoid deposition into other sites (see **Chapter 8**).
- Measurements that have been made of combined skin and s.c. tissue show large variations with respect to body mass index (BMI) at all sites (arm, thigh, abdomen and buttock) hence making truly personalised medicine more difficult.

Intramuscular injection

- There are few studies on potential difference between intramuscular (i.m.) administration of drugs in different age groups, but it is known that the time to reach peak drug levels after i.m. injection of ampicillin, cefalexin, cefaloridine and benzylpenicllin is equivalent in neonates, children and adults.
- Neonates have less muscular mass and subcutaneous fat and a higher water content which may the affect solubility and diffusion of drugs deposited in intramuscular depots.

Transdermal delivery

Patches

- Transdermal administration can provide a non-invasive method for paediatric drug delivery.
- Fentanyl, buprenorphine, clonidine, scopolamine, methylphenidate, and oestrogens have been formulated as patches for paediatric use.

Key point

The evolving skin barrier function in premature neonates represents a significant formulation challenge.

Microneedles

- Microneedles, discussed in **Chapter 8**, have several advantages over conventional systems.
- Microneedles fabricated by one of a variety of techniques are now being used in practice to provide a means of administering drugs or vaccines which may be poorly absorbed across the stratum corneum.

Intranasal delivery

- Intranasal fentanyl has been used for pain relief as an alternative to oral morphine in the treatment of burns and procedures during treatment, such as the removal of dressings in paediatric patients.
- The ideal paediatric analgesic should be potent and have a quick onset, a short duration of action and minimal side effects.

Ophthalmic delivery

- The eye of the newborn is about two-thirds of its adult size; it reaches adult size at around 3–4 years.

Key point

There is a risk of systemic side effects after ocular delivery of drops in infants, as absorption drugs enter a small circulating blood volume. Timolol in young children achieves blood levels from 3.5 to 34 ng/mL, much higher than the average levels of 2.45 ng/mL in adults.

Administration by inhalation

- Drugs can be delivered via the respiratory tract by the methods discussed in **Chapter 8**.
- However, the disparity in the sizes of children and their tolerance to aerosols formed by nebulisers or pressurised devices varies. *Figure 9.6* shows assessments of systems for nebulisation, pMDI's (pressurised metered-dose inhaler) or DPI's (dry powder inhaler) suitability for the different age ranges.
- Spacers (holding chambers) (*Figure 9.7*) are used in inhalation therapy for both adults and children. Spacers are easier to use by children than pressurised MDIs themselves.

Dosage form	Preterm newborn infants	Term newborn infants (0d-28d)	Infants and Toddlers (1m-2y)	Children (pre school) (2-5y)	Children (school) (6-11y)	Adolescents (12-16/18y)
Liquids for nebulisation	Applicable with problems	Probably applicable, not preferred	Good applicability	Best and preferred applicability	Good applicability	Probably applicable, not preferred
pMDI with spacer / holding chamber	Not applicable	Probably applicable, not preferred	Good applicability	Best and preferred applicability	Good applicability	Good applicability
DPI	Not applicable	Not applicable	Probably applicable, not preferred	Good applicability	Best and preferred applicability	Best and preferred applicability

Figure 9.6: *The appropriateness of forms of inhalation for various age groups, a figure modified from the EMA Committee for Medicinal Products for Human Use 2006. From Leiner S. A respiratory product for children - development and submission experiences.* Int J Pharm 2014;469:263–264.

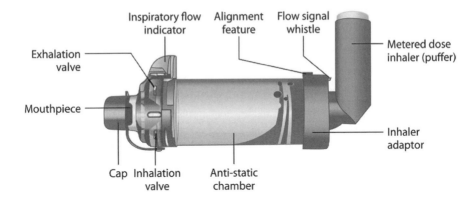

Figure 9.7: *Diagram of a holding chamber or spacer for use with a pMDI, showing the inhalation and exhalation valves and the adapters for the inhaler.*

Key point

It has been shown that beclometasone deposition from an aerosol without a spacer varies from 37% in 5–7 yr olds, through 47% in 8–10 yr olds to 54% 11–14 yr old children. With a spacer deposition in the three groups is 57–58%

The elderly and their medication

Key point

The terms 'elderly' and 'geriatric' cover a much longer span than does the category 'paediatric'. It has been suggested that there are the young elderly (from 70–85 yrs) and the old elderly (from 85 yrs onward).

Changes with age that affect medication

- There are physiological and other changes which occur with ageing that can complicate pharmaceutical care, these are summarised in *Figure 9.8.*

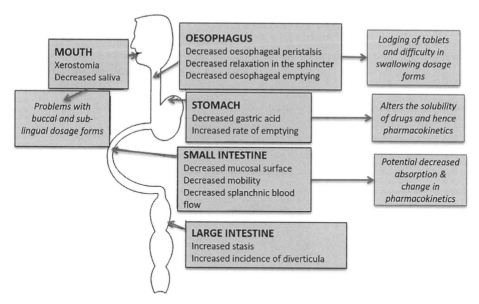

Figure 9.8: *The principal changes in GI function with age and some consequences. Modified from Macdonald ET and Macdonald JB,* Drug Treatment in the Elderly. *John Wiley, Chichester, 1982.*

Complicating factors

- The issues in *Figure 9.8* are in addition to the problems of co-morbidity and consequent polypharmacy, hence there are increased drug-drug interactions and problems of compliance.
- Specific issues include: xerostomia (dry mouth) and dysphagia (difficulty in swallowing). Fast-dissolving formulations administered sublingually can be one solution to the problem of dysphagia; such formulations are frequently bioequivalent to the conventional oral forms. The problems of xerostomia may, however, compromise outcomes.
- Achlorhydria and hypochlorhydria: the absence of production of hydrochloric acid in the stomach and the condition where there are low levels of stomach acid. The incidence of achlorhydria is found in up to 20% of elderly patients and hypochlorhydria in 20% of patients over 70 years of age. Around 11% of elderly subjects have a median fasting gastric pH of above 5.

Key points

- The average patient is a myth, hence prediction of outcomes is rendered difficult. The effects of the changes discussed before may be self-cancelling or may be significant. Much will depend on the drug. It is difficult to predict largely because individual patient data are rarely available.
- The need to adapt drug doses for the elderly relates mostly to changes in cardiovascular, renal and hepatic function.

Drugs and enteral nutrition (EN)

- Enteral feeding is used to enhance nutrition in patients unable to take food normally. Enteral feeding tubes also allow the administration of drugs to such patients.
- Different feeding tubes have different destinations (*Figure 9.9*) hence it is important to choose the correct site for the administration of the drug, depending on the characteristics of the medication.
- Even though drugs may be absorbed maximally in the intestine, bypassing the stomach may result in poor absorption as the drug may not have the opportunity to first dissolve in the acidic environment of the stomach.

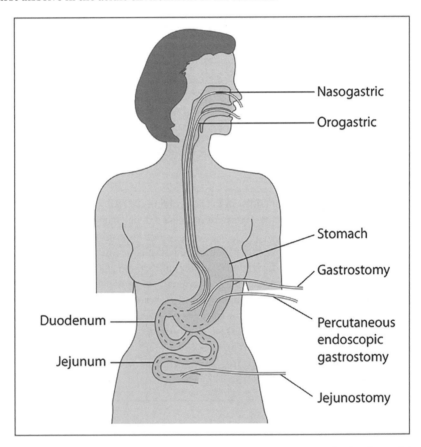

Figure 9.9: *Different types of feeding tubes leading to the stomach. Nasoduodenal, nasojejunal and percutaneous jejunostomy tubes extend to the small intestine.*

Preparation of enteral fluids incorporating existing medications.

This is an important area for study and evaluation and special care has to be taken.

- Conventional-release tablets can be crushed for administration with EN fluids. The finely ground tablet is added as a suspension in water (15–30 mL). Particle size distribution is clearly vital.
- The contents of liquid gelatin capsules are often viscous and it is not easy to remove all of the contents from a single capsule.
- Delayed-release pancreatic enzyme capsules that contain enteric-coated beads can be mixed with apple sauce or juice for administration via feeding tube. Soft-gelatin capsules can be dissolved in hot water and the whole administered.
- Extended-release tablets and capsules have to be treated as special cases: the contents of capsules containing coated pellets can be mixed with EN fluids, but there can be a tendency for these to clump and block narrow-bore feeding tubes.

Drug interactions with enteral fluids

- Liquid formulations and solid dosage forms can be administered with enteral fluids. With caution several medications can be given at the same time. Nevertheless, drug–nutrient interactions can take place, there can be problems with the osmolality of the liquids administered, and there can be blockage of the tubes.
- Drugs may interact with nutrient solutions, perhaps by binding to proteins, or solubility may be affected by electrolytes. Phenytoin absorption has been reported to be reduced by up to 70% on co-administration with enteral feeds. *Table 9.1* records selected examples.

Table 9.1: *The effect of interactions of selected drugs with enteral fluids*

Drug	Interaction/Effect
Ciprafloxacin	Absorption decreased by 25%
Hydralazine	Decreased absorption and concentration
Penicillin V	Unpredictable absorption
Sucralfate	Binds to protein in the feed
Theophylline	Absorption decreased by 60–70%
Warfarin	May interact with vitamin K in feed

From Thomson FC, Naysmith MR and Lindsay A, Hosp Pharm 2000;7:155–164. Available at https://www.pharmaceutical-journal.com/learning/learning-article/managing-drug-therapy-in-patients-receiving-enteral-and-parenteral-nutrition/11097109.article

Osmolality of enteral feeding formulae

- The osmolality of enteral feeding formulae is important because of its influence on the GI tract.
- Osmolality is expressed in mOsm/kg, and is affected by the concentration of amino acids, carbohydrates and electrolytes.
- If quantities of a liquid with a higher osmolality than the gut contents are administered, water is drawn into the intestine; such a process leads to diarrhoea, nausea and distension.
- The osmolality of normal body fluids is 300 mOsm/kg and isotonic formulations have values close to this. *Table 9.2* lists liquid medications that have osmolalities greater than 300 mOsm/kg. The exact osmolalities will vary with the exact formulations used and will often differ between various brands of a formulation.

Table 9.2: *Some liquid medications with osmolalities greater than 300 mOsm/kg*

Acetominophen (paracetamol) elixir, 65 mg/mL
Amantadine HCl solution, 10 mg/mL
Chloral hydrate syrup, 50 mg/mL
Cimetidine solution, 60 mg/mL
Docusate sodium syrup, 3.3 mg/mL
Lactulose syrup, 0.67 mg/mL
Metoclopramide HCl syrup, 1 mg/mL
Promethazine HCl syrup, 1.25 mg/mL

From Dickerson RN and Melnik G, Am J Hosp Pharm 1988;45:832–834.

Key points

- Not all liquid preparations are suitable for administration by enteral feeding tubes.
- Viscous liquids may occlude the feeding tubes.
- Syrups with pH values <4 may be incompatible with enteral nutrition (EN) formulations, which may result in clumping, increase in viscosity and consequent clogging of the feeding tubes.

Memory maps

Some considerations in the dosage of medication of the elderly

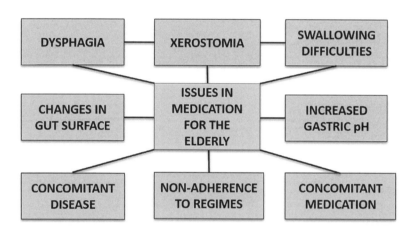

Complexities of the choices for the production of liquid paediatric dosage forms – not only formulation

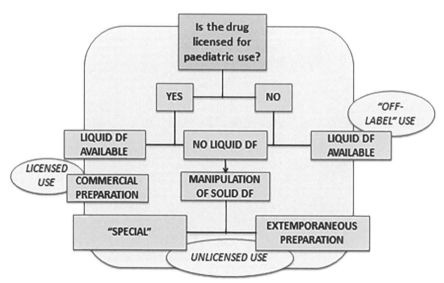

Adapted from Standing JF and Tuleu C. Paediatric formulations – Getting to the heart of the problem. Int J Pharm 2005;300:56–66.

Issues in choice of dose in paediatric patients

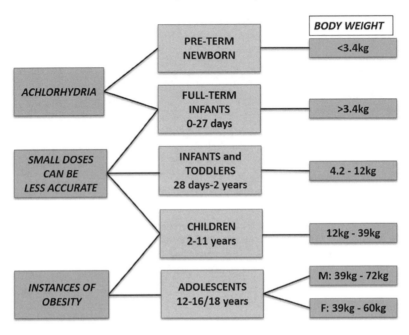

Questions

1. **Indicate which of the following statements are correct in relation to paediatric medication.**
   A: Growth in childhood involves changes in gastric pH and gastric emptying
   B: Modifying adult medicines for use in children is the best option
   C: Excipients used in adult medicines may be contraindicated in children
   D: Low dosage liquids are difficult to administer accurately
   E: A teaspoon provides a standard measure of liquid dose

2. **Indicate which of the following statements are correct in relation to optimising oral dose forms for individual young patients.**
   A: Mini tablets are able to provide a range of precise dosages
   B: Taste masking is a greater problem with liquid dose forms
   C: Solid dose forms may be difficult to swallow
   D: Childhood doses can be extrapolated from adult doses

3. **Indicate which of the following statements are true in relation to extemporaneous preparations.**
   A: These are necessary to achieve the correct dose for individuals when proprietary products are not available
   B: Quality control measures must be applied to the drug used (source and purity)
   C: Quality control measures need not to be applied to the final dose form
   D: Sustained release preparations are a useful source of starting material

4. **Which of the statements below are true for intramuscular injection administration?**
   A: There are many studies on the difference between i.m. administration of drugs in different age groups
   B: The time to reach peak levels of ampicillin, cefalexin and benzylpenicillin after i.m. injection are the same in neonates, children and adults
   C: The smaller muscular mass and subcutaneous fat in neonates may affect the solubility and diffusion of drugs in i.m. depots

5. **Ocular delivery of drugs in infants must be used with caution as:**
   A: The newborn eye is around two-thirds of adult size
   B: The eye reaches adult size at around 1–2 years
   C: The blood levels of timolol after ocular delivery in young children can vary by a factor of ten
   D: Timolol drug levels in adult patients are less than those achieved in young children

6. **In inhalation therapy, which of the following are true in relation to spacers?**
   A: Spacers reduce the velocity of the particles released from metered dose inhalers (MDIs)
   B: Reduction in velocity allows evaporation of the solvent and a reduction in particle size of the droplets emitted from the MDI
   C: The electric charge on the surface of some spacers projects the particles toward the patient via the mouth piece
   D: Spacers lead to enhanced effects due to the greater percentage of inhaled small particles
   E: Some particles can be adsorbed to some plastic spacers

7. **In considering changes with age that affect medication for the elderly, which of the statements below are true?**
   A: There is no 'average patient'
   B: Age alone is a specific enough measure to adapt dosing
   C: Achlorhydria is found in around 20% of the elderly population
   D: Cardiovascular, renal and hepatic changes are important in the older patient
   E: Vital parameters are mostly known for individual patients

8. **Which of the following are generally true in relation to physiological changes on ageing?**
   A: There is increased mucosal surface in the small intestine
   B: There is decreased motility in the small intestine
   C: There is increased oesophageal peristalsis
   D: There is an increased rate of gastric emptying

9. **Adding drugs to enteral nutrition (EN) fluids can be a route of drug administration in the elderly. Drug interactions with components of the fluid may occur. Which of the following are true?**
   A: Drug may bind with proteins in the fluid
   B: Drug solubility can be reduced leading to decreased absorption
   C: Coated drug pellets can avoid the problems of interactions with the fluids
   D: Decreased absorption of drugs in enteral fluids of up to 70% have been measured
   E: Liquid medicines such as cimetidine solution are unlikely to cause problems when added to EN fluids

CHAPTER 10

Physicochemical drug interactions and incompatibilities

LEARNING OBJECTIVES

Upon completion of this chapter you should be able to:
- understand the effect of pH that can lead to drug precipitation
- understand the effect of dilution of formulations that can lead to precipitation
- understand cation–anion interactions forming complexes
- understand salting-in and salting-out processes increasing or decreasing solubility respectively
- understand chelation effects
- understand ion-exchange interactions
- understand adsorption of drugs to excipients and containers, interactions with plastics, all causing loss of drug
- understand the effect of protein binding of drugs on their free concentrations *in vivo*.

Solubility problems

- Some drugs which are administered by the intravenous route cannot safely be mixed with all available intravenous fluids because of the resulting poor solubility and precipitation of the drug.
- If the solubility of a drug in a particular infusion fluid is low, crystallisation may occur (sometimes very slowly) when the drug and fluid are mixed. Microcrystals may be formed which are not immediately visible.
- The mechanism of crystallisation from solution will often involve a change in pH.
- The pH of commercially available infusion fluids can vary within a range of 1–2 pH units. Therefore a drug's compatibility may vary depending on the fluid batch.
- The application of the equations relating pH and pK_a to solubility (see **Chapter 3**) should allow additions of drugs to be safely made or to be avoided.

Key points

- Drug–drug or drug–excipient interactions can take place before administration of a drug. These may result in precipitation of the drug from solution, loss of potency or instability.
- An incompatibility occurs when one drug is mixed with other drugs or agents and produces a product unsuitable for administration. This might be due to some modification of the effect of the active drug, such as an increase in toxicity or conversely a decrease in activity through some physical changes such as decrease in solubility or stability.
- There are several causes of interactions and incompatibilities, which include:
  - changes in pH which may lead to precipitation of the drug
  - change of solvent characteristics on dilution, which may also cause precipitation
  - cation–anion interactions in which complexes are formed
  - the influence of salts on decreasing or increasing solubility, respectively 'salting-out' and 'salting-in'
  - chelation – in which a chelator binds with a metal ion to form a complex
  - ion exchange interactions where ionised drugs interact with oppositely charged resins
  - adsorption to excipients and containers causing loss of drug
  - interactions with plastics and loss of drug
  - protein binding to plasma proteins through which the free plasma concentration of drugs is reduced.

Tip

Remember that the solubility of an ionisable drug is strongly influenced by the pH of the solution because of the effect of pH on the ionisation of the drug. Undissociated drugs cannot interact with water molecules to the same extent as ionised drugs, which are readily hydrated and therefore more soluble. A change of pH can therefore sometimes lead to precipitation of ionised drugs. See **Chapter 3** for equations linking pH to solubility.

Tip

Titratable acidity

Note that, whereas the pH indicates the concentration of hydrogen ions, some ions may be locked into the system and not free. The titratable acidity or alkalinity of a system may be more important than pH itself in determining compatibility and stability. For example, solutions of dextrose may have a pH as low as 4.0, but the titratable acidity in such an unbuffered solution is low, and thus the addition of a drug such as benzylpenicillin sodium or the soluble form of an acidic drug whose solubility will be reduced at low pH may not be contraindicated.

pH effects *in vitro* and *in vivo*

In vitro pH effects

- pH changes often follow from the addition of a drug substance or solution to an infusion fluid. An increase or decrease in pH may then produce physical or chemical changes in the system:
  - For example, as little as 500 mg of ampicillin sodium may raise the pH of 500 cm^3 of some fluids to over 8, and carbenicillin or benzylpenicillin may raise the pH of 5% dextrose or dextrose saline to 5.6 or even higher. Both drugs are, however, stable in these conditions.
- Chemical, as well as physical, instability may result from changes in pH, buffering capacity, salt formation or complexation.
- Chemical instability may give rise to the formation of inactive or toxic products.

In vivo pH effects

Gastric effects

- Gastric fluids have a pH of 1–3 in normal subjects but the measured range of pH values in the human stomach is wide (up to 7) (see **Chapter 9**).
- Changes in the acid–base balance have a marked influence on the absorption and thus on the activity of drugs.
- Ingestion of antacids, food and weak electrolytes will change the pH of the stomach.
- Antacids can also have an effect on gastric emptying rate. Gastric emptying tends to become more rapid as the gastric pH is raised. Magnesium preparations promote gastric emptying. However, antacid preparations containing aluminium or calcium can retard emptying.

Intestinal absorption

- The pH gradients between the contents of the intestinal lumen and capillary blood are smaller than in the stomach.
- Sudden changes in the acid–base balance will, nonetheless, change the concentration of drugs able to enter cells, however pH changes can change the binding of the drug to proteins.

The importance of urinary pH

- Ingestion of some antacids over a period of 24 h will increase urinary pH and hence affect renal resorption and handling of some drugs.
  - Administration of sodium bicarbonate with aspirin reduces blood salicylate levels by about 50%, due to increased salicylate excretion in the urine.
- When a drug is in its un-ionised form it will more readily diffuse from the urine to the blood.
- Change in urinary pH will change the rate of urinary drug absorption (*Figure 10.1*).
- In acidic urine, acidic drugs will diffuse back into the blood from the urine.

- In alkaline urine, acidic drugs such as nitrofurantoin are excreted faster.

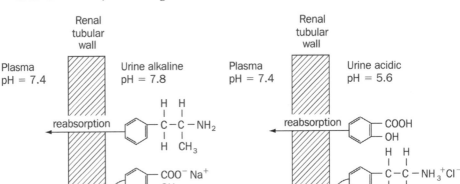

Figure 10.1: *Schematic representation of the influence of urinary pH on the passive reabsorption of a weak acid and a weak base from the urine.*

Precipitation of drugs *in vivo*

- Pain on injection may be the result of precipitation of a drug at the site of injection brought about by either solvent dilution or alteration in pH.
- Precipitation of drugs from formulations used intravenously can lead to thromboembolism.
- The kinetics of precipitation under realistic conditions must be taken into account; if the rate of infusion is sufficiently slow, precipitated drug may redissolve and so this problem can be avoided.
- The flow rate of blood or normal saline (Q) required to maintain a drug in solution during its addition to an intravenous fluid can be predicted from $Q = R/S_m$ where R is the rate of injection of drug in mg min^{-1} and S_m is the drug's apparent maximum solubility in the system (mg cm^{-3}).

Dilution of mixed solvent systems

- Care should be taken when injectable products containing, e.g., phenytoin, digoxin and diazepam, formulated in a non-aqueous, water-miscible solvent (such as an alcohol–water mixture) or as a solubilised (e.g. micellar) preparation are diluted in an aqueous infusion fluid.
- Addition of such formulations to water may result in precipitation of the drug, depending on the final concentration of the drug and solvent.
- When a drug dissolved in a cosolvent system is diluted with water, both drug and cosolvent are diluted. The logarithm of the solubility of a drug in a cosolvent system

generally increases linearly with the percentage of cosolvent present (*Figure 10.2*). On dilution, the drug concentration falls linearly (not logarithmically) with a fall in the percentage of cosolvent. When the drug concentration is high the system may become supersaturated on dilution, causing precipitation.

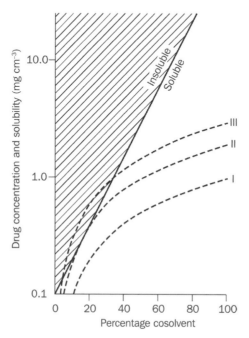

Figure 10.2: *Dilution profiles of solutions (I, II and III) containing 1, 2 and 3 mg cm⁻³ of drug respectively, plotted on a semilog scale along with the solubility line. Reproduced from Yalkowsky SH and Valvani S. Precipitation of solubilized drugs due to injection or dilution. Drug Intell Clin Pharm 1977;11:417–419.*

Cation–anion interactions

- The interaction between a large organic anion and an organic cation may result in the formation of a relatively insoluble precipitate.
- Complexation, precipitation or phase separation can occur in these circumstances; the product is affected by changes in ionic strength, temperature and pH.
- Examples of cation–anion interactions include the following drug pairs:
  - Procainamide and phenytoin sodium, procaine and thiopental sodium, hydroxyzine hydrochloride and benzylpenicillin.
  - Nitrofurantoin sodium and alkyl *p*-hydroxy benzoates (parabens), phenol or cresol, all such mixtures tending to precipitate the nitrofurantoin.

Ion-pair formation

- Ion-pair formation may be responsible for the absorption of highly charged drugs such as the quaternary ammonium salts and sulfonic acid derivatives, the absorption of which is not explained by the pH-partition hypothesis.
- Why? The formation of an ion-pair results in the 'burying' of the charges (*Figure 10.3*).
- Ion-pairs may be considered to be neutral species formed by electrostatic attraction between oppositely charged ions in solution.
- They are often sufficiently lipophilic to dissolve in non-aqueous solvents.

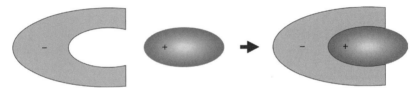

Figure 10.3: *Representation of an organic ion-pair.*

Chelation and other forms of complexation

- The term chelation (derived from the Greek *chele*, lobster's claw) relates to the interaction between a metal atom or ion and another species, known as the ligand, by which a heteroatomic ring is formed.
- Chelation changes the physical and chemical characteristics of the metal ion, and the ligand.
- It is simplest to consider the ligand as the electron pair donor and the metal as the electron pair acceptor, with the donation establishing a coordinate bond (see, for example, the copper–glycine chelate shown below).

- Many chelating agents act in the form of anions which coordinate to a metal ion. For chelation to occur there must be at least two donor atoms capable of binding to the same metal ion, and ring formation must be sterically possible. For example, ethylenediamine (1,2 diaminoethane, NH2CH2CH2NH2) has two donor nitrogens and acts as a bidentate (two-toothed) ligand.
- When a drug forms a metal chelate the solubility and absorption of both drug and metal ion may be affected, and drug chelation can lead to either increased or decreased absorption.
- Tetracycline chelation with metal ions is a well-known example of complex formation leading to decreased drug absorption:
  - Polyvalent cations such as Fe^{2+} and Mg^{2+}, and anions such as trichloracetate or phosphate interfere with absorption in both model and real systems. Ferrous sulfate has the greatest inhibitory effect on tetracycline absorption perhaps because it dissolves in water more quickly than organic iron compounds.
  - All the active tetracyclines form stable chelates with Ca^{2+}, Mg^{2+} and Al^{3+}.
  - It is important to recognise that the antibacterial action of the tetracyclines depends on their metal-binding activity as their main site of action is on ribosomes, which are rich in magnesium.
  - Tetracyclines readily form complexes with divalent metals, but they have a greater affinity for the trivalent metals with which they form 3:1 drug–metal chelates.
  - Therapeutically active tetracyclines form 2:1 complexes with cupric, nickel and zinc ions while inactive analogues form only 1:1 complexes.
  - The site of chelation is the C_{11}, C_{12} enolic system on the tetracycline molecule (below); isochlortetracycline, which lacks this, does not chelate with Ca^{2+} ions.

  - The highly coloured nature of tetracycline chelates such as the uranyl ion–tetracycline complex may be utilised in analytical procedures.
- Therapeutic chelators are used in syndromes where there is metal ion overload. For example, ethylenediaminetetraacetic acid (EDTA) as the monocalcium disodium salt is used in the treatment of lead poisoning; the calcium averts problems of calcium depletion. Deferiprone chelates iron.
- A new therapeutic chelator is the polymer veverimer which binds HCl in cases of metabolic acidosis (see *Figure 10.4*).

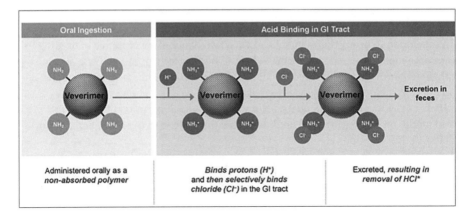

Figure 10.4: *Diagrammatic representation of the polymer veverimer and its interaction with protons and then chloride ions in the GI tract. It is currently awaiting a US licence. From http:// www.tricida.com/ with permission.*

Key points

- Complexes which form are not always fully active, nor is their formation obvious from the ingredients. For example, neomycin sulfate unexpectedly forms a complex when incorporated into Aqueous Cream BP. This is because the Aqueous Cream BP comprises 30% emulsifying ointment which itself contains 10% sodium lauryl sulfate or similar anionic surfactant. The complex that forms is between neomycin sulfate and the anionic surfactant.
- Interactions are not always visible. The formation of visible precipitates depends to a large extent on the insolubility of the two combining species in the particular mixture and the size to which the precipitated particles grow.
- Interactions between drugs and ionic macromolecules are another potential source of problems:
  - Heparin sodium and erythromycin lactobionate are contraindicated in admixture, as are heparin sodium and chlorpromazine hydrochloride or gentamicin sulfate.
  - The activity of phenoxymethylpenicillin against *Staphylococcus aureus* is reduced in the presence of various macromolecules such as acacia, gelatin, sodium alginate and tragacanth.

Tip

If a membrane is considered in its simplest form to be a strip of lipoidal material, then it can reasonably be assumed that only lipid-soluble agents will cross this barrier. The un-ionised form of acids or bases will be absorbed whereas ionised forms will not. This is the basis of the pH-partition hypothesis (see **Chapter 8**).

Other types of complex

- Molecular complexes of many types may be observed in systems containing two or more drug molecules:
  - Generally, association follows from attractive interactions (hydrophobic, electrostatic or charge transfer interactions) between two molecules.
  - The imidazole moiety is involved in many interactions. For example, caffeine and theophylline are frequently implicated in interactions with aromatic species. Caffeine increases the solubility of ergotamine and benzoic acid.
- Cyclodextrin complexes:
  - Complexes can form between modified cyclodextrins and drugs. Such interactions have been utilised to achieve enhanced solubility of poorly soluble drugs, however, there are interesting and clinically useful interactions between the cyclodextrin, sugammadex, and neuromuscular blocking agents rocouronium and vecuronium. The interaction is such that sugammadex is used to reverse the effects of the anaesthetic and hence speed up the recovery of patients at a chosen time point.
  - Such interactions have also been used to reduce anaphylaxis caused by rocuronium in some patients.

Ion-exchange interactions

- Ion-exchange resins are used medicinally and as systems for modified release of drugs.
- Colestyramine and colestipol are insoluble quaternary ammonium anion exchange resins which, when administered orally, bind bile acids and increase their elimination because the high-molecular-weight complex is not absorbed.
  - As bile acids are converted *in vivo* into cholesterol, colestyramine is used as a hypocholesteraemic agent. When given to patients receiving other drugs as well, the resin would conceivably bind anionic compounds and reduce their absorption. For example, phenylbutazone, warfarin, chlorothiazide and hydrochlorothiazide are strongly bound to the resin *in vitro*.
  - Decreased drug absorption can be caused by use of colestyramine or colestipol and has been reported to decrease absorption of thyroxine, aspirin, phenprocoumon, warfarin, chlorothiazide, cardiac glycosides and ferrous sulfate.

Adsorption of drugs

- Adsorbents can be used to remove noxious substances from the lumen of the gut.
- Unfortunately, they are generally non-specific so will also adsorb nutrients, drugs and enzymes when given orally.
- Several consequences of adsorption are possible:
  - If the drug remains adsorbed until the preparation reaches the absorption site, the concentration of the drug presented to the absorbing surfaces will be reduced, resulting in a slower rate of absorption.

— Alternatively, the release of drug from the adsorbent might be complete before reaching the absorption site, possibly hastened by the presence of electrolytes in the gastrointestinal tract, in which case absorption rates may not be affected.

— Loss of activity of preservatives can arise from adsorption on to solid drug substances.

Protein and peptide adsorption

- Adsorption of peptides to glass or plastic may occur because of the amphipathic nature of many peptides. This becomes pharmaceutically important when they are originally present in low concentrations in solution.

- The adsorption of peptides on to glass is ascribed to bonding between their amino groups and the silanol groups of the glass.

Drug interactions with plastics

- The plastic tubes and connections used in intravenous containers and giving sets can adsorb or absorb a number of drugs leading to significant losses in some cases.

- Those drugs which show a significant loss when exposed to plastic, in particular poly(vinyl chloride), include insulin, nitroglycerin, diazepam, clomethiazole, vitamin A acetate, isosorbide dinitrate.

- Preservatives such as the methyl and propyl parabens present in formulations can be sorbed into rubber and plastic membranes and closures, thus leading to decreased levels of preservative and, in the extreme, loss of preservative activity.

- There are particular issues with high molecular weight drugs such as proteins and monoclonal antibodies in terms of their interaction with plastics. Some of these are discussed in **Chapter 12**.

Tips

Note the difference between adsorption and absorption:
- Adsorption is the attachment of a molecule to a surface.
- Absorption involves its penetration into the substance with which it interacts.

Protein binding of drugs

Binding of drugs to proteins is important because the bound drug assumes the diffusional and other transport characteristics of the protein molecule. This may occur spontaneously but the process has been utilised deliberately to devise drug–protein complexes as drug delivery systems with special absorption and distribution characteristics (see **Chapter 12**).

- Drugs bound to albumin (or other proteins) are attached to a unit too large to be transported across membranes. They are thus prevented from reacting with receptors or from entering the sites of drug metabolism or drug elimination, until they dissociate from the protein.

A second important consequence of protein binding is that the free drug concentration is reduced. This is important because it is only free drug that is able to cross the capillary endothelium:

- In cases where drug is highly protein-bound (around 90%), small changes in binding lead to drastic changes in the levels of free drug in the body.
- Both ampicillin (50 mg kg^{-1} every 2 h) and oxacillin (50 mg kg^{-1} h^{-1}) produce similar peak levels in the serum when given as repeated intravenous boluses. Levels of free drug are markedly different, however, as oxacillin is 75% protein-bound and ampicillin is 17.5% bound.
- The level of free drug in serum is important in determining the amount of drug that reaches tissue spaces because it determines the gradient of drug concentration between the serum and the tissues. This relationship is given by:

$$C_t = \frac{C_s f_s}{f_t}$$

where C_t is the total concentration of drug in tissue fluid, C_s is the serum drug concentration, and f_s and f_t are the free fractions of drug in serum and tissue fluid, respectively.

Binding to plasma proteins

- Most drugs bind to a limited number of sites on the albumin molecule.
- Plasma proteins other than albumin may also be involved in binding. Blood plasma normally contains on average about 6.72 g of protein per 100 cm^3; the protein comprises 4.0 g of albumin, 2.3 g of globulins and 0.24 g of fibrinogen.
- Dicoumarol binds to β- and γ-globulins, and certain steroid hormones are specifically and preferentially bound to particular globulin fractions.
- Binding to plasma albumin is generally easily reversible, so that drug molecules bound to albumin will be released as the level of free drug in the blood declines.
- Binding to albumin is a process comparable to partitioning of drug molecules from a water phase to a non-polar phase. The hydrophobic sites, however, are not necessarily 'preformed'.

Lipophilicity and protein binding

- The extent of protein binding of many drugs is a linear function of their partition coefficient P (or log P).
- A linear equation of the form:
  log (percentage bound/percentage free) = 0.5 log P – 0.665 may be applied to serum binding of penicillins. Although there may be an electrostatic component to the interaction, the binding increases with the degree of lipophilicity, suggesting, as is often the case, that more than one binding interaction is in force.

- Muscle protein may bind drugs such as digoxin and so act as a depot. Concentrations of 1.2 ± 0.8, 11.3 ± 4.9 and 77.7 ± 43.3 ng cm^{-3} have been reported for digoxin in plasma, skeletal and cardiac muscle, respectively.
  - Dicloxacillin, which is 95% bound to protein, is absorbed more slowly from muscle than ampicillin, which is only bound to the extent of 20%.
- Protein binding can affect antibiotic action. For example:
  - Penicillins and cephalosporins bind reversibly to albumin. Only the free antibiotic has antibacterial activity.
  - Oxacillin in serum at a concentration of 100 µg cm^{-3} exhibits an antibacterial effect similar to that of 10 µg cm^{-3} of the drug in water. A high degree of serum protein binding may nullify the apparent advantage of higher serum levels of some agents.
- The degree of binding of drug D to protein P may be estimated as follows:
  - Assuming that protein binding can be considered to be an adsorption process obeying the law of mass action:

$$D + P \rightleftarrows (DP)$$
$$(DP = \text{protein–drug complex})$$

  - Then, at equilibrium:

$$D_f + (P_t - D_b) = D_b$$

  where D_f is the molar concentration of unbound drug, P_t is the total molar concentration of protein and D_b is the molar concentration of bound drug (= molar concentration of complex).
  - The ratio, r, of the number of moles bound to the total protein in the system can be shown to be:

$$r = \frac{nKD_f}{1} \quad \text{or} \quad \frac{1}{r} = \frac{1}{n} + \frac{1}{nKD_f}$$

  where n is the number of binding sites per molecule and K is the ratio of the rate constants for association and dissociation.
- The fraction of drug bound, β, generally varies with the concentration of both drug and protein and is given by:

$$\beta = \frac{1}{1 + (D_f/nP_t) + 1/(nKP_t)}$$

Memory maps

Some causes of interactions and incompatibilities

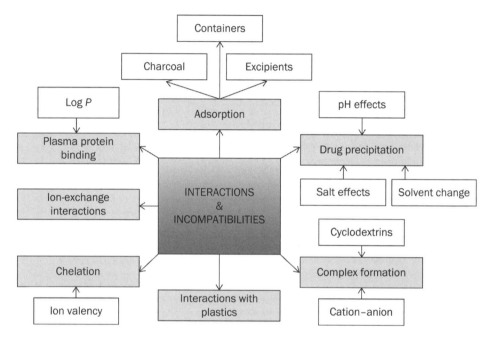

Drug interactions and incompatibilities

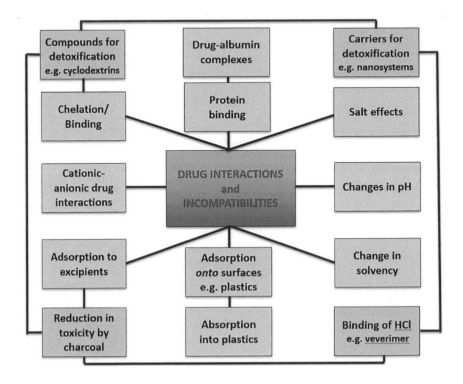

Questions

1. Indicate which of the following statements are true. In general, the administration of antacids would be expected to:
   A: Increase the gastric pH
   B: Affect gastric emptying time
   C: Decrease urinary pH
   D: Decrease the ionisation of acidic drugs in the stomach
   E: Reduce the gastric absorption of acidic drugs

2. Indicate which of the following statements are true. Acidification of the urine:
   A: May result from the administration of antacids
   B: Would be expected to increase the rate of urinary excretion of acidic drugs such as nitrofurantoin
   C: Would be expected to increase the rate of urinary excretion of basic drugs such as imipramine
   D: May cause precipitation of drugs in the urine
   E: Would be expected to increase the reabsorption of a basic drug

3. Indicate which of the following statements are true. Ion pair formation:
   A: Occurs between ions of similar charge
   B: Is a consequence of electrostatic interaction between ions
   C: Decreases the absorption of quaternary ammonium salts
   D: Results in the formation of a neutral species

4. Indicate which of the following statements relating to the formation of chelates are true.
   A: Chelation is the interaction between a large organic anion and an organic cation
   B: Chelation is the interaction between a metal ion and a ligand
   C: The ligand is the electron pair acceptor
   D: Chelation results in the formation of a heteroatomic ring
   E: Tetracyclines form 3:1 drug–metal chelates with magnesium ions

5. Indicate which of the following interactions might be expected to lead to an increased drug absorption.
   A: Ion pair formation
   B: Drug binding to plasma proteins
   C: Adsorption of drug on to antacids
   D: Interaction of drug with the plastic tubing of giving sets
   E: Chelation of tetracyclines with metal ions

6. Indicate which of the following statements relating to the protein binding of drugs are true.
   A: Protein binding to plasma albumin is a reversible process
   B: Protein binding decreases the free drug concentration
   C: Drugs with a low lipophilicity have a high degree of protein binding
   D: Protein binding of antibiotics usually increases antibiotic action

7. If the rate of injection of a drug is 7 mg min^{-1}, and the maximum solubility of the drug is approximately 0.5 mg cm^{-3}, what blood or saline flow rate is required to prevent observable precipitation?
    A: 14 cm^3 min^{-1}
    B: 2 cm^3 min^{-1}
    C: 3.5 cm^3 min^{-1}
    D: 0.29 cm^3 min^{-1}

8. A drug is bound to serum albumin to the extent of 95% bound. What is the percentage effect on the free levels of the drug of a reduction in binding to 92%?
    A: 3% increase
    B: 8% increase
    C: 160% increase
    D: 3% decrease

CHAPTER 11

Adverse events – the role of formulations and delivery systems

Adverse events and adverse drug reactions

Adverse reactions following administration of a medicine or use of a device can be discussed in terms of adverse events (where the causality is not known) or adverse reactions (where the causative factor is the drug itself or a specific component of a formulation).

- When both drug and its formulation are involved, or when an excipient is implicated, the term adverse event is possibly the more accurate.
- It is often assumed when an adverse reaction or adverse event occurs that the drug is the causative agent. It is generally the case that the drug itself is the cause of most adverse reactions and effects, but there are instances when formulation factors come into play.
- Sometimes, as we discuss later in this chapter, excipients may have their own biological effect, and sometimes the way in which the product is constructed and behaves in the body may cause the drug to have enhanced toxicity.
- *Figure 11.1* shows both product and patient factors in the causation of adverse events. Errors of choice of product or drug aside, when the correct drug and formulation has been administered, there are still many opportunities for unwanted effects.
- The wider range of causations include:
  - abnormal (high or low) bioavailability caused by a product or manufacturing defect or change
  - sensitivities to formulation ingredients
  - reactions to impurities and breakdown products of drug or excipients
  - aggregation of protein and peptide drugs in devices such as pumps
  - device failure, for example with medicated stents or infusion pumps

— the nature of the formulation or dosage form, for example adhesive tablets lodging in the oesophagus, or drug precipitating from administered injections.

- *Figure 11.1* categorises adverse events as those dependent on patient factors and those related to formulations and devices. Adverse events include allergic reactions, local toxicities, systemic effects or idiosyncratic reactions. We cannot here recount patient-related factors in detail, although there are of course dosage form–patient interactions (see **Chapter 10**) that make these of interest. Changed physiology in the postnatal growth period in childhood and physiological changes in the elderly (see **Chapter 9**) means that dosage forms can behave differently in certain patient groups. The following sections deal with some product-related adverse effects.

- The variety of adverse events that have occurred in the recent past is illustrated in *Table 11.1*. Historical or 'classic' cases are valuable as they can provide clues to adverse events occurring with new therapeutic agents or delivery systems.

- In the case of the indomethacin osmotic tablets (see **Chapter 7** – see section on osmotic pumps) three factors conspired to produce the adverse effects: the nature of the drug itself, the nature of the osmotic core (potassium chloride) and the localised release of both close to oesophageal tissue. There were instances of oesophageal perforation! The product was withdrawn.

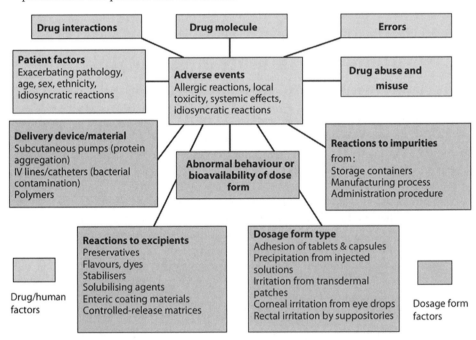

Figure 11.1: *Drug/human factors and dosage form factors in adverse events following medication administration. Modified from Uchegbu IF, Florence AT. Adverse drug events related to dosage forms and delivery systems. Drug Safety 1996;14:39–67, with kind permission from Springer Science and Business Media.*

Table 11.1: *Some 'classic' adverse events as a result of use of formulations*

Dosage form	Trade name	Adverse event
Indometacin osmotic minipump tablets	Osmosin	Intestinal perforation
Fluspirilene IM injection	Redeptin	Tissue necrosis at site of injection
Epidural injection of prednisolone injection containing benzyl alcohol as preservative	Depo Medrol	Mild paralysis
Inhalation of nebulised ipratropium bromide solution containing benzalkonium chloride as preservative	Atrovent	Paradoxical bronchoconstriction
Povidone iodine solution for vaginal application		Anaphylactoid reaction
Application of timolol eye drops	Timoptic	Bronchoconstriction
Fentanyl transdermal patch	Duragesic	Respiratory depression and death

From Uchegbu IF and Florence AT. Adverse drug events related to dosage forms and delivery systems. Drug Safety 1996;14:39–67, with kind permission from Springer Science and Business Media.

Key points

- Detecting the causes of adverse events is not an easy task, especially when drugs or drug products are novel.
- It is essential that we look for analogies, reliable reports on closely related drugs and similar formulations.
- The older literature should not be disregarded as it may reveal clues which might have relevance to new medicines and treatments.

Key questions

Is the recorded event:
- due to the drug molecule (its chemistry, pharmacological activity or physical properties?)
- linked to the use of concomitant medication?
- due to an excipient, a vehicle or matrix effect?
- a result of the physical nature of the dosage form?
- the result of concomitant pathologies?
- unrelated to the medication as can occur with placebos? This is termed the 'nocebo' effect.*

*A nocebo is a procedure or medicine that harms a patient due to a psychological effect and not a physiological effect. A nocebo is said to harm because patients believe it will harm them, not because of any chemical or biological reaction stemming from the procedure or medicine itself.

Excipient effects

- Excipients are not always the inert substances that we presume. Some cases and reports of the adverse action of excipients are discussed here. While labelling requirements insist on the listing of ingredients in some products, the plethora of trade names (e.g. for surfactants, polymers, lipids and other excipients) can make ready accurate identification of materials difficult.

- Batch-to-batch variation of some excipient raw materials adds another layer of complexity in tracking down and comparing case histories. A case in point would be polymeric substances which are not monodisperse.

- Preservatives and dyes are used widely in formulation. Methylparaben, propylparaben, sodium benzoate, and sodium metabisulfite are some of the most frequently encountered preservatives. There are many available dyes with widely varying structures.

- It is not possible to generalise about the effects of excipients with all their structural diversity and uses.

- Many polymeric materials are complex (see **Chapter 7**), not only because of the existence in any one sample of a range of molecular weights, but also because many contain plasticisers to adjust their physical properties or agents to aid their production.

- Plasticisers such as diethyl phthalate can leach from plastic giving sets into infusions, particularly those that have ingredients (such as surfactants) that might aid the solubilisation of the phthalate. Dioctyl phthalate and dioctyl adipate have been found in some silicone tubing.

- With polymers and other macromolecules one needs to know their molecular weight, or more likely their molecular weight distribution, and about the presence of impurities, such as catalysts and peroxides. The latter is found in some polysorbate 80 samples (see **Chapter 5** –polysorbate 80 is a synthetic non-ionic surfactant where such residues may be found).

- Excipients are not always produced to the extremely high standards of purity that apply to drug substances. There may be batch differences or brand differences in excipients.

- The presence of impurities rather than the material itself might be the cause of any adverse event, in some cases producing the culprit by inducing degradation of the drug.

- Some problems with excipients are shown in *Table 11.2*.

Table 11.2: *Excipients that have caused problems in paediatric and adult medicines*[a]

Excipient or class	Selected observed reactions
Sulfites	Wheezing, dyspnoea, anaphylactoid reactions
Benzalkonium chloride	Paradoxical bronchoconstriction, reduced forced expiry volume
Aspartame	Headache, hypersensitivity
Saccharin	Dermatological reactions; avoid in children with sulfa allergies
Benzyl alcohol	In high concentrations can cause neonatal death
Various dyes	Reactions to tartrazine, similar to aspirin intolerance; patients with the 'classic aspirin triad' reaction (asthma, urticaria, rhinitis) may develop similar reactions from other dyes such as amaranth, erthyrosin, indigo, carmine, Ponceau, Sunset Yellow, Brilliant Blue
Lactose	Problem in lactose-sensitive patients (those with lactase deficiency)
Propylene glycol	Localised contact dermatitis topically; lactic acidosis after absorption

[a]*Data from American Academy of Pediatrics. Pediatrics 1997;99:266–278.*

> ### Key point
>
> The clinical literature does not always detail formulations or product brands used in clinical studies.

> ### Key point
>
> The route of administration and sometimes the mode of administration (for example, a particular device such as a nebuliser) and the excipient concentration will affect the appearance or severity of many adverse effects.

E-numbers

- The primary classification system codifies additives both in food and in pharmaceuticals in terms of E-numbers.
- The general numbering system for several classes of ingredients is:
  - E100–E199 (colours)
  - E200–E299 (preservatives)
  - E300–E399 (antioxidants, acidity regulators)
  - E400–E499 (thickeners, stabilisers, emulsifiers)
  - E500–E599 (acidity regulators, anti-caking agents)
  - E600–E699 (flavour enhancers)

- It is useful when trying to detect cross-reactivity and sensitivities to know the E-numbers of dyes, preservatives, and other ingredients. Each additive has a number within the classifications shown before. The structures of some dyes are quite complex and, perhaps not surprisingly, some do have pharmacological effects as shown in *Table 11.3*.

Table 11.3: *Observed adverse effects of dyes and colouring agents*

Compound	Structure	Adverse effects
Sunset Yellow		Urticaria exacerbation
Indigo carmine		Urticaria exacerbation
Tartrazine		Headache, gastrointestinal disturbance, exacerbation of asthma, dangerous in aspirin-intolerant individuals
Amaranth		Potential carcinogenicity (banned)
Brilliant Blue		Hypersensitivity reactions

Reproduced from Pifferi G and Restani P. The safety of pharmaceutical excipients. Il Farmaco 2003;58:541–550. Copyright Elsevier 2003.

Cross-reactivity

- Cross-reactivity can be defined as a reaction to different compounds which may or may not have some structural similarity.
- Cross-sensitisations between azo dyes and *para*-amino compounds can partially be explained on the basis of structural similarities, as may be seen from the structures below.

para aminoazobenzene (PAAB)   Disperse Yellow 3

Disperse Blue 124

Chemical structures of three azo dyes.

Surfactants

- Non-ionic surfactants are widely used in formulations as wetting agents and solubilising agents as discussed in **Chapter 5**. Surfactants accumulate at air–water and oil–water interfaces and crucially in this regard at the biological membrane–water interface. They can influence the fluidity of these membranes, and at higher concentrations, above their critical micelle concentrations, they can cause membrane damage through solubilising structural membrane lipids and phospholipids.
- While non-ionic surfactants allow poorly water-soluble drugs to be formulated as injectables, some have side-effects that are by now well known.
- The two most commonly used, and therefore often cited as causing adverse events, are polysorbate 80 (Tween 80; E433) and the polyoxyethylated castor oil, Cremophor EL. Anaphylactic reactions are the most frequently noted, although these occur in a minority of patients.

- Cremophor EL is a component of some formulations of teniposide, ciclosporin and paclitaxel. Docetaxel and etoposide formulations contain polysorbate 80. Product details should always be ascertained because of the possibility of combined effects of the ingredients.

Polyoxyethylene glycols (PEGs)

- Polyoxyethylene glycols (PEGs) (macrogols) are not of course surface-active, but they can exert adverse effects when used as suppository bases through being hygroscopic, absorbing water from the rectal tissues causing irritation. This can be minimised by first moistening the PEG base before insertion.
- This affinity for water is the result of the interaction of water molecules with the oxygen of the repeating $-CH_2CH_2O-$ units; a macrogol of molecular weight 44 500 Da has approximately 1000 such ethylene oxide units, each interacting with up to four H_2O molecules. Macrogols 4000 and 3350 are used to sequester water in the bowels (Idrolax (Ipsen) or Laxido (Galen)).
- PEG presence in laxative formulations aids the penetration of water into the faecal mass. Paediatric powder formulations of PEGs are available for faecal impaction and constipation (Movicol Paediatric, Norgine) with a dose of 6.56 g of Macrogol 3350.

Adjuvants as therapeutic substances

- This section emphasises the fact that adjuvants can be biologically active.

Nonoxynol-9

Nonoxynol-9 is used as a spermicide because, being a non-ionic surface-active agent, it interacts with spermatozoal membranes and reduces their mobility. It has also some activity against HIV but it is suspected to increase viral access through the vaginal wall as it not only interacts with the spermatozoa but also the vaginal membrane.

Poloxamers

- Poloxamers are ABA block copolymer surfactants (see **Chapter 5**). The properties of the poloxamers depend on the length of each chain. ABA block copolymer surfactants such as poloxamer 199 are wetting, solubilising and emulsifying agents, but some like poloxamer 188 (Pluronic F68) have interesting biological activity, for example, it reduces endothelial adherence and improves the rheology of sickle erythrocytes.
- Poloxamer 118 has some haemorheological activity, improving microvascular blood flow by reducing blood viscosity.

Active excipients in multiple therapies

- Several non-ionic surfactants have been found to inhibit P-glycoprotein mediated drug transport.
- When such an excipient in one formulation is administered along with another product whose absorption is P-gp-dependent, then interpretation of interactions can be difficult if the influence of the excipients in both products are not taken into account.

Influence of dosage form type

Adhesion of tablets

- Oesophageal damage can be caused by tablets or other oral dose forms. In some cases the pyloris can be blocked by dose forms.
- Two cases of this are shown in *Figure 11.2*. *Figure 11.2(a)* shows a tablet of pantoprazole (Protonix) 'perched' in the oesophagus of a 57-year-old woman with oesophageal dysmotility and (b) an enteric-coated aspirin tablet, its coating still intact, in an ulcer in the gastric antrum of another patient. In this case as with many others a combination of pathology and dose form conspired to cause a problem.
- The manner in which dosage forms behave in the presence of aqueous media, in the oesophagus or later in the stomach, are varied.
- Simple *in vitro* studies can be illuminating. *Figure 11.3* illustrates the unusual disintegration properties of two tablet formulations, (b) being typical of emepronium bromide tablets (once marketed as Cetiprin) for the treatment of nocturnal enuresis. The tablet is seen to break apart, exposing a core of pure drug, which has surfactant properties as can be seen from its structure (below *Figure 11.3*). In this case the combination of adherence and the presence of a potentially irritant drug is the problem.
- The oesophagus is a primary site for such adverse events, since tablets and capsules will generally not have disintegrated during their oesophageal transit and thus retain their bulk.
- Other drugs that have been reported to cause oesophageal injury are listed in *Table 11.4*.
- Formulations have other effects and influences in modulating or causing adverse events, apart from the influence they have on pharmacokinetics and bioavailability.
- Precipitation of drugs from injection solutions is one prime example. *Figure 11.1* reminds us of others:
  - irritation caused by the adhesives of transdermal patches,
  - corneal irritation from eye drops.

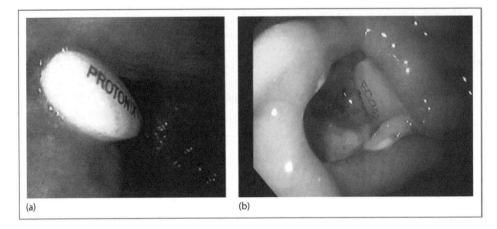

Figure 11.2: *Tablets adhering to the oesophageal mucosa. (a) Pantoprazole (Protonix™). From Singh MK et al. Another reason to dislike medication. Lancet 2008;371:1388. (b) An enteric-coated aspirin tablet with coating still intact within an ulcer of the gastric antrum of a 76-year-old woman. From Levy DJ. An Aspirin Tablet and a Gastric Ulcer. N Engl J Med 2000;343:863.*

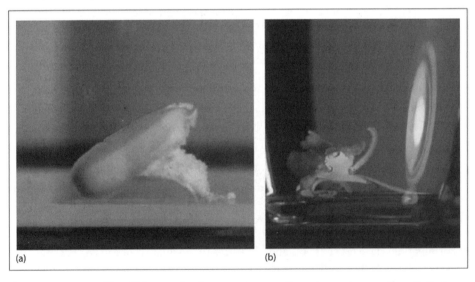

Figure 11.3: *Two tablets disintegrating in an aqueous medium at room temperature. Both show the splitting of the coating layer on the tablets, but (b) shows a now-discontinued tablet of emepronium bromide (Cetiprin) that is unravelling to expose the core of pure drug, irritant to the oesophageal lining. From Florence AT and Salole EG, Formulation Factors in Adverse Reactions. London: Wright., 1990.*

Structure of emopronium bromide, showing its surfactant-like nature.

Table 11.4: *Some drugs that have caused oesophageal injury*

Alendronate	Ferrous salts
Alprenolol	Indometacin
Aspirin	Potassium chloride
Clindamycin	Risendronate
Doxycycline	Tetracycline
Emepronium bromide	Thioridazine

Tear films and eye drops

- Eye drops can disrupt the natural tear film, e.g. through surface-active additives such as benzalkonium chloride (BKC).
- The component surfactant molecules adsorb onto the corneal surface in dry eye syndrome (xerostomia), rendering it more hydrophobic. The tear film can then de-wet the surface exposing the corneal epithelial cells. The process may start at a given point on the corneal surface. The tear film break-up time (BUT) (see *Figure 11.4*) is measured in the clinic and is a useful measure to compare artificial tear fluids or severity of the syndrome of dry eye.

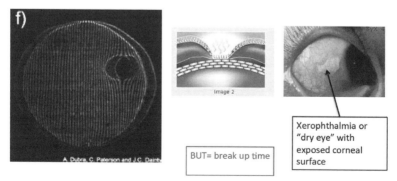

Figure 11.4: *Tear film break up (from L-R) Reproduced with permission from Dubra A et al. Double lateral shearing interferometer for the quantitative measurement of tear film topography. Applied Optics 2005;44(7):1191-1199 © The Optical Society; a diagrammatic representation of the process and a photograph of exposed corneal surface, from a series of which break-up times (BUT) can be assessed.*

Fluoroquinolone eye drops
- Drugs can behave differently in tear fluid depending on their degree of solubility.
- The pH of the tear film for the first 15 minutes after instillation is determined by the pH of each formulation. Rapid precipitation of ciprofloxacin has been seen to occur 8 min after dosing owing to the supersaturation of the drug in the tear fluid, but not so with ofloxacin and norfloxacin whose tear concentrations remain below saturation solubility.
- Such findings may explain the reports of pre-corneal deposits following the use of ciprofloxacin and related drugs.

Reactions to impurities

- Reactions to impurities generally involve breakdown products of the active, which may be initiated by moisture or acidity, excipients or materials leached from containers and packaging.
- Acute sensitivity to penicillins occurs in a minority of patients, although the reaction is well known. Nevertheless, the source of at least some adverse reactions is not always appreciated.
- Impurities in amoxicillin samples can include 2-hydroxy-3-(4-hydroxyphenyl)pyrazine, 4-hydroxyphenylglycine, 4-hydroxyphenylglyclamoxicillin, 6-aminopenicillanic acid, amoxicilloic acid and seven others not including its dimer and trimer. These latter and other oligomers are possibly prime culprits in penicillin allergies as they are formed with peptide bonds and resemble peptides.

Structure of amoxicillin

Delivery devices and materials

- Problems can arise with the materials used in delivery, such as syringes and giving sets, or with the manner in which the device as a whole behaves (system plus active material) as below:
  - Protein aggregation in insulin pumps is accompanied by a significant loss of biological activity.

- — Insulin aggregation (when insulin fibrils form) can occur owing to agitation of the pump during use or to temperature fluctuations.
- — Stability is influenced by the type of insulin, the solvent and concentration.
- — Metal ion contamination has also been implicated and the use of EDTA has been recommended to sequester ions in formulations.
- — Insulin aggregates will at times block delivery channels.
- The diffusion of insulin from sites of administration is important for its activity; retention of insulin and its degradation at the site of deposition might reduce biological activity. Pharmacokinetic differences between different modes of administration might be found.
- Proteins may also degrade physically in pumps: interleukin 2 can lose 90% of its activity over a 24-hour period of infusion. Insulin adsorbs to glass, so that in low concentration formulations free drug levels can be reduced.

Drug eluting stents

- The first drug eluting stents to appear were those with non-biodegradable (or durable) polymer coats as the drug reservoir (see **Chapter 8**).
- Whether so-called durable and biodegradable coated stents are equivalent therapeutically has been debated. There have been concerns that the former may induce inflammation. Biodegradable polymers on stents were suggested to be safer because when degraded the bare metal stent is left, reducing any inflammation caused by the polymer.
- Some adverse effects might be due to the drug involved, such as paclitaxel, and the lactams sirolimus, everolimus, and zotarolimus.
- Sirolimus for example, is formulated in a controlled release polymer. *Figure 11.5* shows the proximity of the polymer-drug layer on a drug eluting stent to the tissues being treated.

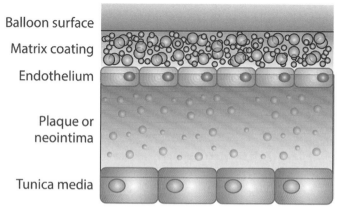

Balloon surface
Matrix coating
Endothelium
Plaque or neointima
Tunica media

Figure 11.5: *Diagram showing the proximity of the polymer drug layer on the stent surface to the endothelial cells, plaque or neointima.*

Transdermal patches as devices

- Transdermal patches can be considered to be devices.
- Adverse reactions have been reported due to the adhesive used in the patches. Allergic contact dermatitis caused by hydroxymethylcellulose has been reported with an estradiol patch.
- Too strong adhesion may lead to pain on removal.
- Cases of burning have been reported when medicated patches containing even small amounts of aluminium are worn during magnetic resonance imaging, a result of overheating of the patch.

Crystallisation

- The situations in which the drug solid state is important clinically include crystalluria and of course the precipitation of drugs before or after injection, and clearly in inhalation therapy (see **Chapter 9**).
- Individual crystals can cause tissue inflammation and large deposits can cause structural changes.
- Aciclovir is a drug that has caused crystalluria. With pK_a values of 2.27 and 9.25 it has a solubility in water at 25°C of >100 mg/mL. At physiological pH, aciclovir sodium is un-ionised and has a minimum solubility in water (at 37°C) of 2.5 mg/mL. However the concentration of aciclovir in human urine after oral administration of 200 mg reaches 7.5 µg/mL, clearly not exceeding its aqueous solubility. So why does the drug precipitate? Urine is concentrated as it passes along nephrons, thus urine drug concentrations increase sometimes to exceed critical concentrations of drug.

Key points

- Knowledge of the solution properties of drugs and the pH at which drugs might precipitate or become saturated in body fluids and compartments is essential if one is to make contributions to patient care using physicochemical principles.
- Biological systems are of course complex. Urine and blood are more complex than water, so simple theories of solution cannot often be applied directly. Nevertheless, theory and applications give clues as to what might be happening *in vivo*. Without them we only guess.

Abnormal bioavailability and adverse events

- Classic examples where the bioavailability of a product has changed after a period when patients have been stabilised and physicians accustomed to responses from a particular dose form or brand, include that of Lanoxin (digoxin). In the 1970s a change in the milling process led to a marked diminution of drug bioavailability through an increase in particle size, resulting from a change in the processing of the drug. When without notice the former process was reintroduced patients titrated on the earlier batches often were overdosed. Some deaths occurred.

- A change in the main excipient in a brand of phenytoin sodium from calcium carbonate to lactose led to a marked increase in bioavailability and overdosing. The calcium was clearly forming a poorly soluble salt of the drug, decreasing its intrinsic solubility and its rate of dissolution. Its removal led to faster absorption and thus toxic effects in patients titrated on the earlier version.
- Other examples of formulation-related effects are discussed in **Chapter 8**.

Testing for adverse effects

How can we become more adept at identifying the causes of adverse effects and reactions related to dosage forms and devices? This depends on:

- a thorough knowledge of the nature of the ingredients and their purpose in the medication concerned
- understanding the nature of the drug substance and its likely interactions with excipients
- understanding the structure of systems such as controlled release preparations
- carrying out straightforward tests to investigate potential problems
- improving the scoring of severity and adopting more quantitative approaches to this.

Contact dermatitis testing

- Contact dermatitis is a skin reaction resulting from exposure to allergens (allergic contact dermatitis) or irritants (irritant contact dermatitis). Phototoxic dermatitis occurs when the allergen or irritant is activated by sunlight. Contact dermatitis can occur from contact with jewellery but also from drugs and devices such as transdermal patch adhesives.
- Suspected contact dermatitis is usually tested for by application of a series of patches containing putative causative agents. The formulation of these materials has often been fairly crude (for example by dispersing nickel sulfate in a paraffin base) and this might affect the outcome. Poor attention to pharmaceutical principles of release, poor choice of vehicle and lack of consideration of particle size all contribute to imprecision.

Photochemical reactions and photoinduced reactions

- There are a variety of light-induced drug effects comprising:
  - Photoallergy: an acquired immunological reactivity dependent on antibody- or cell-mediated hypersensitivity. (Chlorpromazine and promethazine)
  - Photosensitivity: a broad term used to describe an adverse reaction to light after drug administration, which may be photoallergic or phototoxic in nature. (Hexachlorobenzene, chlorophenols)

    — Phototoxicity: the conversion of an otherwise non-toxic chemical or drug to one that is toxic to tissues after absorption of electromagnetic radiation. (Nalidixic acid, Psoralens, Tetracyclines)

    — Photodynamic effects: photoinduced damage requiring the presence of light, photosensitiser and molecular oxygen, and the positive dynamic effect.

    — Photodynamic therapy (PDT): therapy in which photoactive drugs inactive in the unexcited state are administered and activated at particular sites in the body, as discussed below.

- Many drugs decompose *in vitro* after exposure to light, but the consequences depend on the nature of the breakdown products. Some derivatives of nifedipine have a very short photochemical half-life, sometimes of the order of a few minutes, while others decompose only after several weeks' exposure.

- A drug may not decompose after exposure to light, but may be the source of free radicals or of phototoxic metabolites *in vivo*. Adverse reactions occur when the drug or metabolites are exposed to light and the absorption spectrum of the drug coincides with the wavelength of light to which it is exposed (the wavelengths of UV-A are 320–400 nm; of UV-B 280–320 nm; and of UV-C 200–290 nm).

- To behave as a photoallergen, a drug or chemical must be able to absorb light energy present in sunlight and on absorption of the light generate a chemical species capable of binding to proteins in the skin, either directly or after metabolism.

Photodynamic therapy (PDT)

- Porfimer sodium (Photofrin) is a photosensitising drug used in photodynamic therapy and radiation therapy in various carcinomas.

- The cautions given in the *British National Formulary* for porfimer are to 'avoid exposure of the skin to direct sunlight or bright indoor light for at least 30 days', and for the related drug temoporfin 'for at least 15 days.' Avoid prolonged exposure of the injection site to direct sunlight for 6 months after administration.

Chemical photosensitivity

- In chemical photosensitivity, patients develop redness, inflammation, and sometimes brown or blue discoloration in areas of skin that have been exposed to sunlight for a brief period.

- This reaction occurs after ingestion of drugs such as tetracycline, or the application of compounds topically in consumer products such as perfumes or aftershaves. These substances (*Table 11.5*) may make some skin more sensitive to the effects of ultraviolet (UV) light. Some develop hives with itching, which indicates a type of drug allergy triggered by sunlight.

Table 11.5: *Some substances that sensitise skin to sunlight*

Type	Examples
Anxiolytics	Alprazolam, chlordiazepoxide
Antibiotics	Quinolones, sulfonamides, tetracyclines, trimethoprim
Antidepressants	Tricyclics
Antifungals (oral)	Griseofulvin
Antihypertensives	Sulfonylureas
Antimalarials	Chloroquine, quinine
Antipsychotics	Phenothiazines
Diuretics	Furosemide, thiazides
Chemotherapeutics	Dacarbazine, fluorouracil, methotrexate, vinblastine
Antiacne drugs (oral)	Isotretinoin
Cardiovascular drugs	Amiodarone, quinidine
Skin preparations	Chlorhexidine, hexachlorophene, coal tar, fragrances, sunscreens

Nanosystems and new biological entities

- Undoubtedly adverse effects will arise from the use of nanosytems (**Chapter 13**). Much has still to be learned about the toxicity of nanomedicines; further assurances are needed *inter alia* on the safety of the materials from which they are made.
- Each system will have to be examined and tested. One can rarely generalise.
- New biological entities such as monoclonal antibodies and stem cells are not without some adverse clinical effects but to date there is not the possibility to interpret all of these.

Conclusions

The determination or, better, the prediction of potential adverse reactions is an important and sometimes complex task. It requires:
- constant attention to the clinical literature
- knowledge of the chemistry of offending drugs or drugs in the same chemical class and pharmacological class
- familiarity with the potential influence of the formulation and its physical form
- awareness of the potential of excipients to act biologically and physically
- understanding the mechanisms of events - if possible
- searching for trends and patterns, and analogies in a quest for prediction and assignment of cause in cases of adverse reactions and adverse events.

Distractors such as the placebo effect and the nocebo effect complicate practice. Placebo effects are those reported by patients after receiving a drug-free dosage form, as in a clinical trial. Nocebo effects are those reported by patients who believe that their medicine has changed when it is in fact identical to their previous medication. These are false trails. The final figure (*Figure 11.6*) below charts the many causes of the events discussed in this chapter.

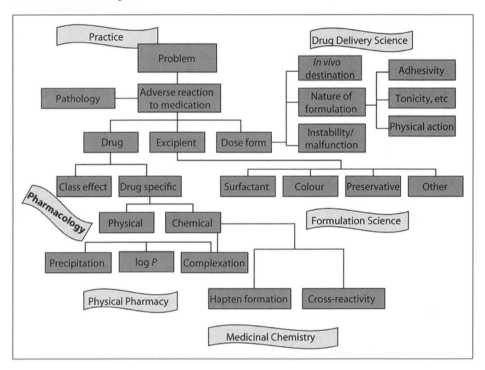

Figure 11.6: *Charting the causes of adverse reactions to medications. The many causes are shown in relation to drug, excipient, nature of formulation, the dosage form or device and their nature.*

Memory map

Sources of adverse reactions and events from delivery systems

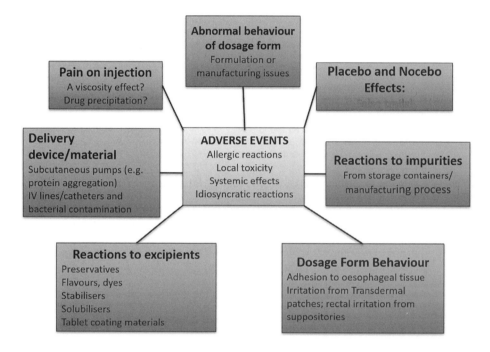

Questions

1. Which of the following are true in relation to biological effects of non-ionic surfactants?

   A: They may at higher concentrations damage biomembranes by interacting with lipid membrane components

   B: Evidence of their side effects completely precludes their use in all formulations

   C: Inhibition of p-glycoprotein dependent drug absorption will increase drug levels

   D: All non-ionic surfactants behave in the same general manner

2. Which of the following in relation to oesophageal injury are correct?

   A: Emepronium bromide, tetracycline and indomethacin have all been implicated

   B: The cause of the effect is always adhesion of a solid dose form to the oesophageal tissue

   C: A potential cause is oesophageal dysmobility in the patient

   D: Perforation of the oesophagus has been observed in extreme cases

   E: Excipients may play a part in the injury

3. Which of the following are true in connection with adverse reactions with ophthalmic drug delivery?

   A: Eye drops can disrupt the natural tear film

   B: One cause of such an effect can be due to the effect of benzalkonium chloride due to its surfactant properties

   C: Amoxicillin eye drops can cause sensitivity and allergies due to the presence of protein-like oligomers

   D: The pH of the treated tear film remains constant due to buffering effects

   E: The solubility of administered drugs may be exceeded in tear fluid

4. Light-induced reaction may be implicated in adverse effects. Which of the following are correct?

   A: Photoxicity involves the conversion of a non-toxic chemical into a toxic form after absorption of electromagnetic radiation

   B: Photosensitivities arise from phototoxic or photoallergic reactions

   C: Drugs may not decompose after exposure to light and thus will not produce adverse effects

   D: Photoallergenic materials not only absorb light energy from sunlight but generate chemicals which bind to skin proteins

   E: Drugs given orally cannot cause skin allergies as a result of chemical photosensitivity

5. Adverse reaction to administered medicines can arise from which of the following?

   A: Reactions to enteric coating materials

   B: Irritation due to adhesives in transdermal patches

   C: Pain on administration of viscous injections

   D: The nature of suppository vehicles

   E: Low bioavailability of oral dose forms

   F: Precipitation of drugs in the GI tract

6. **Which of the following are classified as adverse drug reactions?**
   A: Synergistic effects caused by two drugs administered together
   B: Responses observed when the dose of a drug is increased to achieve a certain outcome
   C: Chemical interaction between two drugs used to treat the same symptoms
   D: When the causality of an event is not known
   E: The effect of impurities in the product concerned

CHAPTER 12

Peptides, proteins and monoclonal antibodies

LEARNING OBJECTIVES

Upon completion of this chapter you should be aware of:
- some of the basic properties of peptides and proteins and understand how their physical properties are dictated not only by the properties of their individual amino acids but also by the spatial arrangement of the amino acids in their polypeptide chains
- the physical and chemical stability of protein pharmaceuticals and formulation procedures for their stabilisation
- the formulation and properties of some therapeutic proteins and peptides and of DNA
- some aspects of therapeutic monoclonal antibodies; and
- the issues in the delivery of proteins, peptides and monoclonal antibodies occasioned by their molecular size, physical properties and stability.

Structure and solution properties of peptides and proteins

Definitions

Peptide: a short chain of amino acid residues with a defined sequence (e.g. leucoproteins).

Proteins: polypeptides which occur naturally and have a defined sequence of amino acids and a three-dimensional structure (e.g. insulin).

Key points

- Most peptides and proteins are not absorbed to any significant extent by the oral route and most available formulations of protein pharmaceuticals are therefore parenteral products for injection or inhalation.
- DNA, RNA and various oligonucleotides are increasingly used in gene therapy. These share some of the problems of proteins as therapeutic agents.

Structure of peptides and proteins

Proteins have in increasing order of complexity (*Figure 12.1*):

- Primary structure – the order in which the individual amino acids are arranged.
- Secondary structures – including coiled α-helix and pleated sheets.
- Tertiary structure – the three-dimensional arrangement of helices and coils.
- Quaternary forms – the association of ternary forms (e.g. the hexameric form of insulin).

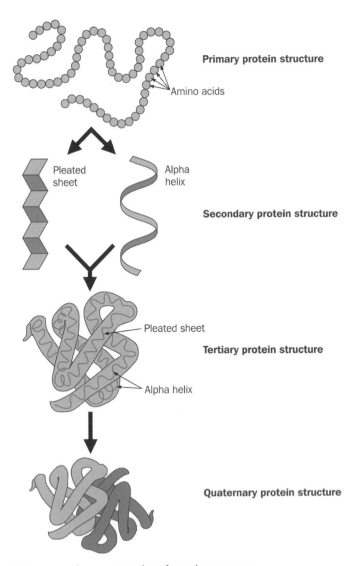

Figure 12.1: *Diagrammatic representation of protein structure.*

> **Key point**
>
> Loss of the unique tertiary or quaternary structure, through denaturation, can occur from a variety of insults that would not affect smaller organic molecules. Formulations must be designed to preserve the protein structure.

Hydrophobicity of peptides and proteins

- Amino acids have a range of physical properties, each having a greater or lesser degree of hydrophilic or hydrophobic nature.
- If amino acids are spatially arranged in a molecule so that distinct hydrophobic and hydrophilic regions appear, then the polypeptide or protein will have an amphiphilic nature.

> **Definition**
>
> **Polypeptide**: a longer amino acid chain, usually of defined sequence and length (e.g. vasopressin).

Solubility of peptides and proteins

- The aqueous solubilities of proteins vary enormously, from the very soluble to the virtually insoluble.
- The solubility of globular proteins increases as the pH of the solution moves away from the isoelectric point (IP), which is the pH at which the molecule has a net zero charge (*Figure 12.2*).
- At its IP a protein has a tendency to self-associate.
- As the net charge increases, the affinity of the protein for the aqueous environment increases and the protein molecules also exert a greater electrostatic repulsion.
- Proteins are surrounded by a hydration layer, equivalent to about $0.3\,g\ H_2O$ per gram of protein (about 2 water molecules per amino acid residue).
- Aqueous solutions of proteins sometimes exhibit phase transitions (*Figure 12.3*). The phase behaviour of protein solutions is affected by pH and ionic strength.
- Addition of electrolytes such as NaCl, KCl and $(NH_4)_2SO_4$ decreases solubility.
- At high ionic strengths proteins precipitate – a salting-out effect.
- Organic solvents tend to decrease the solubility of proteins by lowering solvent dielectric constant.

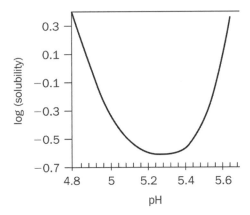

Figure 12.2: *A plot of the logarithm of aqueous solubility of β-lactoglobulin versus pH.*

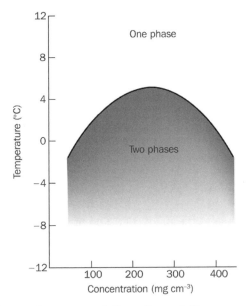

Figure 12.3: *Phase diagram for aqueous solutions of γ-crystallin.*

The stability of proteins and peptides

> **Key points**
>
> Protein pharmaceuticals can suffer both physical and chemical instability:
> - Physical instability results from changes in the higher-order structure (secondary and above).
> - Chemical instability is modification of the protein via bond formation or cleavage.

Physical instability

Denaturation
- Is the disruption of the tertiary and secondary structure of the protein molecule.
- Can be reversible or irreversible:
  - It is reversible if the native structure is regained, for example on decreasing the temperature when temperature has caused the initial changes.
  - It is irreversible when the unfolding process is such that the native structure cannot be regained.

Aggregation
- Some proteins self-associate in aqueous solution to form oligomers.
- Insulin, for example, exists in several states:
  - The zinc hexamer of insulin is a complex of insulin and zinc which slowly dissolves into dimers and eventually monomers following subcutaneous administration, so giving it long-acting properties.

Surface adsorption and precipitation
- Adsorption of proteins such as insulin can occur on surfaces such as glass or plastic in giving sets therefore:
  - reducing the amount of agent reaching the patient
  - leading to further denaturation, which can then cause precipitation and the physical blocking of delivery ports e.g. in protein pumps.
- Denaturation is facilitated by the presence of a large headspace in the container allowing a greater interaction of proteins with the air–water interface.

Formulation and protein stabilisation

Stability testing
- Stability testing of protein-containing formulations often involves subjecting the solutions to shaking for several hours and the subsequent assessment of the protein configuration.

Improving the physical stability of proteins through formulation

Prevention of adsorption
- Additives can be used either to coat the surface of glass or bind to the proteins to prevent adsorption.
- Serum albumin can be included in the formulation to compete with the therapeutic protein for the binding sites on glass and thus reduce adsorption.
- A similar effect can be achieved by the addition of surfactants such as poloxamers and polysorbates to the protein solution.

Minimisation of exposure to air
- Significant denaturation of proteins can occur when protein solutions are exposed at the air–solution interface.
- Agitation of protein solutions in the presence of air or application of other shear forces (e.g. in filters or pumps) may lead to denaturation.
- The inclusion of surfactants can reduce denaturation arising from these processes.

Addition of cosolvents
- Some excipients and buffer components added to the protein solution are able to minimise denaturation through their effects on solvation.
- These include polyethylene glycols and glycerol, and are referred to as cosolvents.
- These act either by causing the preferential hydration of the protein or alternatively by preferential binding to the protein surface (*Figure 12.4*):
  - Preferential hydration results from an exclusion of the cosolvent from the protein surface due to steric effects (as in the case of polyethylene glycols) or surface tension effects (as with sugars, salts and amino acids). As a result more water molecules pack around the protein in order to exclude the additive and the protein becomes fully hydrated and stabilised in a compact form.
  - Alternatively, the cosolvent may stabilise the protein molecule by preferentially binding to it either non-specifically or to specific sites on its surface.

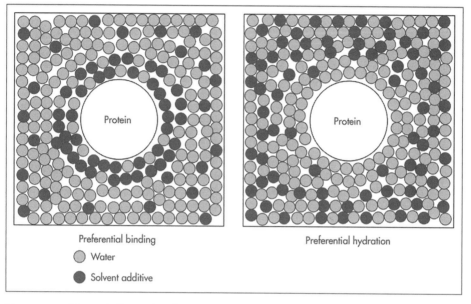

Figure 12.4: *Schematic illustration of preferential binding and preferential hydration by solvent additives. In preferential binding the additive occurs in the solvation shell of the protein at a greater local concentration than in the bulk solvent, while preferential hydration results from the exclusion of the additive from the surface of the protein. Reproduced with permission from Timasheff SN, Arakawa T. In: Creighton TE (ed.)* Protein Structure: A Practical Approach. *Oxford: IRL Press; 1989: 331–345.*

Optimimisation of pH
- To avoid stability problems arising from charge neutralisation and to ensure adequate solubility, a pH must be selected which is at least 0.5 pH units above or below the IP.
- Since a pH range of 5–7 is usually required to minimise chemical breakdown, this frequently coincides with the IP.

Characterisation of degradation
- If the formulation does not prevent denaturation and aggregation of the protein, then the pharmacology, immunogenicity and toxicology of the denatured or aggregated protein must be studied to determine its safety and efficacy.
- If the aggregates are soluble there may be a significant effect on the pharmacokinetics and immunogenicity of the protein.
- Insoluble aggregates are generally unacceptable.

Chemical instability

Deamidation
In deamidation the side-chain linkage in a glutamine (Gln) or asparagine (Asn) residue is hydrolysed to form a free carboxylic acid.

Prevention of deamidation

- If the deamidation occurs by a general acid–base mechanism then the optimum pH for a peptide formulation will usually be about 6, where both rates are at their minimum.
- If the deamidation occurs through the cyclic imide intermediate it is preferable to formulate at a low pH since this type of deamidation is base-catalysed.

Oxidation

- Oxidation is one of the major causes of protein degradation.
- The side chains of histidine (His), methionine (Met), cysteine (Cys), tryptophan (Trp) and tyrosine (Tyr) residues in proteins are potential oxidation sites.
- Methionine is very susceptible to oxidation and reacts with a variety of oxidants to give methionine sulfoxide ($RS(OO)CH_3$) or, in highly oxidative conditions, methionine sulfone ($RS(O)CH_3$).
- The thiol group of cysteine readily reacts with oxygen to yield, successively, sulfenic acid (RSOH), a disulfide (RSSH), a sulfinic acid (RSO_2H) and, finally, a sulfonic (cystic) acid (RSO_3H) depending on reaction conditions.
- An important factor determining the extent of oxidation is the spatial positioning of the thiol groups in the proteins.
- Histidine is susceptible to oxidation in the presence of metals, primarily by reaction with singlet oxygen, and this constitutes a major cause of enzyme degradation.
- Both histidine and tryptophan are highly susceptible to photooxidation.

Prevention of oxidation

- In most cases oxidation results in a complete or partial loss of activity.
- Minimising protein oxidation is essential for maintaining the biological activity of most proteins and avoiding the immunogenic response caused by degraded proteins.
- A variety of measures may be employed in order to prevent protein oxidation:
  - Temperature reduction, either by refrigeration or by freezing.
  - Control of pH if the rate of oxidation is pH-dependent.

Racemisation

All amino acid residues except glycine (Gly) are chiral at the carbon atom bearing the side chain and are subject to base-catalysed racemisation.

Proteolysis

Proteolysis involves the cleavage of peptide (–CO–NH–) bonds:

- Asp is the residue most susceptible in proteolysis.
- The cleavage of the peptide bonds in dilute acid proceeds at a rate at least 100 times that of other peptide bonds.

Beta-elimination

High-temperature treatment of proteins leads to destruction of disulfide bonds as a result of β-elimination from the cysteine residue:

- The inactivation of proteins at high temperatures is often due to β-elimination of disulfides from the cysteine residue.
- Other amino acids, including Ser, Thr, Phe and Lys, can also be degraded via β-elimination.
- The inactivation is particularly rapid under alkaline conditions and is also influenced by metal ions.

Disulfide formation

The interchange of disulfide bonds can result in incorrect pairings with consequent changes of three-dimensional structure and loss of catalytic activity.

Accelerated stability testing of protein formulations

- The mechanisms of degradation at higher temperatures may not be the same as at lower temperatures and the application of the Arrhenius equation in the prediction of protein stability will be more uncertain than with small-molecule drugs.
- Deviation from the Arrhenius equation occurs, however, if the protein exists in multiple conformational forms that retain activity during unfolding.

Protein formulation and delivery

Protein and peptide transport

- It can be shown that, for a series of 11 model peptides in an *in vitro* intestinal cell monolayer system, there is a good correlation between the permeability coefficient, P, and the log of the partition coefficient of the peptides between heptane and ethylene glycol (rather than octanol and water).
- Molecular volume (or size) will increasingly be a factor influencing transport as the molecular weight of the peptide increases.
- The rate of translational movement depends on the size of the molecule, its shape and interactions with solvent molecules.

Tips

- The rate of translational movement is often expressed by a frictional coefficient, f, defined in relation to the diffusion coefficient, D, by:

  $f = k_B\, T/D$

  where k_B is the Boltzmann constant and T is the absolute temperature.
- Many proteins are nearly spherical in solution but if their shape deviates from sphericity this is reflected in a frictional ratio, f/f_0, above unity, where f_0 is the rate of diffusion of a molecule of the same size but of spherical shape.
- The frictional ratio of lysozyme is 1.24, and trypsin 1.187, compared to globular proteins, which have values of f/f_0 in the range of 1.05–1.38.

Lyophilised proteins

- Proteins such as insulin, tetanus toxoid, somatotropin and human albumin aggregate in the presence of moisture, which can lead to reduced activity, stability and diffusion.
- Because of their potential instability in solution, therapeutic proteins are often formulated as lyophilised powders.
- Even in this state several suffer from moisture-induced aggregation.

Controlled delivery of proteins and peptides

A wide range of biodegradable polymers are used for the controlled delivery of proteins and peptides, including:

- natural substances, starch, alginates, collagen
- a variety of proteins such as cross-linked albumin
- a range of synthetic hydrogels, polyanhydrides, polyesters or orthoesters, poly(amino acids) and poly(caprolactones). Poly(lactide-glycolide) is one of the commonest polymers used in microsphere form to deliver proteins and peptides.

Tip

Lyophilisation is a method of drying proteins without destroying their physical structure. The protein solution is frozen and then warmed in a vacuum so that the ice sublimes.

Definition

Poly(amino acids): random sequences of varying lengths, generally resulting from non-specific polymerisation of one or more amino acids (e.g. glatiramer).

Routes of delivery

Invasive and non-invasive routes of delivery for peptides and proteins involve direct injection of solutions, depot systems and a variety of nasal, inhalation, topical and other formulations.

Therapeutic proteins and peptides

Some examples of therapeutic proteins and peptides, including their size and use or action, are given in *Table 12.1*.

Table 12.1: *Some therapeutic proteins and peptides, their molecular weights and use/ actions*

Protein/peptide	Size (kDa)	Use/action
Oxytocin	1.0	Uterine contraction
Vasopressin	1.1	Diuresis
Leuprolide acetate	1.3	Prostatic carcinoma therapy
LHRH analogues	~1.5	Prostatic carcinoma therapy
Somatostatin	3.1	Growth inhibition
Calcitonin	3.4	Ca^{2+} regulation
Glucagon	3.5	Diabetes therapy
Parathyroid hormone (1–34)	4.3	Ca^{2+} regulation
Insulin	6	Diabetes therapy
Parathyroid hormone (1–84)	9.4	Ca^{2+} regulation
Interferon-gamma	16 (dimer)	Antiviral agent
TNF-α	17.5 (trimer)	Antitumour agent
Interferon α-2	19	Leukaemia, hepatitis therapy
Interferon β-1	20	Lung cancer therapy
Growth hormone	22	Growth acceleration
DNase	~32	Cystic fibrosis therapy
α₁-Antitrypsin	45	Cystic fibrosis therapy
Albumin	68	Plasma volume expander
Bovine IgG	150	Immunisation
Catalase	230	Treatment of wounds and ulcers
Cationic ferritin	400+	Anaemias

LHRH, luteinising hormone-releasing hormone; TNF-α, tumour necrosis factor-α; IgG, immunoglobin G. Reproduced from Niven RW. Pharm Technol 1993; July: 72.

Insulin

There are three main types of insulin preparation:

1. Those with a short duration of action which have a relatively rapid onset (soluble insulin, insulin lispro and insulin aspart).
2. Those with an intermediate action (isophane insulin and insulin zinc suspension).
3. Those with a slower/slow action, in onset and lasting for long periods (crystalline insulin zinc suspension).

Precipitation of insulin and other proteins

- Precipitation of insulin in pumps due to the formation of amorphous particles, crystals or fibrils of insulin can lead to changes in release pattern.
- 'Amorphous' or 'crystalline' precipitates can be caused by the leaching of divalent metal contaminants or lowering of pH (due to CO_2 diffusion or leaching of acidic substances).
- Interactions leading to fibril formation result from change in monomer conformation and hydrophilic attraction of the parallel β-sheet forms.
- Fibril formation is also encouraged by contact of the insulin solution with hydrophobic surfaces.
- Chemical modifications to an endogenous protein, however minor, can lead to significant differences in properties and activity.
- Recombinant human protein analogues may be subtly different.
- There is as yet no simple way to predict the consequence of subtle changes in structure.

Calcitonin

- Calcitonin, a peptide hormone of 32 amino acids, has a regulatory function in calcium and phosphorus metabolism and is therefore used in various bone disorders such as osteoporosis.
- Salmon, human, pig and eel calcitonin are used therapeutically to regulate levels of calcium in the blood.
- Source species differences may be significant – salmon calcitonin is 10 times more potent than human calcitonin.
- Human calcitonin has a tendency to associate rapidly in solution and, like insulin, forms fibrils, resulting in a viscous solution. The fibrils are 8 nm in diameter and often associate with one another.

DNA and oligonucleotides

DNA

- DNA of varying molecular weights (base pairs) is used in gene therapy.
- As a large hydrophilic, polyanionic and sensitive macromolecule, successful delivery to target cells and the nucleus within these cells is an issue.
- Shearing of high-molecular-weight DNA while stirring in solution can lead to breakdown of the molecule.
- One approach to delivery is to complex the DNA with polymers or particles of opposite charge to produce more compact species.
- DNA can be condensed to form nanoparticles with cationic polymers (such as polylysine and chitosan), cationic liposomes and dendrimers. These retain an overall positive charge and are able to transfect cells more readily than native or naked DNA.

Oligonucleotides

- Antisense oligonucleotides (used for the sequence-specific inhibition of gene expression) are polyanionic molecules with between 10 and 25 nucleotides, which resemble single-stranded DNA or RNA.
- They have molecular weights ranging from 3000 to 8000 Da and are hydrophilic, having a log P of approximately -3.5.
- Like DNA, they clearly do not have the appropriate properties for transfer across biological membranes.
- They are also sensitive to nucleases and non-specific adsorption to biological surfaces.

Monoclonal antibodies

An increasing number of antibodies produced from a single clone of cells (monoclonal antibodies, MAbs) are now in clinical use (see *Table 12.2*). *Figure 12.5* shows their general structure.

- The nomenclature of therapeutic antibodies has been devised so that the name of individual MAbs transmits information on their cell source and their therapeutic use.
- *Figure 12.6* shows some examples.

Table 12.2: *Some of the MAbs marketed for clinical use*

Antibody	Trade name	Primary indication
Adalimumab	Humira	Rhumatoid arthritis
Bevacizumab	Avastin	Colorectal, lung, breast cancer
Certolizumab pegol	Cimzia	Crohn's disease
Ranibizumab	Lucentis	Macular degeneration
Tositumab	Bexxar	Non-Hodgkin's lymphoma
Trastuzumab	Herceptin	Breast cancer

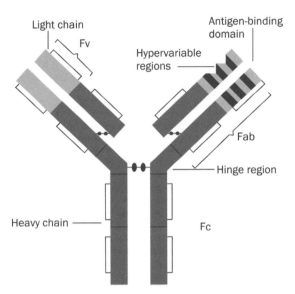

Figure 12.5: *Diagrammatic representation of a monoclonal antibody showing the complex nature of the high-molecular-weight molecule with its light and heavy chains and the important antigen-binding domain.*

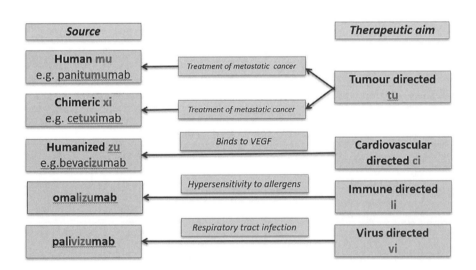

Figure 12.6: *Aspects of monoclonal antibody nomenclature – source and therapy. Guidelines for nomenclature are changing see e.g. Manis JP. Overview of therapeutic monoclonal antibodies. Available at https://www.uptodate.com/contents/overview-of-therapeutic-monoclonal-antibodies.*

There are facets of this class of therapeutic agents that are shared with other macromolecular agents, not least that:

- Their poor biodistribution and tissue penetration is due principally to their large molecular size.
- MAbs have molecular weights of the order of 150 kDa and thus they diffuse slowly in tissues, and especially in tumours or inflamed sites.
- The intravenous route has been commonly used for their delivery, so formulation has often concentrated on the development of stable solutions.
- Absorption following i.m. or s.c. administration is slow and in some cases it is dose dependent.
- Physical chemistry can explain in part their mechanism of action, which includes (a) blocking the action of target antigens, or (b) binding to an antigen.
- Typical MAbs include:
  - the anti-HER2 monoclonal antibody trastuzumab (Herceptin) for breast cancer
  - the anti-CD20 monoclonal antibody rituximab (Rituxan) for malignant lymphoma.
- Antibodies with a molecular size larger than 150 kDa are prevented from passage through the blood–brain barrier.
- The cerebrospinal fluid level of rituximab in patients is reported to be only 0.1% of that of serum levels.
- Many monoclonal antibodies are low-potency molecules in spite of their specificity. Doses are in the range of mg/kg by the i.v. or s.c. routes.
- Many MAbs have a short *in vivo* half-life.
- Pegylation can enhance MAb circulation, as with certolizumab pegol, a pegylated derivative of a recombinant humanised FAb′ fragment.
- When the s.c. route is used it is necessary to inject concentrated solutions to reduce the volume of injection administered.
- Concentrated solutions can be viscous and the antibodies are prone to aggregation. Even small amounts of silicone oil used as lubricant for syringes can lead to antibody aggregation.
- The production processes of monoclonal antibodies for clinical use are complex. These involve several key steps each with a degree of variability which leads to small molecular differences in products, which in turn leads to the nomenclature used in comparing products from different manufacturers not as bioequivalent but 'biosimilar'.
- Biosimilarity means that the product has the same mechanism of action in the medical condition for which the originator product was approved, and the same route of administration, dose form and strength.
- Biosimilars can be safely substituted for the reference product.

Factors affecting degradation of MAbs

- The factors below influence the production, storage and handling of these agents:
  - Temperature
  - Freezing
  - pH extremes

- — Surfactants
- — Pressure/Shearing
- — Light
- — Metals
- — Interfaces (MAbs interact with surfaces e.g. of containers, syringes and tubing).
- ● Many of the above influences can be predicted from our knowledge of the behaviour of proteins.

Antibody–drug conjugates (ADCs) in anticancer therapy (*Figure 12.7*)

- ● An ADC comprises of an antibody linked to a cytotoxic drug via a linker.
- ● The ADC is delivered intravenously and localises by binding to tumour-specific antigens.
- ● After internalisation, proteases and hydrolases digest the antibody and linker to release free drug.
- ● The drug then should bind to its molecular target, leading to apoptosis.

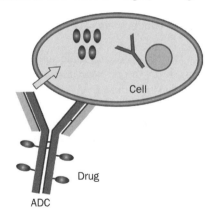

Antibody–Drug Conjugate (ADC)

Figure 12.7: *A diagram of a monoclonal antibody–drug complex (ADC) showing the drug which is carried to the target by the monoclonal antibody (MAb). Note that the physical properties of the MAb are altered considerably by the attached drug molecules.*

Memory maps

Aspects of injectable protein and macromolecule formulations

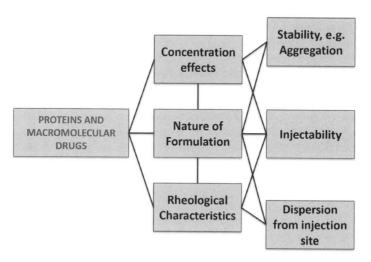

Physical modes of protein degradation, causes and consequences

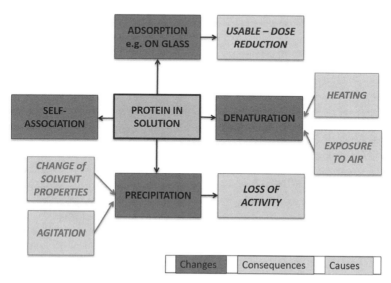

Chemical aspects of protein instability

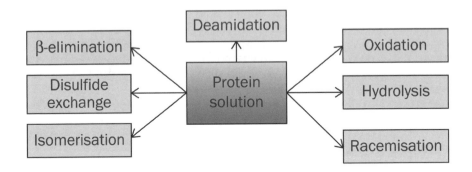

Differentiation between low molecular weight drugs and monoclonal antibodies

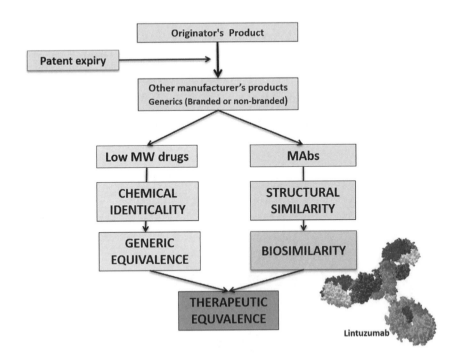

Questions

1. Indicate which of the following statements are true. The solubility of globular proteins:
   A: Is minimum at the IP
   B: Decreases when the dielectric constant of the solvent is decreased
   C: Is increased by addition of electrolytes
   D: Is independent of pH
   E: Is higher in organic solvents than in water

2. Indicate which of the following statements are true. Denaturation of proteins:
   A: Is the result of disruption of the tertiary and secondary structure
   B: Occurs more readily in the presence of cosolvents such as glycerol
   C: Cannot be reversed
   D: Can be caused by agitation of protein solutions in the presence of air
   E: Is increased by the presence of surfactants in the solution

3. Indicate which of the following statements are true. The surface adsorption of proteins:
   A: Can be reduced by including serum albumin in the formulation
   B: Is increased when surfactants are present in the formulation
   C: Can be prevented by using plastic containers
   D: Can lead to protein denaturation
   E: Can be minimised by reducing the headspace in the container

4. Indicate which of the following statements relating to the properties of insulin are true. Insulin can:
   A: Associate in aqueous solution to form oligomers
   B: Form amorphous or crystalline precipitates at high pH
   C: Form fibrils due to the hydrophobic attraction of the parallel β-sheet forms
   D: Form fibrils on contact with hydrophobic surfaces
   E: Be formulated as an insulin zinc suspension to give rapid onset of action

CHAPTER 13

Pharmaceutical nanotechnology

LEARNING OBJECTIVES

Upon completion of this chapter you should be able to:
- outline the characteristics of nanosystems and the rationale for the design of nanoparticles for drug delivery and targeting
- understand the influence of particle size on the properties and behaviour of nanoparticles
- outline the methods used to prepare nanoparticulate systems
- outline the physicochemical properties determining the fate of nanoparticles.
- appreciate the complexity of the behaviour of nanoparticles *in vivo*.

Introduction

- Pharmaceutical nanotechnology is concerned with the preparation and processing of systems with dimensions ranging from several nanometres to around 100–150 nm that are designed as carriers for drugs and other actives, their characterisation, their applications and biological evaluation. When drugs are encapsulated in, or attached to, nanoparticles the fate of the particles determines to a large extent the fate of the drug. Colloid science (see **Chapter 6**) and nanotechnology overlap considerably as nanoparticles are colloids.
- Examples of pharmaceutical nanosystems include:
  - Surfactant or polymer micelles used for solubilising drugs have diameters of about 1–3 nm.
  - Microemulsions (nanoemulsions), comprising droplets in the size range of 10–100 nm.
  - Nano-sized carrier systems include nanoparticles formed from polymers or lipids, nanosuspensions of poorly soluble drugs, dendrimers, fullerenes and carbon nanotubes as well as the smallest liposomes.
- Nanosystems can be divided into two types:
  - Soft systems include nanoemulsions and polymeric micelles. These can deform and reform, and are thus better able to navigate constricted capillary beds and tissue extracellular spaces.
  - Hard systems include polymeric nanoparticles, nanosuspensions or nanocrystals, dendrimers and carbon nanotubes. These are neither flexible nor elastic and may block spaces and fenestrae that have similar dimensions as the particles.

- Physiochemical characterisation of nanosystems includes investigation of:
  - drug loading capacity
  - drug release rate
  - chemical and physical stability of both drug and carrier
  - particle size and shape
  - flexibility or elasticity of particles
  - surface charge and character (whether the surface is hydrophilic or hydrophobic).
- Biological evaluation of nanosystems involves knowledge of:
  - the absorption, distribution and excretion of both the drug and the carrier along with its load of encapsulated or attached drug
  - the mode and speed of the biodegradation of the nanoparticle.
- The main areas of focus of pharmaceutical nanotechnology are summarised in *Figure 13.1*.

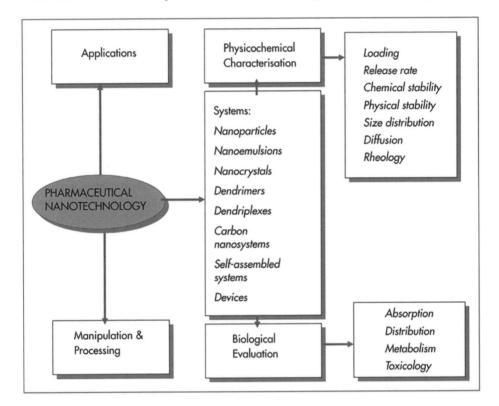

Figure 13.1: *Pharmaceutical nanotechnology's main areas of focus, namely, applications, manipulation and processing, physicochemical characterisation and biological evaluation. An understanding of the relevance of the physicochemical properties of these systems and biological barriers and environments they encounter is essential. Absorption, distribution, metabolism and toxicology refer to both the drug once released from the delivery system and the delivery system itself, the two being intertwined.*

Nanoparticles for drug delivery and targeting

Challenges in targeting

- There are many potential advantages and exciting opportunities in deploying nanocarriers to achieve, for example, enhanced accumulation in particular pathological sites.
- It should be noted, however, that such efforts have led to date to not more than 5–10% accumulation of nanoparticles in tumour sites. This translates to often very low drug levels as nanoparticles cannot be comprised of drug alone. This presents three main challenges involving:
  - the compatibility of drugs, macromolecules and proteins with the materials that make up the nanosystems,
  - ensuring the optimal timing and rate of release of the encapsulated drug, and
  - the changing physical and genetic nature of tumours as they grow and the biological complexities of other targets. That is, the target is a moving target.

Rationale and design

The rationale for the encapsulation of drugs in nanoparticles or their adsorption onto the surface of nanoparticles is:

- To transport the active molecules to the required site of action, e.g. the liver or spleen, or tumours in various organs.
- To protect the active molecules from the external environment until such time as they are released, when they then behave as free drug molecules.
- To modify the pharmacokinetics of the active by its slow release from the carrier and its trajectory, which may lead to reduction in toxicity.

It is important to design and formulate systems which are stable *in vitro* but which can also survive dilution in blood, mixing and shearing forces in flow. Particular issues include:

- Compatibility of drug and carrier system – vital to the even distribution of drug throughout the nanoparticle and to avoid premature release, which occurs when the drug migrates to the particle surface.
- Loading of the drug into the particles depends not only on the nature of the drug but also on the nature of the carrier material.
- The intravenous route results in mixing of the nanoformulation with blood, perhaps particle adsorption onto erythrocytes, opsonisation (which is the adsorption of the proteins or opsonins onto the surface of the nanoparticles which then cause the particles to be recognised as foreign and taken up by the liver and spleen), and partial escape from the circulation by extravasation.
- Positive interaction with target receptors.

Application of nanoparticles in drug delivery

- Nanoparticles can potentially be used to deliver drugs, genes and radiolabels by a variety of routes – ocular, oral, intravenous, intraperitoneal, intraluminal, subcutaneous, intramuscular, nasal, respiratory and intratumoural.
- Nanoparticles carrying radioactive agents may also be used to aid diagnosis and to locate tumours; some may carry therapeutic agents and are termed 'theranostics'.
- Administration of empty carriers (for example liposomes) may be a method of absorbing excess drug in the circulation as a means of detoxification.
- To be successful therapeutically, systems must:
  - have optimal size and surface characteristics
  - have a narrow size distribution; size polydispersity complicates the achievement of targeting because particles of different sizes have potentially different fates
  - have a high loading capacity efficiency
  - have a high degree of chemical and physical stability
  - have appropriate release characteristics at the target site
  - be biodegradable and biocompatible.
- Not all drug (active)–polymer (carrier) combinations can be readily formulated, because of
  - the low affinity of the drug for the carrier, or
  - incompatibility between drug and carrier: for example, proteins do not always mix with polymers without phase separation. Formulations where drug and carrier material do not produce an isotropic mixture or where the production process (e.g. drying) leads to a movement of drug towards the surface of the particles often show undesirable burst release of drug.

Particle structures

- The general features of systems for selective delivery of drugs to cells, organs and tissues are drawn in *Figure 13.2*, which summarises the complex structural nature of such a nanoparticulate system comprising eight aspects of design, namely:
  1. Nature of the interior space
  2. Nature of the shell
  3. Nature of the surface
  4. Interior payload levels
  5. Shell payload level
  6. Surface payload
  7. Surface coating
  8. Targeting ligands.
- It may be that the particle is solid, formed from a single polymer without a shell. What is then important is the distribution of the drug throughout the system.

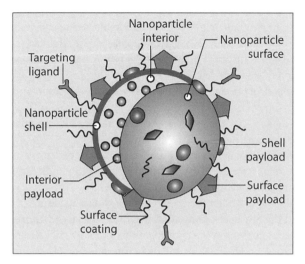

Figure 13.2: *General elements of nanoparticles designed for targeting, using targeting ligands to interact with appropriate receptors on target cells or tissues. Surface coatings are used to modify nanoparticle behaviour in vivo. Interior, surface or shell-based payloads with the characteristics of the nanoparticle surface and the nature of the particle interior and shell, if present, are other factors in design and characterisation. Reproduced with permission from Mieszawska AJ et al. Multifunctional gold nanoparticles for diagnosis and therapy of disease. Mol Pharm 2013;10:831–847.*

Importance of particle size

- Nanosystems are defined principally by their size (or their size range) and surface character.
- Some, like dendrimers, are synthesised as discrete chemical entities of identical size.
- Particle size influences many of the properties and behaviour of nanoparticles, including:
  - Drug release: the large surface area per unit weight of nanoparticles leads to potentially high release rates compared to the same weight of larger particles, as solvent penetration and release will be a function of $n\pi r^2$, where n = number of nanoparticles per unit weight and r is the particle radius.
  - Oral uptake: although drugs must be in their molecular form to be taken up by epithelial cells, there is a mechanism for particle uptake. The main site involves the membranous epithelial cells (M-cells) of the gut-associated lymphoid tissue (GALT). Smaller particles (i.e. those 5–150 nm) with the appropriate surface properties are taken up more readily than the equivalent larger particles (>300 nm), and above a certain size (around 500 nm) particles will not be absorbed, at least not intact.
  - Flow in capillaries: once injected, nanoparticles flow in the blood and particle diameter is important.

— Embolisation: nanoparticles are too small to block blood vessels and capillaries, but if they aggregate then blockage (embolisation) might occur.
— Surface erosion is involved in many degradation and drug release processes, and is a function of surface area.
— Adsorption: adsorption of proteins, whether from the blood or deliberately attached to alter the surface properties of nanoparticles, will depend on the available surface area per particle, the area/molecule of the adsorbing molecule, the charge and hydrophobicity of the surface.
— Endocytosis (uptake of particles by cells) is size-dependent.
— Extravasation (escape of particles from the circulation into target cells or tissues) occurs more readily with small particles.
— Physical (colloid) stability is dependent on radius, the nature of the material, its charge and the presence of any adsorbed molecules (see **Chapter 6**).
— Diffusion is important in the translocation of nanoparticles and their transport through mucus and tissues, as well as in tumours and other targets. In a simple fluid medium the diffusion coefficient is inversely proportional to particle radius (Stokes–Einstein equation – see **Chapter 3**). Movement in complex media, e.g. cells and gels, will be represented by more complex equations.

Key points

- Nanosystems have a size range of several nanometres up to about 150 nm.
- Typical nano-sized carrier systems include 'soft systems' such as micelles and nanoemulsions (microemulsions) and 'hard systems' such as polymeric nanoparticles, dendrimers and nanosuspensions or nanocrystals of drugs themselves.
- The main pharmaceutical interest of nanosystems is as carriers for drugs, which may be encapsulated in or attached to the nanoparticles. This provides two main advantages: the drug is protected from the external environment until it is released, and the fate of the drug *in vivo* is determined by the fate of the carrier rather than the characteristics of the drug itself.
- The important characteristics of nanoparticles are their size and surface characteristics. The size influences a wide range of properties, including drug release, M-cell uptake, capillary flow, embolisation, surface erosion, adsorption of ligands, endocytosis, extravasation, physical stability and diffusion.
- Their formulation involves investigation of drug loading capacity, drug release rate and the chemical and physical stability of both the carrier and encapsulated drug. An important requirement of the formulation is that it should have a narrow size distribution with an even distribution of drug throughout the carrier; it should be stable *in vitro* and be able to survive dilution in blood and the passage through tissues.
- Their biological fate requires knowledge of the absorption, distribution and excretion of both the drug and the carrier.

Preparing nanoparticles

There are a large number of methods to prepare nanoparticulate systems (see *Table 13.1*), depending to a large extent on the material which will form the carrier, which can include polymers, proteins, metals (e.g. gold) or ceramics.

Table 13.1: *Methods of manufacturing polymeric or protein nanoparticles*[a]

Method	Relevant physical events
1. Solvent displacement	Mixing of solvents to cause the material to come out of solution
2. Salting-out	Reducing solvency: as above but using another component to salt-out the material
3. Emulsion-diffusion	Diffusion of solvent from emulsion droplets leaving behind the nanoparticle material
4. Emulsion-solvent evaporation	Evaporation of solvents: material in the droplets is revealed by removing solvent
5. Supercritical fluid technology (SCT)	Solvent phase behaviour: utilising SCT to produce nanoparticles
6. Complexation, coacervation	Macromolecular interactions to create a complex mixture of e.g. polymers in the micro- or nano-size range.
7. Reverse micellar methods	Solubilisation of monomers in inverse micelles and polymerising the monomers by a variety of techniques
8. *In situ* polymerisation	Growth of polymers in suspension
9. Synthesis (e.g. dendrimers)	Covalent growth from a core molecule, by layer by layer addition of linking groups

[a]*Some of the above methods are outlined in the text. A fuller account can be found in Florence AT. Pharmaceutical aspects of nanotechnology. In: Florence AT, Siepmann J (eds). Modern Pharmaceutics, 5th edn, vol. 2, chapter 12. New York: Informa Healthcare; 2009.*

The main approaches to nanoparticle manufacture are:
- by comminution (in the case of solids, milling, and in the case of liquids, emulsification)
- molecular self-assembly of units (e.g. polymeric micelles)
- precipitation from a solution of the polymer
- polymerisation of monomers dissolved in either micelles or emulsion droplets
- supercritical fluid technology.

These form the basis of the following methods used to prepare nanosystems:
- Solvent displacement method. This is perhaps the simplest means of preparing polymeric nanoparticles. The polymer is dissolved along with the drug to be encapsulated in commonly used water-miscible solvents – ethanol, acetone or

methanol. The polymer solution is then diluted in the presence of stabilisers such as poly(vinyl alcohol) (PVA) or polysorbate 80, and the change of solvent causes the formation of stabilised nanoparticles with narrow size distributions as shown in *Figure 13.3*.

- Salting-out method. A variant on the above technique includes a polymer plus a drug dissolved in a water-miscible organic solvent which is added to a stirred aqueous gel containing a salting-out agent and a stabiliser. The polymer–drug combination is salted out as nanoparticles.

- Emulsion-diffusion method. A partly water-miscible solvent in which the drug and polymer are dissolved forms an emulsion on dilution in an aqueous phase containing a stabiliser. Because of the partial miscibility of the first solvent, it diffuses from the dispersed drops into the bulk reducing their size and so providing polymer nanoparticles containing drug as shown in *Figure 13.4*.

- Emulsion-solvent evaporation method. This involves the dissolution of the drug–polymer mix in an organic solvent that is immiscible with water, so that on addition to an aqueous phase an emulsion is formed in the presence of emulsifiers. On heating, the internal organic phase can be evaporated in a controlled fashion leaving the polymer–drug nanoparticles, whose size is dependent on the nature of the emulsion (see *Figure 13.5*).

- Using supercritical fluid technology. A supercritical fluid (SCF) is a substance at a temperature and pressure above its thermodynamic critical point (T_c) (see *Figure 13.6*). In this state it can diffuse through solids like a gas, and dissolve materials like a liquid. Carbon dioxide and water are the most commonly used supercritical fluids. A drug and polymer are dissolved in an organic solvent or carbon dioxide. Under certain conditions of pressure and temperature (see *Figure 13.6*) the liquid phase is transformed into the supercritical state, which for CO_2 occurs at pressures >74 bar (atmospheric pressure = 1.013 bar (101.3 kPa)) and temperatures >31°C (T_c). The rapid expansion of this supercritical solution on exposure to atmospheric pressure causes the formation of microspheres or nanospheres.

- Coacervation and complexation techniques. A coacervate is a gel-like liquid state of matter that can be treated to produce solid microparticles or nanoparticles. There are several possibilities:

  - In complex coacervation suitable quantities of positively and negatively charged macromolecules are mixed under specified conditions of temperature and ionic strength, resulting in phase separation to form coacervate nanoparticles.

  - In simple coacervation the conditions for the formation of coacervate nanoparticles of single macromolecules of either charge are created by solvent change or salting-out methods.

- *In situ* polymerisation. Synthesis of polymeric nanoparticles (e.g. of polybutylcyanoacrylates) involves dispersing monomeric materials (e.g. butylcyanoacrylate) in a suitable solvent which is emulsified. An initiator is generally added to the system; the monomers condense to form a polymeric matrix.

- Synthetic and semi-synthetic processes: dendrimers and carbon nanotubes.

- — Dendrimers are synthesised 'generation' by 'generation' from a multivalent core molecule as demonstrated in the model in *Figure 13.7.*
- — Carbon nanotubes are obtained from soot and processed to form single-walled nanotubes (SWCNTs) or multiwalled nanotubes (MWCNTs) shown in *Figure 13.8.*
- Polymeric fibres and tubes. These are produced by electrospinning (see **Chapter 7**) and are being studied for a variety of delivery challenges.
- Drug nanocrystals.
  - — Nanocrystals of poorly water-soluble drugs can be prepared by precipitation, homogenisation, sonochemical techniques and combinations of these technologies.
  - — Their greatly reduced particle size increases the surface area per unit weight and hence, as seen from the Noyes–Whitney equation (see **Chapter 1**), increases the rate of dissolution of the drug, all things being equal. There may be a degree of supersaturation, but the equilibrium solubility is unaffected by particle size until very small particle sizes are reached, as shown in *Figure 13.9.* The critical value depends on the surface energy of the material in question.
  - — The combination of increased intrinsic solubility and increased surface area has the potential to enhance absorption dramatically if the absorption of the drug is dissolution rate-limited. Plasma level versus time plots of danazol as a nano-sized suspension shows equivalence to solubilisation of the drug in a cyclodextrin and a great enhancement over a conventional suspension.
  - — If nanocrystals are used as suspensions they must be stabilised, for example by surface adsorption of non-ionic surfactants. The ratio of any stabiliser to the drug content must be carefully titrated as in any stability study.
  - — Nanocrystals can be used not only as suspensions but also as freeze-dried powders for reconstitution, they can be incorporated into liposomes, used as aerosols, incorporated in gels or in microspheres, adsorbed onto microparticles, dispersed in soft gelatin capsules, or used as mini-depot tablets.

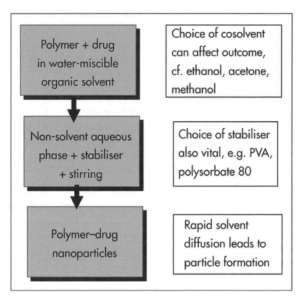

Figure 13.3: *A summary of the solvent displacement method. The poly(vinyl alcohol) (PVA) or polysorbate 80 stabilises the particles as they precipitate following the dilution of the non-aqueous solvents. The rapid diffusion of solvent from the polymer phase allows rapid formation and hence a small size distribution.*

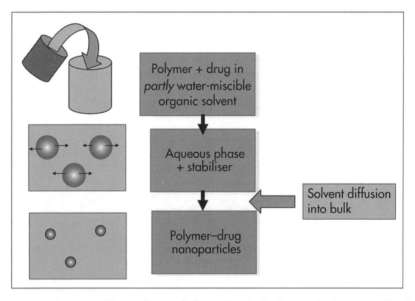

Figure 13.4: *Schematic of the emulsion technique wherein the drug and polymer are dissolved in a partly water-miscible solvent. This is then added to an aqueous phase in the presence of surfactant or other stabiliser. Emulsion particles are formed. The solvent, being partly miscible in the water phase, diffuses from the emulsion droplets to form nanoparticles.*

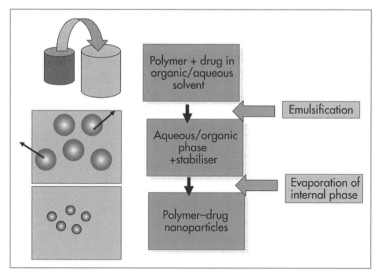

Figure 13.5: *A process similar to that in Figure 13.4. The polymer/drug organic solution is emulsified in water as an oil-in-water system, or the polymer and drug are dissolved in an aqueous phase, which when added to an organic phase forms a water-in-oil emulsion. The internal phase in both cases is evaporated, leaving the polymer–drug particles.*

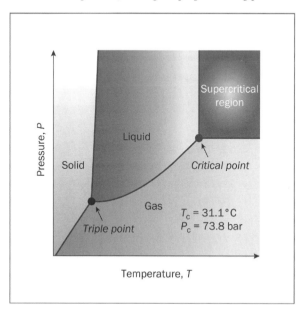

Figure 13.6: *The pressure–temperature phase diagram of CO_2 showing the T_c and P_c at the supercritical region.*

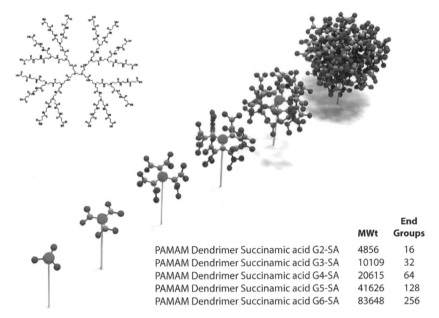

	MWt	End Groups
PAMAM Dendrimer Succinamic acid G2-SA	4856	16
PAMAM Dendrimer Succinamic acid G3-SA	10109	32
PAMAM Dendrimer Succinamic acid G4-SA	20615	64
PAMAM Dendrimer Succinamic acid G5-SA	41626	128
PAMAM Dendrimer Succinamic acid G6-SA	83648	256

Figure 13.7: *Scheme of the stepwise synthesis of dendrimers to form spherical or quasi-spherical nanocarriers. Top left: second-generation polyamidoamine (PAMAM) dendrimers; bottom right: the molecular weights and number of end-groups on second- to sixth-generation PAMAM dendrimers.* **Chapter 7** *has more details. Model, Deutsches Museum, Munich, 2009.*

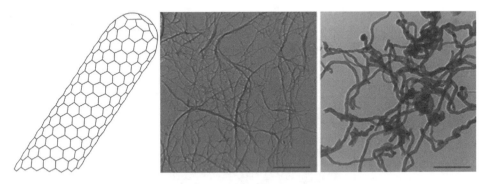

Figure 13.8: *Representation of a single-walled carbon nanotube (CNT). In the photomicrograph on the left the native state of carbon nanotubes is seen, and on the right, double-walled nanotubes at the same magnification. The surface of the CNTs can be altered through adsorption of desired molecules or by covalent attachment of molecules for the purpose of stabilisation (for example, to prevent aggregation) or by addition of drug molecules or targeting moieties. Reproduced with permission from Mérard-Moyen C et al. Functionalized carbon nanotubes for probing and modulating molecular functions. Chem Biol 2010;17:107–115. Copyright Elsevier 2010.*

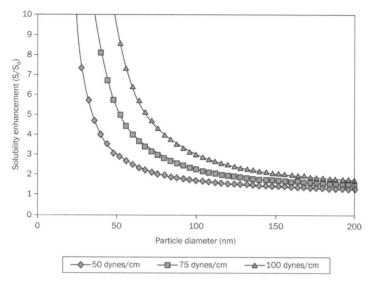

Figure 13.9: *Solubility enhancement as a function of particle diameter for three hypothetical compounds with surface energies of 50, 75 and 100 m Nm^{-1} (dyn cm^{-1}). It can be seen that, where S_O is the solubility of a large crystal, and S is the solubility of the crystal of a specific size, the solubility enhancement (S/S_O) does not increase significantly until particle diameters reach below around 75 nm. Reproduced from Kipp JE. The role of solid nanoparticle technology in the parenteral delivery of poorly water-soluble drugs. Int J Pharm 2004;284:109–122.*

Key points

The general approaches to the manufacture of nanoparticles include:
- comminution, as in the milling of solids or the emulsification of liquids
- molecular self-assembly, as in the formation of some dendrimers and polymeric micelles
- precipitation from solution
- polymerisation of monomers dissolved in micelles or emulsion droplets.

The choice of method is influenced by the nature of the material that forms the basis of the carrier. The main methods of manufacture include:
- solvent displacement
- salting-out
- emulsion-diffusion
- emulsion-solvent evaporation
- use of supercritical fluid technologies
- coacervation and complexation techniques
- *in situ* polymerisation
- nanocrystal formation by a variety of techniques of size reduction.

Physicochemical properties determining the fate of nanoparticles

Complexity of particle flow

Particles must translocate from the site of injection to distant organs and accumulate at the target sites.

- To an extent this depends on the flow patterns of nanoparticles in the blood and in interstitial spaces: the small size of nanoparticles allows freer movement than that of, say, microspheres in the circulation, lymph and tissues.
- Polydispersity of size may lead to particle segregation during flow because the flow rates across the diameter of the vessels are not constant; the larger particles are unable to approach close to the capillary wall and remain predominantly closer to the centre of the capillary vessels where the flow rate is fastest and hence they move more rapidly.
- Particle aggregation may be induced by flow, which will alter flow patterns and interaction with receptors.
- Particle size, flow rate, forces of interaction between particles and receptors, and the density of receptors can all influence the adhesion of the nanoparticles onto receptors.

Aggregation of nanoparticles

Due to of their large surface to volume/weight ratios, nanoparticles are prone to aggregate.

- Aggregation:
  - changes the hydrodynamic size of the particles
  - decreases their diffusion
  - restricts extravasation
  - reduces the effective surface area for interactions with receptors.
- The tendency to aggregate can be reduced by the covalent attachment of polyoxyethylene glycol (PEG) chains to the surface of the nanoparticles (PEGylation) as shown in *Figure 13.10*.
- This procedure stabilises the nanoparticles by:
  - creating a hydrated surface on hydrophobic particles, which allows for both steric and enthalpic stabilisation
  - reducing opsonin adsorption, leading to increased circulation times and the enhanced statistical possibility of nanoparticle uptake after multiple passages through the circulation.

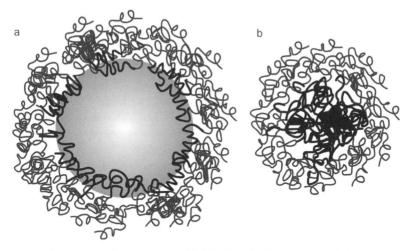

Figure 13.10: *A representation of (a) a particle PEGylated with a polyoxyethylene-based block copolymer and (b) a block copolymer micelle with the external hydrophilic chains. The hydrophilic polymer chains on adjacent particles provide both a physical and a thermodynamic barrier to aggregation.*

The diffusional properties of nanoparticles

These are important in the translocation towards targets in tissues.

- The Stokes–Einstein equation (**Chapter 3**) relates the diffusion coefficient, D, of a molecule or object to the continuous phase viscosity, η, and the radius of the diffusing particle, r, in the form $D = kT/6\pi\eta r$. Note that the diffusion coefficient of spherical particles is inversely related to their radius.

- Diffusion is important in free solution, in cell culture media, in the gel-like interior of cells, even perhaps in the cell nucleus and in the extracellular matrix. In the brain, for example, diffusion of drugs from nanoparticles or implants is slow and the radius of spread of a drug like paclitaxel after release from implants or nanoparticles is of the order of only millimetres.

- Gels have been used as models for diffusion of nanoparticles in complex media: in gels the viscosity in the equation is not the bulk viscosity but the so-called microscopic viscosity, η_0, which is actually close to that of water, as it is the viscosity of the medium in which nanoparticles move between the entangled chains of the macromolecular gels. When the diameter of the particles reaches a critical size in gels, a size approaching the nominal diameter of the pores, diffusion asymptotically approaches zero.

- Diffusion within cells is complex: the cytoplasm is a molecularly crowded zone, a complex gel with structural obstacles such as actin and myosin fibrils and strands. There is the additional tortuosity as the moving particle avoids the regions of the macromolecular chains and the obstruction effects from the impenetrable regions of the cytoplasm. If we designate by D_e the effective diffusion coefficient and by D_0 the coefficient in water we can write,

$$D_e/D_0 = \varepsilon/\tau$$

τ is the tortuosity factor approximately equal to $(1 + \varphi_v)$, where φ_v is the volume fraction of anything in the path of the diffusing material, and ε is the fraction of the volume available to the diffusing solute, thus $\varepsilon \sim (1 - \varphi_v)$. The binding of particles to components of cells and tissues reduces the number of free particles and hence further reduces flux.

- Nanoparticle size is important in diffusion in complex media because the diffusional space may be restricted when the diameter of the particle exceeds the 'pore' diameter of the membrane. Adsorption, obstruction and entrapment occur, and at a certain particle radius diffusion virtually ceases.

Uncertainty about nanoparticle destination and fate

- The randomness of movement of nanoparticles free in solution (Brownian motion) leads to a degree of uncertainty of, for example, an individual particle extravasating on its passage along a capillary, or the chance of a nanoparticle ligand adhering to the appropriate receptor. Such events are said to be stochastic processes.

Regulatory challenges: characterisation

Regulatory challenges generally have evolved for good reasons to ensure reproducibility and quality *in vitro* and *in vivo*. Parameters and questions that must be addressed before clinical use of nanosystems include:

- Can there be a standardised procedure for measuring mean particle diameter and size distribution?
- Is there assurance of stability of size *in vitro*, that is, lack of aggregation/flocculation?
- Standardisation of surface characteristics: what specific methodology is used (zeta potential measurements may be nonspecific)?
- The distribution on surfaces and properties of ligands on the surfaces of targeted systems.
- The determination or prediction of stability *in vivo* (esp. of particle diameter).
- The measurement and validation of the release rate of active from the systems and the choice of suitable experimental media.
- Biocompatibility: is the system compatible with blood?
- Biodegradability: is there evidence of biodegradation of the system to nontoxic products?
- Toxicity of nanosystems: what are reasonable predictive animal or tissue culture tests?

Key points

Physicochemical properties are important in determining the biological fate of nanoparticles:

- The particle size of the nanoparticle influences its flow in blood and interstitial spaces. Polydispersity of size may lead to particle segregation during flow; particle aggregation may be induced by flow, which will alter flow patterns and interaction with receptors. Particle size, flow rate, forces of interaction between particles and receptors, and the density of receptors can all influence the adhesion of the nanoparticles onto receptors.
- Particle aggregation increases the hydrodynamic size of the particles, decreases their diffusion, restricts extravasation and reduces the effective surface area for interaction with receptors.
- Covalent attachment of PEG chains to the nanoparticle surface allows for steric and enthalpic stabilisation and reduces opsonin adsorption.
- The diffusional properties of the nanoparticles are important in their translocation towards their targets in tissues. Diffusion within complex media such as cells is not only determined by the diameter of the nanoparticle, but is also strongly influenced by the tortuosity of its path through the cytoplasm, the void volume available for diffusion and any adsorption or entrapment of the particles. Gels have been used as models of diffusion through such complex environments.
- Stochastic processes evident in many stages of nanoparticle movement and behaviour lead to there being a degree of uncertainty about particle destination and fate.

Memory maps

Properties of nanoparticles

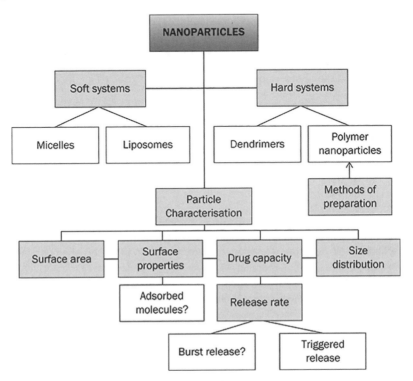

Vital elements of nanoparticle delivery

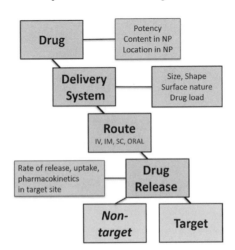

Questions

1. Indicate which of the following statements are true with regard to the properties of nanoparticles.

   A: Nanosystems have particle sizes ranging from a few nanometres to several micrometres

   B: Dendrimers are examples of 'soft' nanoparticles

   C: Drug nanocrystals are examples of 'hard' nanoparticles

   D: Nanoparticle suspensions are colloidal systems

   E: Microemulsions have particle sizes within the range of nanosystems

2. Indicate which of the following statements are true concerning the size and surface area of nanoparticles.

   A: The large surface area per unit weight of nanoparticles leads to high release rates of encapsulated drug

   B: The large surface area per unit weight of nanoparticles increases the possibility of adsorption of proteins from the blood

   C: Decrease of particle size of nanoparticles decreases their flow rate in the blood

   D: Decrease of particle size of nanoparticles increases their uptake by cells

   E: Decrease of particle size of nanoparticles decreases their extravasation

3. Indicate which of the following statements are true in relation to the production of nanoparticles.

   A: The formation of dendrimers is an example of molecular self-assembly

   B: Nanoparticle formation by emulsification of liquids is an example of comminution

   C: Salting-out is an example of a precipitation method of nanoparticle formation

   D: In complex coacervation a coacervate nanoparticle is formed when a charged macromolecule is salted out of solution

   E: Nanoparticle formation by milling of solids is an example of comminution

4. Indicate which of the following statements are true with regards to the physicochemical properties of nanoparticles.

   A: Aggregation of nanoparticles decreases the rate of their diffusion through tissues

   B: Aggregation of nanoparticles increases extravasation

   C: Aggregation of nanoparticles decreases their ability to interact with receptors

   D: PEGylation of nanoparticles decreases their physical stability

   E: PEGylation of nanoparticles increases opsonin adsorption

5. Indicate which of the following statements are true concerning the diffusion of nanoparticles.

   A: Diffusion increases as the size of the nanoparticles decreases

   B: The viscosity of the medium through which the nanoparticles move is greater than the bulk viscosity of the medium

   C: Diffusion increases as the viscosity of the medium decreases

   D: The effective diffusion coefficient increases as the tortuosity factor increases

6. **Indicate which of the following statements are true with regard to the desirable characteristics of nanoparticles.**
   A: They should have a wide distribution of sizes
   B: The drug should be distributed mainly near the surface of the nanocarrier
   C: They should have a high-loading capacity for the drug
   D: They should be non-biodegradable

CHAPTER 14

In vitro assessment of dosage forms

LEARNING OBJECTIVES

Upon completion of this chapter you should be able to:
- understand the basics of some *in vitro* tests which can be applied to pharmaceutical products
- understand how some of the key parameters of pharmaceutical systems such as particle size, viscosity, adhesion or formulation can be estimated *in vitro*
- outline the importance of *in vitro* testing in formulation development, in batch-to-batch control and in assessing defects in products
- understand that *in vitro* tests might be preferred to *in vivo* measures when there is an established good correlation between *in vitro* and *in vivo* behaviour.

Dissolution testing of solid dosage forms

Key points

- *In vitro* tests provide the opportunity to make precise and reproducible release measurements to distinguish between different formulations of the same drug or the same formulation after ageing or processing changes or during production, i.e. batch-to-batch variation.
- They do not replace the need for clinical work, but an *in vitro* test can pinpoint formulation factors during development which are of importance in determining drug release.
- Physiological verisimilitude is not essential for validity in quality control, where reproducibility of a product is in itself a goal.
- *In vitro* tests have a role in identifying counterfeit pharmaceutical products which are an issue now not only in the developing world (see the example of Cialis).

The rate of solution of a solid drug substance from a granule or a tablet is dependent to a large extent on its solubility in the solvent phase and its concentration in that phase. The physicochemical factors which point to the need for dissolution testing include:
- low aqueous drug solubility

- poor product dissolution – evidence from the literature that the dissolution of one or more marketed products is poor
- drug particle size – evidence that particle size may affect bioavailability
- the physical form of drug – when polymorphs, solvates and complexes have poor dissolution characteristics
- presence of specific excipients which may alter dissolution or absorption
- tablet or capsule coating which may interfere with the disintegration or dissolution of the formulation.

Key points

- With drugs of very low solubility it is sometimes necessary to consider the use of *in vitro* tests which allow sink conditions to be maintained. This generally involves the use of a lipid phase into which the drug can partition; alternatively it may involve dialysis or physical replacement of the solvent phase.
- Mixed-solvent systems such as ethanol–water or surfactant systems may have to be used to enhance the solubility of sparingly soluble drugs, but some prefer the use of flow-through systems in these cases.

In vitro methods may be divided into two types:

1. Natural convection in which, for example, a pellet of material is suspended from a balance arm in the dissolution medium. Because there is no agitation, the conditions are not representative of *in vivo* conditions.
2. Forced convection in which a degree of agitation is introduced, so making this method more representative of *in vivo* conditions. Most practical methods fall into this category. There are two types of forced convection methods: those that employ non-sink conditions and those that achieve sink conditions in the dissolution medium.

Tips

- If released drug is not removed from the dissolution medium during dissolution testing, i.e. if testing is performed under non-sink conditions, the drug concentration in this medium may, in some cases, approach saturation level and thus the rate of release of the drug will be significantly reduced (see Noyes–Whitney equation, **Chapter 1**).
- Sink conditions normally occur when the volume of the dissolution medium is at least 5–10 times the saturation volume.

Experimental methods of testing tablet dissolution

Pharmacopoeial and compendial dissolution tests

- The *British Pharmacopoeia* method involves a rotating wire mesh basket in which tablets or capsules are placed (*Figure 14.1*). The mesh is small enough to retain broken pieces of tablet but large enough to allow entry of solvent without wetting problems. The basket may be rotated at any suitable speed but most *United States Pharmacopeia* monographs specify 50, 100 or 150 rpm.
- In all methods the appropriate pH for the dissolution medium must be chosen and there should be a reasonable degree of agitation.

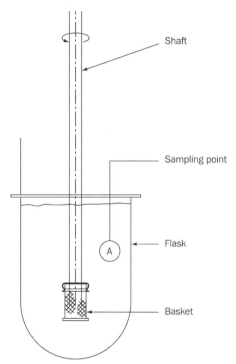

Figure 14.1: *The rotating basket method.*

Flow-through systems

A variant of the dissolution methods discussed uses convection achieved by solvent flow through a chamber. Dissolution data obtained from such a system with continuous monitoring of drug concentration must be interpreted with care as the concentration–time profile will be dependent on the volume of solvent, its flow rate and the distance of the detection device from the flow cell, or rather the void volume of solvent.

Key points

- There is no absolute method of dissolution testing.
- Whatever form of test is adopted, results are only really useful on a comparative basis – batch versus batch, brand versus brand, or formulation versus formulation. For example, in the fight against counterfeit products, dissolution testing of Cialis tablets and copies of this has found wide divergences in release rate *(Figure 14.2)*.

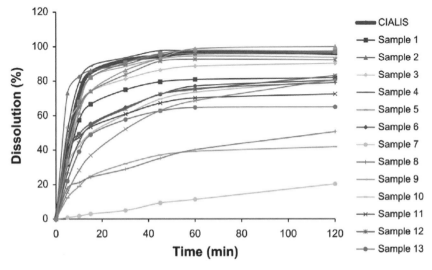

Figure 14.2: *Dissolution test data for the genuine Cialis® brand of tadalafil and 13 samples collected by authorities showing the wide variation in rates and indeed final endpoints, indicating both formulation and content issues. From Deconinck E et al. Comparative dissolution study on counterfeit medicines of PDE-5 inhibitors. J Pharm Analysis 2014;4:250–257.*

In vitro evaluation of non-oral systems

Suppositories

- Suppositories are difficult to study *in vitro*, because it is not easy to simulate the conditions in the rectum.
- One system employs a suppository placed in a pH 7.8 buffer in a dialysis bag which is then placed in a second dialysis bag filled with octanol and the whole is suspended in a flow system at 37°C. The amount of drug released into the outer liquid is monitored.

In vitro release from topical products and transdermal systems

- *In vitro* testing of the lot-to-lot uniformity of semisolid dosage forms of creams, ointments and lotions is important in quality control.

- Ointments and transdermal systems encounter little water in use but useful data can be obtained by measuring release into aqueous media, which can sometimes be predictive of *in vivo* performance.
- Alternatively, a liquid biophase can be simulated using isopropyl myristate (*Figure 14.3*).
- A rotating bottle apparatus has been used to measure the release of nitroglycerin from Deponit transdermal patches.
- The *British Pharmacopoeia* specifies a distribution (release) test for transdermal patches based on the paddle apparatus for tablets and capsules.

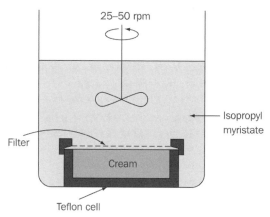

Figure 14.3: *An apparatus for examination of the release of drug from a cream formulation using isopropyl myristate as the receptor phase.*

Rheological characteristics of products

- The terms 'soft and unctuous' and 'hard and stiff' are used to describe dermatologicals but are difficult to quantify.
- Viscosity monitoring can be used as a quality control procedure, and some very practical rheological tests may be carried out. For example, the injectability of non-aqueous injections, which are often viscous and thus difficult to inject, can be assessed by a test for syringeability. Sesame oil, a commonly used liquid phase, has a viscosity of 56 cP, but added drugs and adjuvants may increase the viscosity.

Adhesivity of dosage forms

Formulation aspects

- Adhesive preparations have been formulated, for example, for the topical treatment of stomatitis.
- The adhesive nature of transdermal patches is important.

- The adhesion of film coats to tablet surfaces is a key quality issue.
- Rubbery polymers which have partly liquid and partly elastic characteristics are employed as adhesives in surgical dressings and adhesive tapes.
- Peeling tests for film coats are routinely used in pharmaceutical development and similar tests for the adhesion of transdermal particles to skin have been used.

Experimental testing for adhesivity

Several current methods of testing oral dosage forms for adhesivity include:

- Measurement of the force of detachment of a solid dosage form by raising the dosage form through an isolated oesophagus.
- Assessment of the adhesion of a moistened capsule or tablet to a surface using a strain gauge. The effects of polymer concentration and composition and of additives on the adhesivity of film coating materials can be studied using this apparatus, and the force required to separate tablet from substrate measured.

Adhesion of coated tablets to mucosal surfaces

The variables likely to affect the process of adhesion of coated tablets to mucosal surfaces (generally an unwanted effect) include:

- film coat thickness
- the nature of the film coat, for example, its hydrophobicity
- the nature of the contacting surface
- rate of coat hydration or dissolution during the adhesion process
- the rheology of the solution of film coating material formed during adhesion, its surface tension and its elongational characteristics.

Particle size distribution in aerosols

Key points

- Analysis of particle size distribution of aerosol formulations during formulation development, clinical trial or after storage is of obvious clinical relevance.
- Aerosols are not easy to size, primarily because they are dynamic and inherently unstable systems.

> **Tip**
>
> Remember that an aerosol is a type of colloidal dispersion in which the liquid or solid particles are dispersed in a continuous phase (air). According to Stokes' law:
>
> $$v = \frac{2ga^2(\rho_1 - \rho_2)}{9\eta}$$
>
> Consequently the rate of sedimentation (v) of the particles will increase with increase of the particle radius (a), and the difference between the density of the particles (ρ_1) and the continuous phase (ρ_2), and decrease with increase of the viscosity (η) of the continuous phase.

Methods of sampling may be divided into:

- Techniques which utilise an aerosol cloud. Sedimentation techniques based on Stokes' law (see Tip box) are applied and the usual detection system is photometric.
- Dynamic methods in which particles are carried in a stream of gas. Instruments utilise both sedimentation and inertial forces and depend on the properties of particles related to their mass.

Particle sizing devices

- The Royco sizer is a commercially available instrument which measures individual particles in a cloud (it is used to monitor the air of 'clean rooms'). This instrument can be used to size particles in aerosol clouds provided that the particle size distribution does not change during the time of the analysis either by preferential settling of larger particles or by coagulation.
- The cascade impactor is probably the most widely used instrument in categorising airborne particles. In this instrument:
  - Large particles leave the airstream and impinge on baffles or on glass microscope slides.
  - The airstream is then accelerated at a nozzle, providing a second range of smaller-sized particles on the next baffle and so on.
  - Progressively finer particles are collected at the successive stages of impingement owing to jet velocity and decreasing jet dimension (*Figure 14.4*).
- 'Artificial throat' devices are useful for comparative studies of the behaviour of medicinal aerosols. In these devices:
  - The particles are segregated according to size.
  - Analysis of the collecting layers at the several levels of the device allows the monitoring of changes in released particle size.
  - Where an artificial mouth is used, washing is carried out to reveal the extent of fall-out of large particles.
  - The smallest particles of all reach the collecting solvent.

- The *British Pharmacopoeia* and other compendia have adopted detailed specifications for two impinger devices. These operate by dividing the dose emitted from an inhaler into the respirable and non-respirable fractions.

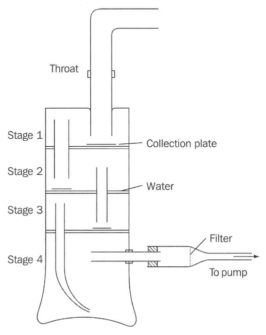

Figure 14.4: *A multistage liquid impinger. Reproduced from Hallworth GW (1987). In: Ganderton D, Jones T (eds). Drug Delivery to the Respiratory Tract. Chichester: Horwood.*

Apparatus A (glass) (*Figure 14.5*)

- Apparatus A employs the principle of liquid impingement and has a solvent in both chambers to collect the aerosol.
- Air is drawn through the system at 60 L min^{-1} and the inhaler is fired several times into the device.
- There are several impaction surfaces at the back of the glass throat about 10 cm away from the activator (similar to human dimensions).
- The upper impinger (stage 1) has a cut-off at a particle size of ~6.4 μm.
- The last impact surface is in the lower impinger (stage 2) and is considered to be the respirable fraction.

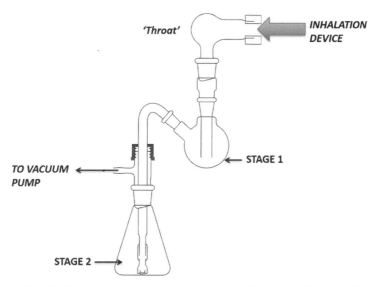

Figure 14.5: British Pharmacopoeia *impinger Apparatus A. Reproduced from British Pharmacopoeia (2007) vol. IV, appendix XIIF. A291 Aerodynamic assessment of fine particles, fine particle dose and particle size distribution.*

Apparatus B

- Apparatus B is made of metal and can be engineered to finer tolerances than the glass Apparatus A.
- Apparatus B is considered to be a superior apparatus for quality control testing and product release.

In vitro–in vivo correlations

- *In vitro* tests do not have to mimic the *in vivo* situation, but realistic parameters are important if useful data are to be achieved.
- The validity of the data from laboratory-based tests in predicting performance in the patient, however, depends on good *in vitro–in vivo* correlations.
- There are other *in vitro* tests that have been devised to measure key parameters of novel dosage forms, such as the flotation of floating oral tablets used to control the site of release of drugs, or the properties of film coats when applied to tablet cores, which are not covered here but are discussed in *Physicochemical Principles of Pharmacy.*

Key points

- We have seen a selection of tests which can be conducted to measure the key parameters of a variety of formulations.
- These tests are not necessarily predictive of performance *in vivo*, but can be used in a comparative sense, testing one product against others or different batches of a product to ensure batch-to-batch consistency.
- Release tests can be applied to rectal and transdermal products by adapting the method used for oral products, altering the receptor phase to mimic the medium in which the formulation resides *in vivo*.
- Key parameters are different for different routes of delivery and different formulations: particle size is a key factor in inhalation products and in topical preparations where the drug is dispersed rather than dissolved in the vehicle.
- Adhesivity of oral dosage forms may be a factor in determining their efficacy (buccal delivery) or in causing adverse events (as in oesophageal injury); adhesion of transdermal patches to the skin is clearly important.
- The rheological properties of topical preparations and formulations for nasal delivery are important, and a key factor is the syringeability of injectables.

Key point

Sometimes simple tests in practice situations can reveal interesting characteristics of dosage forms as demonstrated in the photograph below *(Figure 14.6)*.

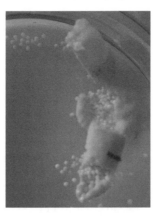

Figure 14.6: *Disintegration of two brands of tamsulosin capsules showing the release of the sustained-release beads.*

In vitro testing of new delivery systems and devices

There is continuing invention and development of drug delivery systems which may require bespoke *in vitro* techniques to define and measure their active agent release characteristics. Two examples are drug-eluting coronary artery stents and biodegradable implants such as those used for drug delivery to the brain (see **Chapter 8**).

- Coated stents to treat occluded arteries and localised tumours contain drugs such as sirolimus and paclitaxel, the drug being applied to the bare metal stent structure in polymer coats such as polyethylene carbonate and poly(lactic-glycolic acid) (see *Figure 14.7*). Slow release of drug is required in coronary artery stenosis and *in vitro* methods must be used to compare systems and to determine the effect of design on release rates over long periods, up to 60 days. There is no standard test and considerable ingenuity is required to devise such diverse designs.
- Polymeric implants embedded in the brain release their drug content but any *in vitro* method of assessment must take into account the limiting slow diffusion of the drug in brain tissue.

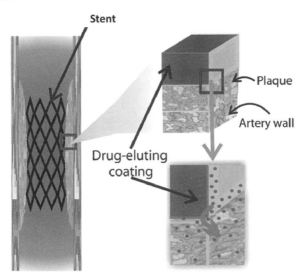

Figure 14.7: *A polymer-coated metallic stent with a drug-eluting coating of a polymer.*

Key point

These systems emphasise the point made earlier in this chapter that *in vitro* tests do not necessarily mimic *in vivo* conditions but are valuable in assessing possible differences in behaviour of batches of the products concerned.

Memory maps

In vitro testing of oral products

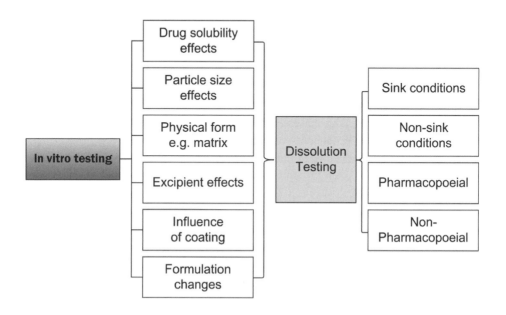

In vitro testing of parenteral products

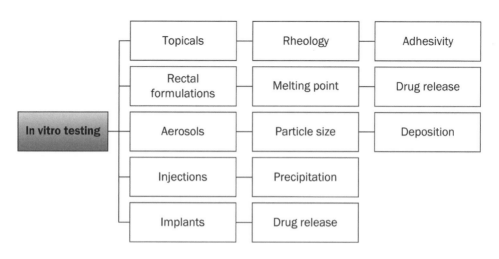

Features and means of *in vitro* testing of pressurised inhalers

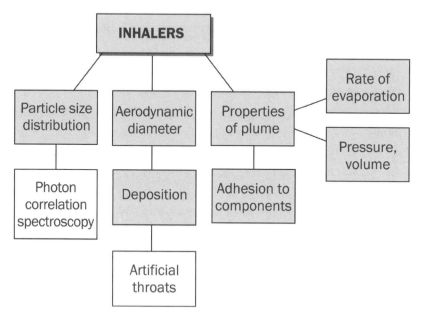

Questions

1. **Indicate which of the following factors might lead you to consider applying dissolution testing to a pharmaceutical formulation.**
    A: Small particle size
    B: High drug solubility
    C: Presence of polymorphs with poor dissolution characteristics
    D: Evidence for a relationship between particle size and bioavailability

2. **Indicate which of the following statements relating to *in vitro* testing methods are true.**
    A: In natural convection methods there is no agitation
    B: Forced convection methods cannot be used under sink conditions
    C: Natural convection methods are representative of *in vivo* conditions
    D: The *British Pharmacopoeia* rotating basket method is a forced convection method

3. **Indicate which of the following statements are true. Sink conditions:**
    A: Can be achieved by physical replacement of the solvent phase
    B: Can be achieved by using a lipid phase into which the drug can partition
    C: Allow the drug to achieve saturation levels in the dissolution medium
    D: Should be used for drugs of very low aqueous solubility

4. **Indicate which of the following statements relating to the adhesion of coated tablets to mucosal surfaces are true. The force of adhesion:**
    A: Is independent of film thickness
    B: Depends on the rate of coat hydration
    C: Depends on the hydrophobicity of the film coat
    D: Is independent of the nature of the contacting surface

5. **Indicate which of the following statements relating to the analysis of particle size distribution in aerosols using the cascade impactor are correct. This apparatus:**
    A: Is routinely used to monitor the air in clean rooms
    B: Is a dynamic method of sizing
    C: Separates particles by impingement on to baffles
    D: Depends on both sedimentation and inertial forces

CHAPTER 15

Generic medicines and biosimilars

LEARNING OBJECTIVES

Upon completion of this chapter you should be able to:
- define generic medicines and biosimilars and describe the similarities and differences between them
- define both chemical equivalence and therapeutic (or bio-) equivalence
- outline possible variables between the originator branded product and the one or several generic products
- outline the regulatory requirements for generic products
- outline the use of generics in specific medical conditions
- describe some of the issues with biomolecular generics arising from their manufacture and processing.

Definitions and characteristics of generic medicines and biosimilars

- The WHO defines a generic product as 'a pharmaceutical product, usually intended to be interchangeable with an innovator product, that is manufactured without a licence from the innovator company and marketed after the expiry date of the patent or other exclusive rights.'[1]
- Generic medicines contain low molecular weight drug products marketed after the expiration of patents on the originator's product. Their bioequivalence with the original medicine is determined in volunteers or patients by pharmacokinetic parameters (such as AUC, C_{max}, and t_{max}).
- Generic forms of conventional (i.e. small-molecule) medicines contain the same drug as the original product (although the molecule may have been prepared by a different route), and the formulation (and appearance) may differ.
- Generic drugs are subject to strict guidelines for licensing so that, within the limits possible with modern analytical techniques and the variability of subjects, they will be bioequivalent, again with certain limits.

1. World Health Organization and Health Action International (2008). Measuring medicine prices, availability, affordability and price components – Glossary, 2nd edn. Available at https://www.who.int/medicines/areas/access/NPrices_Glossary.pdf?ua=1

- Biosimilars are macromolecular or protein-based drugs and monoclonal antibodies whose sources and production processes cannot always be identical to that of the originator's product, hence they are termed 'similar' and not 'equivalent'.
- Biosimilarity has been defined to mean that 'the biological product is highly similar to the reference product notwithstanding minor differences in clinically inactive components' and that 'there are no clinically meaningful differences between the biological product and the reference product in terms of safety, purity and potency'.[2]
- Generic drugs and biosimilars differ as defined in *Table 15.1*.

Table 15.1: *Differences between generic drugs and biosimilars, modified from amgenbiosimilars.com*

Properties	Generics	Biosimilars
Molecular weight	c 150–400 Daltons	c 4500–150 000 Daltons
Structure	Simple, well-defined	Complex with potential structural variations
Manufacturing	Predictable chemical process to make identical copy	Specialised biological process to make similar copy
Complexity	Easy to characterise	Difficult to characterise
Stability	Relatively stable	Sensitive to storage and handling conditions
Adverse immune reactions	Low potential	High potential
Manufacturing quality tests	≤50	≥250

Key points

- Bioequivalence is important to optimise and maintain constancy of therapy (in a variable population), as generic products should be as consistent as possible and inter-changeable.
- Sustained- (extended-) release generic products require special attention, as it is not simple to define degrees of 'sustained' release of the drug.

---

2. Section 351(i) of the PHS Act, US DHHS 2015.

Regulatory requirements

In this section we consider the necessary requirements for generic products to gain regulatory approval by US and European authorities, and some of the issues raised by these. To gain regulatory approval, a generic drug must:

- contain the same active ingredients as the innovator drug (inactive ingredients may vary)
- meet the same batch requirements for identity, strength, purity and quality
- be manufactured under the same strict standards of good manufacturing practice (GMP) regulations required for innovator products
- be identical in strength, dosage form, and route of administration
- have the same use indications
- be bioequivalent.

Issues in determining equivalence

The range of issues in determining the equivalence of formulations is illustrated in (*Figure 15.1*).

- Bioequivalence and therapeutic equivalence. The question of bioavailability can be considered in several ways. Products can be bioequivalent yet not therapeutically equivalent, perhaps because the rate of absorption of the drug differs in the first 30 min or so. If bioavailability is measured by the area under the plasma concentration–time curve (AUC) over 24 or 48 h, then such measures of bioavailability might not show up subtle differences.
- Chemical and therapeutic equivalence. Equivalence between medicinal products can be at two levels, both important, namely:
  - Chemical equivalence, which refers to dosage forms containing the same amount of the same drug in similar dose forms. Pharmacopoeias provide limits on impurities in the drug. Chemical equivalence is a prerequisite for therapeutic equivalence. Limits are set for drug content, e.g. tetracycline products must contain ≤96% and ≥102.0% of the drug. Because of its known toxicity 4-epi-anhydrotetracycline is limited in tetracycline products.
  - Therapeutic equivalence, refers to medicines having not only the same bioavailability (as measured by the AUC), but the same clinical effects. For therapeutic equivalence, the product should have essentially the same safety profile as the comparator product. Regulations do not speak of identicality between products, but essential similarity.

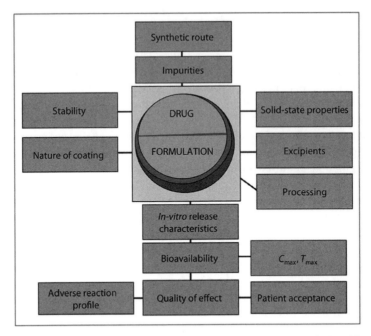

Figure 15.1: *The range of issues in determining the equivalence or essential similarity of formulations.*

Figure 15.2 and *Figure 15.3* demonstrate the limits of bioequivalence and non-bioequivalence. *Figure 15.3* shows how, while two generic products may be equivalent to the first branded product, the two generics may not be equivalent to each other, which may pose problems in practice.

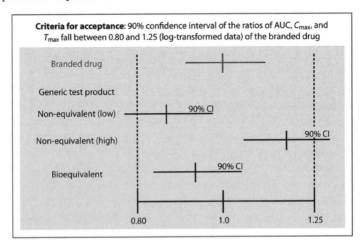

Figure 15.2: *The issue of variability in branded and generic products with their 90% confidence limits and the definition of non-equivalence and equivalence in visual form. Reproduced from Medscape.*

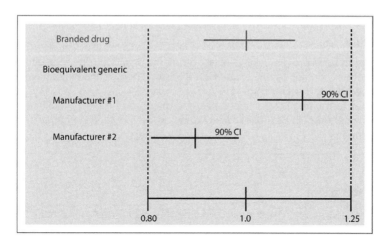

Figure 15.3: *Visual demonstration of bioequivalence between generics and branded drugs, which demonstrates clearly, that while generic 1 can be equivalent to the brand, generic 2 may not be equivalent to generic 1. From Medscape.*

Use of generics in specific medical conditions

- In the treatment of some conditions differences in the performance of products are relevant.
- There are also some medical conditions where additional care has to be taken in titrating patients and maintaining therapeutic levels closely throughout treatment. This has been shown, for example, in relation to antiepileptic drugs as seen in *Figure 15.4.*

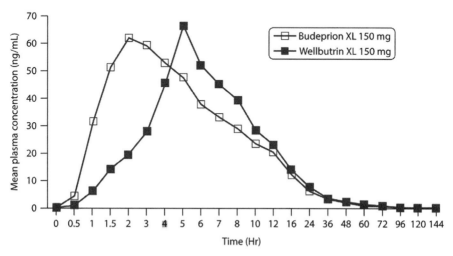

Figure 15.4: *Mean plasma concentration of bupropion (Budeprion XL and Wellbutrin XL) as a function of time in 24 fasting healthy volunteers. See details in Woodcock MD et al. Withdrawal of generic budeprion for nonbioequivalence.* N Engl J Med 2012;367:2463–2465.

Key points

- Drugs that have proven bioavailability problems or which require special formulation techniques and drugs with a narrow therapeutic index have to be considered with special care.
- Complex formulations, e.g. liposomal, and micro- and nano-particulate systems, e.g. of amphotericin B, are less likely to be equivalent to the originator's preparations.

Discussion point

The true measure of quality is not minor differences in drug peak plasma levels or AUCs but therapeutic outcome. Outcomes can of course differ, as we have discussed, between individuals being administered identical products.

Bioequivalence of parenteral medicines

The large majority of generic medicines are oral products but there are of course many parenteral medicaments, as discussed in other chapters of this book (e.g. **Chapter 8** – see Routes of administration). Biologicals such as those discussed below are almost exclusively given by injection, hence the section below indicates some of the issues in determining equivalence.

Biosimilars: proteins and monoclonal antibodies

- Generic forms of biologicals, especially of recombinant proteins, present other issues as the active molecule may possess say, subtle differences in amino acid sequence due to the often inevitable differences in the mode of production and processing. Such molecules encompass hormones such as insulin and human growth hormone, cytokines, clotting factors, monoclonal antibodies, vaccines, and enzymes.
- As we discuss below the manufacture and processing of many biologically active macromolecules can lead to differences in their physical state as well as their composition or conformation.
- The term 'biosimilars' has been adopted for generic forms of such biologicals; alternative terms include 'follow-on biologics' (FOBs) or 'biogenerics'.
- *Table 15.2* lists some approvals in Europe of biosimilars.

Table 15.2: *Some biosimilars approved in Europe*

Insulin glargine	Abasaglar	2014	Elli Lilly/Boehringer Ingelheim
	Ladsuna	2017	Merck (MSD)
Filgrastim	Accofil	2014	Accord Healthcare
		2009	Hexal
	Grastofil	2013	Apotex
	Nivestim	2010	Hospira
	Ratiograstim	2008	Ratiopharm
	Tevagastim	2008	Teva Generics
	Zarzio	2009	Sandoz
Infliximab	Flixabi	2016	Samsung Bioepis
	Inflectra	2013	Hospira
	Remsima	2013	Celltrion
Enoxaparin sodium	Inbixa	2016	Techdow Europe
	Thorinane	2016	Pharmathen

From *http://www.gabionline.net/Biosimilars (updates on recently approved biosimilars can be found on this website).*

Key points

- For biologics, 'the product is the process'. Complex processes starting with cell lines cannot be exactly duplicated by another manufacturer.
- The complexity of proteins as drugs is well known (see **Chapter 12**). Peptides and proteins are subject to a variety of chemical and physical instabilities in aqueous solution and at interfaces, and can also suffer during the stresses of some manufacturing processes.

Issues with biomolecular generics

- The impurities in proteins are often very similar to the parent compound and, although present in low concentrations, may be pharmacologically or immunologically active.
- Small changes in the complex manufacturing processes (see **Chapter 12**) may lead to final products that are not identical to the originator's product. Aggregation, protein folding and glycosylation may be affected, any of which can lead to differences in pharmacokinetics, immunogenicity or indeed efficacy.
- Aggregation of biologicals such as monoclonal antibodies during manufacturing processes is a key problem because if the correct form of the MAb is not retained then

biological activity will be compromised. Aggregation during processing includes the events shown in *Figure 15.5*.

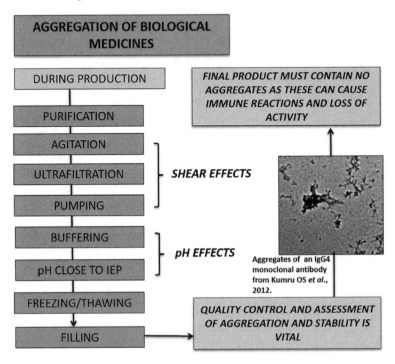

Figure 15.5: *Factors in the aggregation of biologicals during production and filling into vials. The inset photomicrograph of aggregates of IgG4 is from Kumru OS et al. Compatibility, Physical Stability, and Characterization of an IgG4 Monoclonal Antibody After Dilution into Different Intravenous Administration Bags. J Pharm Sci 2012;101:3636–3650.*

Biosimilars: generic biologicals

Methods used to show that small-molecule therapeutics are nearly identical to each other are not sufficient for biologicals. Bioequivalence is usually defined in terms of areas under the curve (AUCs), but this is only part of the story with biological products:

- The nature of impurities is different. These impurities might indeed be analogues with a single amino acid difference, and may be potent. If this is the case, this can lead to clinical problems.
- Impurities might be more difficult to detect in biological products if they are analogues of the main agent, so there is the risk of immunological and other side-effects.
- It is also possible that the formulation may be the cause of differences in protein products, as with recombinant human erythropoietin (Eprex). A change of stabiliser from albumin to sorbitol resulted in the formation of anti-erythropoietin antibodies

and hence pure red cell aplasia.

PEGylated proteins

- Attachment of long-chain polyoxyethylene glycols (PEGs) to proteins is the basis of pegylation (see also **Chapter 12**).
- This can increase the circulation time of proteins with short half-lives and can reduce immunogenicity.
- Filgrastim and pegfilgrastim (see *Figure 15.6*) are available in the clinic, e.g. to reduce neutropenia induced by chemotherapy. The latter has a longer half-life than the native molecule so that filgrastim is administered daily for up to 14 days, while pegfilgastrim is given once for each chemotherapy cycle. They are considered to be biosimilar.

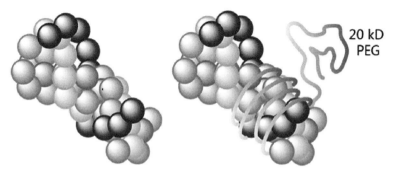

Figure 15.6: *L) Filgrastim and R) Pegfilgrastim, which is filgrastim modified with a 20 kDa polyoxyethylene glycol chain covalently bound as shown in this simplified representation.*

Conclusions

For the majority of conventional oral medicinal products the initial brand and the subsequent generic products are therapeutically equivalent.

- There are of course differences such as the shape, colour and size of capsules and tablets or the appearance of liquids, which can influence patient compliance and adherence to regimes.
- There are drugs that have a narrow therapeutic index or that are perhaps poorly soluble, which perhaps suggests that they might not be used interchangeably, but these are few in number, and experts do not always agree.
- There is however a practical problem in that both generic A and generic B will be bioequivalent to the brand leader, but this does not necessarily mean that the two are equivalent.
- The source of generics is important.

With subsequent versions of biologicals or biosimilars the issues can become somewhat more complex.

- Developments in analytical methods will assist in elucidating the similarity or otherwise of this growing array of drugs in the future.

With both conventional drugs and biological drugs, wherever a formulation has been devised to alter the rate of release or delivery of the active agent, it is not automatic that generic versions will produce identical results.

- The extended action of pegfiligastrim is determined by its structure with its intrinsic long half-life and not by its formulation.

Discussion point

Can all pegylated biomolecular drugs be considered to be biosimilar? What factors need to be known about them? *Figure 15.7* gives clues.

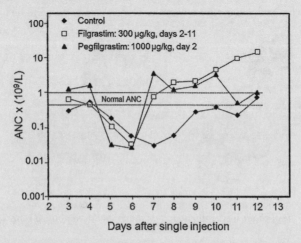

Figure 15.7: *Comparison of Absolute Neutrophil Counts (ANC) after filgrastim administered daily from days 2-11 and pegfilgrastim injected on day 2 in restoring normal ANC's in mice after a single dose of 5-fluorouracil at day zero. Molecular weight of filgrastim = 18,800 Da; of pegfilgrastim 39,000 Da. Figure from Molineux G et al. A new form of Filgrastim with sustained duration in vivo and enhanced ability to mobilize PBPC in both mice and human.* Exp Hematol *1999;27:1724–34. Permission: Elsevier.*

Key point

To be able to make informed decisions on generics and biosimilars, pharmacists, physicians and Drugs and Therapeutics Committees need access to the facts about such products and in particular their biopharmaceutical profiles in patients or volunteers. However, few practitioners have access to appropriate data.

Memory maps

Key differences between generic drugs, complex formulations and biosimilars

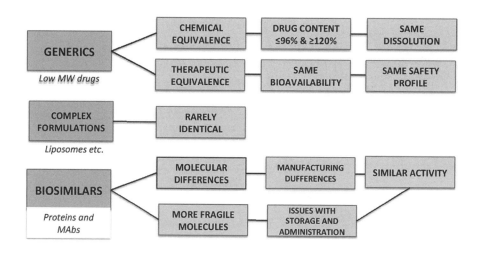

Equivalence of dosage forms of low molecular weight drugs

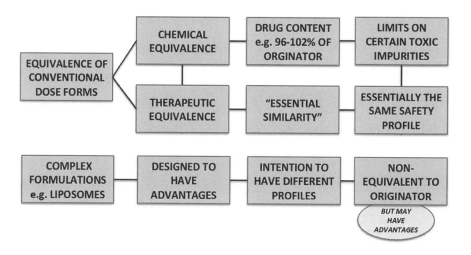

Some of the differences between high MW biologicals and low MW drugs

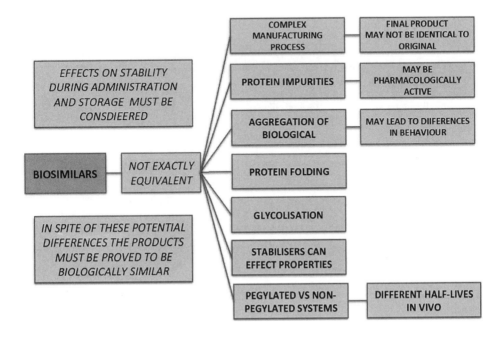

EFFECTS ON STABILITY DURING ADMINISTRATION AND STORAGE MUST BE CONSDIEERED

BIOSIMILARS — NOT EXACTLY EQUIVALENT

IN SPITE OF THESE POTENTIAL DIFFERENCES THE PRODUCTS MUST BE PROVED TO BE BIOLOGICALLY SIMILAR

COMPLEX MANUFACTURING PROCESS — FINAL PRODUCT MAY NOT BE IDENTICAL TO ORIGINAL

PROTEIN IMPURITIES — MAY BE PHARMACOLOGICALLY ACTIVE

AGGREGATION OF BIOLOGICAL — MAY LEAD TO DIIFERENCES IN BEHAVIOUR

PROTEIN FOLDING

GLYCOLISATION

STABILISERS CAN EFFECT PROPERTIES

PEGYLATED VS NON-PEGYLATED SYSTEMS — DIFFERENT HALF-LIVES IN VIVO

Questions

1. **Bioequivalence of generic dosage forms has which of the following attributes?**
   - A: Non-sustained release generic dosage forms have identical bioavailability
   - B: Generic forms of sustained release dosage forms must demonstrate identical rates and extents of drug absorption (C_{max} and t_{max})
   - C: The drugs involved have molecular weights below circa 500 Daltons
   - D: *In vitro* dissolution tests are insufficient to determine differences between standard generic forms

2. **Which one of the statements below refers to generic oral dosage forms?**
   - A: Inactive ingredients must be identical
   - B: All licensed generic products are therapeutically equivalent
   - C: The equivalence of generics can be measured by determination solely of areas under the plasma concentration–time plots (AUCs)
   - D: The drug molecules concerned are synthesised by identical routes

3. **Biosimilars are biological products generally with high molecular weights. Which of the following statements are true?**
   - A: Biosimilarity between such biological products does not mean identicality
   - B: Their comparison is made difficult because of differences in processing methods
   - C: They must be produced from the same biological sources
   - D: The physical stress on the product during administration can lead to physical changes which may influence the molecular behaviour and biological reactions
   - E: Biosimilarity guarantees a low potential for adverse immune responses in patients

4. **Some biologicals are available in their primary form and as pegylated entities. Which of the following are true?**
   - A: All pegylated biological molecules should be considered to be biosimilar to the parent biomolecule
   - B: Filgrastim (MW 18 800 Da) and pegfilgrastim (MW 39 000 Da) are considered to be biosimilar
   - C: Pegylation can reduce the immunogenicity of the parent biological
   - D: Pegylation decreases the circulation time of the parent molecule
   - E: The dosage of a pegylated biomolecule is the same as that of its non-pegylated form

5. **The accuracy and reliability of reports of adverse reactions to generic medicines can be compromised by which of the following?**
   - A: Placebo effects
   - B: Nocebo effects
   - C: Differences in the nature of excipients of products being compared
   - D: Knowledge of the chemical structures of drugs with known adverse effects
   - E: Deselection from trials of patients with known sensitivities

6. The physicochemical behaviour of biological agents differs considerably from that of low molecular weight entities. Which of the following statements are true?

A: Production processes used for biologicals may be the cause of biological differences

B: Their chemical complexity results in the need for more varied and detailed chemical characterisation

C: Differences in efficacy can occur because of changes during administration of biosimilars

D: Impurities in proteins may be immunologically active

E: Physicochemical assessment of products alone is of little relevance

Chapter 1: Solids

1. **B**
   See *Figure 1.1*.
2. **A and D**
   See *Figure 1.1*.
3. **C**
   Applying the rules to determine Miller indices: taking reciprocals of intercepts gives 1/3, ½ and 0; clearing fractions by multiplying by the lower common denominator which is 6 gives 2, 3, 0; therefore the Miller indices are 230.
4. **B and D**
   See description of pseudopolymorphic solvates in text.
5. **A and C**
   Wetting of a solid surface is called spreading wetting, which to be spontaneous requires a zero contact angle, a zero or positive value of the spreading coefficient and a low surface tension of the wetting liquid.
6. **D and E**
   The type of spreading is called immersional wetting and for effective wetting of the powder the contact angle should be between 0° and 90°, i.e. the surface tension of the liquid should be low and the surface should be hydrophilic.
7. **B, C and E**
   From the Noyes-Whitney equation: dissolution coefficient *D* is decreased when viscosity is increased so answer option A is incorrect; reduction of particle size increases surface area of particles so answer option B is correct; agitation of liquid reduces thickness of diffusion layer so answer option C is correct; decrease of saturation solubility reduces ($c_S - c$) and so answer option D is incorrect; removal of drug from solution decreases c so answer option E is correct.
8. **C and E**
   Reference to *Figure 1.8* shows that below the eutectic temperature the system is a microcrystalline mixture of A and B in solid form so answer option A and answer option B are incorrect

and answer option C is correct; on cooling a solution which has a higher concentration of A than B will cause crystals of A to appear so answer option D is incorrect; by definition the eutectic mixture will have the lowest melting point so answer option E is correct.

Chapter 2: Solid dosage forms

1. **A, C and D**
   Refer to section on formulation of tablets and capsules.
2. **A, B and E**
   Refer to section on flow properties of powder mix.
3. **A, C and D**
   Refer to section on granulation.
4. **B, D and E**
   Refer to section on tablet manufacture.
5. **B and E**
   Refer to section on capsule membrane and capsule manufacture.

Chapter 3: Solubility and solution properties of drugs

1. **B**
   Refer to section on concentration units.
2. **C**
   Refer to section on concentration units.
3. **C**
   Refer to section on concentration units.
4. **B and D**
   Apply Raoult's law and convert to psig as explained in section on solvents for pharmaceutical aerosols.
5. **A, B, and D**
   Refer to section on factors influencing solubility.
6. **A and D**
   Refer to section on factors influencing solubility.
7. **A, C, D and E**
   Refer to section on ionisation of drugs in solution.
8. **B and D**
   Refer to section on ionisation of drugs in solution. Note that sodium in a drug name means a salt of the strong base sodium hydroxide; hydrochloride

implies the salt of the strong acid hydrochloric acid; maleate implies the salt of the weak acid maleic acid.

9. **B**
   Refer to section on ionisation of drugs in solution.

10. **C**
    Use equation for pH of an acidic drug given in section on pH of drug solutions.

11. **B**
    Use equation for pH of a basic drug given in section on pH of drug solutions.

12. **C**
    Use the Henderson-Hasselbalch equation for the pH of a buffer of a weak acid and its salt given in section on buffers.

13. **A and C**
    Refer to section on osmotic properties of drugs.

14. **D**
    Use the equation for the calculation of the composition of isotonic solutions given in section on osmotic properties of drugs.

15. **B and D**
    Refer to section on partitioning of drugs between immiscible solvents.

16. **A, C and E**
    Refer to section on diffusion of drugs in solution.

Chapter 4: Drug stability

1. **A and D**
   Refer to section on kinetics of chemical decomposition in solution.

2. **A and B**
   Refer to section on kinetics of chemical decomposition in solution.

3. **D**
   Refer to section on kinetics of chemical decomposition in solution.

4. **C and E**
   Refer to section on factors influencing drug stability of liquid dosage forms.

5. **A, D and E**
   Refer to section on factors influencing drug stability of liquid dosage forms.

6. **A and D**
   Refer to section on factors influencing drug stability of liquid dosage forms.

7. **B and C**
   Refer to section on factors influencing drug stability of liquid dosage forms.

8. **D**
   Use first-order rate equation given in section on kinetics of chemical decomposition in solution.

9. **B**
   Use first-order rate equation given in section on kinetics of chemical decomposition in solution.

Chapter 5: Surfactants

1. **A**
   When applying Traube's rule note that for every extra C atom you require 3 times less of the compound and so for 2 extra C atoms you need 9 times less compound.

2. **A**
   Apply Gibbs equation as given in section on reduction of surface and interfacial tension, assuming $x = 1$.

3. **B, D and E**
   Refer to section on reduction of surface and interfacial tension.

4. **A and E**
   Refer to section on Factors affecting the CMC and micellar size noting that this is a non-ionic surfactant.

5. **A, B and E**
   Refer to section on micellisation.

6. **A and D**
   Refer to section on factors affecting adsorption.

7. **C and E**
   Refer to section on insoluble monolayers.

8. **B, C and D**
   Refer to section on formation of liquid crystals and vesicles.

9. **B**
   Refer to section on micellisation. The entropy increase is due to the loss of the ordered structure of water molecules around the hydrophobic group as the surfactant molecule is transferred into the micelle.

10. **C**
    Refer to section on solubilisation.

Chapter 6: Emulsions, suspensions and other dispersed systems

1. **A and B**
   Refer to Stokes' law equation as given in section on colloid stability.
2. **C**
   Refer to section on DLVO theory of colloid stability.
3. **B**
   Refer to section on DLVO theory of colloid stability.
4. **B and D**
   Refer to section on effect of electrolytes on stability.
5. **B, C and D**
   Refer to section on repulsion between hydrated surfaces.
6. **A and C**
   Refer to section on stability of oil-in-water and water-in-oil emulsions.
7. **C**
   Refer to section on HLB.
8. **A, C and D**
   Refer to section on microemulsions.
9. **A and B**
   Refer to section on stability of suspensions.
10. **C**
    Apply equation HLB = $(E + P)/5$ using weight percentages of ethylene oxide E and sorbitol P given.
11. **B, D and E**
    Refer to section on Newtonian flow.
12. **A, B and C**
    Refer to section on non-Newtonian flow.

Chapter 7: Polymers

1. **C**
   Refer to section on polymer structure.
2. **D and E**
   Refer to section on polymer structure.
3. **C, D and E**
   Refer to section on viscosity.
4. **D and E**
   Refer to section on properties of polymer gels.

5. **B, D and E**
   Refer to section on properties of polymer gels.
6. **B, D and E**
   Refer to section on water-insoluble polymers.
7. **A and C**
   Refer to section on matrices.
8. **A and D**
   Refer to section on microcapsules and microspheres.

Chapter 8: Drug absorption and delivery

1. **C and D**
   The percentage of drug absorbed increases with log P, but reaches a maximum as seen in *Figure 8.2* which indicates that there is an optimum value for each drug.
2. **B and D**
   See Lipinski's rules in the section on molecular weight and drug absorption.
3. **B**
   Drugs are affected by their degree of ionisation as they need to be lipophilic to be absorbed across membranes, hence ionised drugs are not absorbed. Weakly acidic drugs have their optimal lipophilicity below their pK_a values. Note the equation for calculating percentage ionisation of acidic and basic drugs.
4. **C, D, F and G**
   Refer to section on the oral route and oral absorption.
5. **A, C and E**
   Absorption by the buccal and sublingual routes is subject to the same criteria for membrane transfer: hence answer option C and answer option E are correct. Answer option A is factual. Drugs administered by this route have direct access to the systemic route.
6. **A, D and E**
   Binding to muscle protein would decrease absorption; hydrophilic drugs are unlikely to bind to protein. Answer option D is factual. Oily

vehicles are widely used to extend the duration of action of lipid soluble drugs such as fluphenazine decanoate.

7. **A, B, D and E**
See *Figure 8.7* and the section on routes of skin penetration.

8. **A and B**
Answer option A and answer option B are factual. Answer option C and answer option D are counter-intuitive. Answer option E is incorrect as drug absorbed by the conjunctiva enters the systemic circulation.

9. **A and D**
The lung comprises a large absorbing surface; particle size is key to the depth of deposition; larger particles fall out from the air stream leaving smaller particles to reach the alveoli for absorption. See *Figure 8.10* and *Figure 8.11*. Note difference between diameter and aerodynamic diameters (see Tips box).

10. **D and E**
Addition of drugs to a suppository base lowers the melting point of the base, hence bases with melting points >36–37°C must be selected. The rectal route does not necessarily avoid the liver. The rate of absorption is determined by the dispersion of the base: surfactants will aid this.

Chapter 9: Paediatric and geriatric medicines

1. **A, C and D**
Dosage of paediatric patients must be as accurate and appropriate as possible. Children's medicines should not be reduced forms of adult dose-forms which may for example contain excipients which are inappropriate for children and also children are not a homogenous group (C). Liquid dosage forms are not readily measured as there is no definition of a teaspoon (D).

2. **A, B and C**
Answer options A, B and C are factual. There are difficulties in extrapolation

of adult doses as discussed in the text, thus answer option D is incorrect. See *Figure 9.3*.

3. **A and B**
See extemporaneous formulations section.

4. **B and C**
Perhaps for ethical reasons few such studies as are referred to in answer option A have been conducted. Changes during growth of children are discussed in the text showing the reasons for answer option B and answer option C to be correct.

5. **A, C and D**
The eye of a child reaches adult size at the age of 3–4 years. See the section on delivery via the eye.

6. **A, B, D and E**
The electric charge on some spacers attracts drug to their surface, hence reducing dosage. See *Figure 9.6* and *Figure 9.7*.

7. **A, C and D**
Adults of all ages cannot be defined by one parameter such as age (A), as explained for example in the point about achlorhydria (C), and in point on cardiovascular, renal and hepatic changes in the elderly (D). Unfortunately, individual patient's profiles are rarely available in general practice in the UK.

8. **B and D**
See *Figure 9.8*. Increased difficulty in swallowing as a result of decreased oesophageal peristalsis with ageing is a problem with both food and dosage form intake. See also **Chapter 11**.

9. **A, B and D**
Drug pellets can cause problems in the behaviour of enteral fluids and the release of drug, while liquid medicines can interact with components of the enteral fluid; drug solubility can be reduced, leading to significant lowering of the percentage of drug being absorbed.

Chapter 10: Physicochemical drug interactions and incompatibilities

1. **A, B and E**
   Antacids neutralise some of the acidity of gastric fluids (A), raising the pH of the stomach and in turn increasing the rate of gastric emptying (B). This reduces gastric absorption (E) because the drugs concerned are, as a result of the interactions, less lipid soluble.

2. **C and D**
   Figure 10.1 and related text discusses the change in the rate of urinary drug absorption and the importance of pH. Drug in un-ionised form diffuses from urine to the blood; drug may precipitate in the urine.

3. **B and D**
   Positive and negative ions attract and thus interact, while those of similar charge repel each other. Ion-pairing results in neutral species by burying the charges.

4. **B and D**
   See examples in the text e.g. tetracycline-metal complexes and the structure of the chelates formed. Tetracyclines form 2:1 complexes with magnesium ions and this chelation reduces absorption.

5. **A**
   Ion-pairs have a zero charge and hence increased hydrophobic properties; drug binding to plasma reduces the free drug concentration as does adsorption onto antacids and adsorption to giving sets. Chelation: see the answer explanation for Q4.

6. **A and B**
   Drugs must have a certain threshold of lipophilicity to bind to proteins; protein binding reduces the free concentration of drugs and results in lower absorption and reduces activity.

7. **A**
   Solubility of drug is 0.5 mg cm^{-3} thus for 7 mg requires 14 cm^3 min^{-1}.

8. **C**
   The reduction in binding leads to 8 free units of drug as opposed to 5, which is a 160% increase.

Chapter 11: Adverse events – the role of formulations and delivery systems

1. **A and C**
   Surfactants at higher concentrations may damage biomembranes by interacting with lipid membrane components. As a range of non-ionic surfactants are used in formulations, they cannot be considered as a single entity with the same biological effects or physicochemical characteristics. However, all have *some* ability to some extent (hence they 'may' in the statement). They do this by solubilising membrane lipids. Some have side effects that others do not possess (A). Inhibiting p-glycoprotein dependent drug absorption will increase drug levels (C).

2. **A, C, D and E**
   It is clear from the text that there are multiple causes for oesophageal injury. Certain drugs as in answer option A have been shown to cause clinical problems; adhesion of the product to the oesophagus is but one cause. It is the result in many cases of both drug and formulation components.

3. **A, B, C and E**
   The nature of the tear film will clearly be affected through dilution by the administration of drops. The surfactant properties of benzalkonium is one cause. Like other penicillin derivatives amoxicillin can form polymers. Drugs may cause the pH to change and the solubility of drugs may be exceeded in tear fluid.

4. **A, B and D**
   Phototoxicity involves the conversion of a non-toxic agent into a toxic entity after absorption of electromagnetic radiation. Drugs absorbed orally can thus result in skin allergies after their distribution *in vivo* (A and B).

Photoallergenic materials can also generate chemical produce which bind to proteins in the skin (D).

5. **A, B, C and D**

Adverse reactions result from many sources during medication, including reactions to enteric coating materials (A). Irritation caused by adhesives is a reality (B) as in pain resulting during injection of viscous formulations (C). Suppository vehicles can absorb water and cause irritation in the rectum (D).

6. **A, D and E**

Sometimes the combined activity of co-administered drugs can cause adverse reactions (A) and sometimes the causes of such interactions are not readily recognised, but are nonetheless adverse events (D). Impurities in excipients or the drug substance are known to have caused adverse reactions (E).

Chapter 12: Peptides, proteins and monoclonal antibodies

1. **A and B**

Electrolytes will reduce protein solubility, which is also dependent on pH (see *Figure 12.2*). Solubility in organic solvents is low.

2. **A and D**

Denaturation can be reversed if the native structure is regained if temperature was the initial cause. Surfactants and cosolvents protect proteins from denaturation.

3. **A, D and E**

See comments above. Proteins adsorb onto plastics leading to denaturation. See sections on improving physical stability of proteins, the effect of cosolvents and exposure to air *inter alia*.

4. **A and D**

See section on therapeutic proteins and peptides. Insulin zinc suspensions have a lower onset of action. Amorphous forms appear at low pH. Fibrils can be formed on interaction with hydrophobic surfaces as discussed under precipitation of insulin.

Chapter 13: Pharmaceutical nanotechnology

1. **C, D and E**

Drug crystals with diameters in the nanometre size range are classified as nanocrystals with the properties of solids (C). Suspensions of nanoparticulate materials obey the laws of colloidal systems (D). Microemulsions have been studied since before the terminology of nanotechnology was applied. Having particle sizes in the nano size range they are now referred to as nanoemulsions (E).

2. **A, B and D**

Small particle size enables uptake of particles through tissues and enhances the possibility of extravasation.

3. **A, B, C and E**

Dendrimers are formed synthetically by chemical reaction between appropriate smaller molecular structures (A). Nanoparticles can be formed by emulsifying appropriate materials and reducing the particles to the nanoparticle size range (B). Nanoparticles may also be formed by salting out of macromolecules (C). Nanoparticles can also be prepared from material in the solid state (e.g. drug molecules) by comminution procedures (E).

4. **A and C**

Particle diffusion is defined by particle radius (see text for relationship between *D* and *r*): larger particles move more slowly. Aggregated particles result in the loss of effective surface area of the involved individual particles with their accompanying receptors hence decreases their interactions.

5. **A and C**

The viscosity of the medium in which particles diffuse is defined by the medium in which they move and not by the bulk viscosity. As tortuosity increases, the effective diffusion coefficient decreases.

6. **C**

As so much depends on particle diameter it is important that there is a narrow and defined size. The factors affecting drug release are crucial to performance. Rapid release caused by answer option B would result in drug lost before reaching target sites. Biodegradable but stable particles are essential.

Chapter 14: *In vitro* assessment of dosage forms

1. **C and D**
   Small particle size and high drug solubility are positive factors encouraging dissolution. Polymorphs should be tested, as their solubility cannot always be predicted. Specific tests should be done to establish particle size-bioavailability relationships.
2. **A and D**
   Forced convection can be used in sink conditions; *in vivo* conditions involve agitation as can be imagined.
3. **A, B and D**
   If the drug is left to achieve saturation, then sink conditions no longer exist.
4. **B and C**
   Adhesion of tablets via the film coating is dependent on its thickness as water entry forms a gel. Hydrophobic coating materials will not gel in water. The mucosal contact surfaces have different characteristics and thus are important.
5. **B, C and D**
   See section on particle size distribution in aerosols. Air in clean rooms monitored by particle counters specifically designed for the task.

Chapter 15: Generic medicines and biosimilars

1. **C and D**
   Regulations speak of 'essential similarity' between approved products, not identicality. The question of identicality is discussed in the chapter (see *Figure 15.2* and *Figure 15.3*). Limits of variation are laid down for generic products of conventional medicines with drug MWs below c 500 Da.

2. **B**
   In generic products approved additives can be chosen to optimise the final product. The route of synthesis of the active does not have to be identical provided the final product has the same therapeutic profile. Therapeutic equivalence is evaluated within certain limits.
3. **A, B and D**
   The complexity of production is discussed in the chapter leading to the correct answer options A, B and D. The large molecular weight and protein structure of biologicals means they are susceptible to degradation which in turn affects immune responses. It is a developing field.
4. **B, C and E**
   Pegylation can improve the solubility of the biological and decrease immunogenicity. It can increase solubility. The effects cannot be generalised hence answer option A is incorrect. Answer option B is correct as the products have been shown to be biosimilar. Pegylation increases circulation times. Aspects of pegylation are discussed in **Chapter 13**.
5. **A, B, C and E**
   Placebo and nocebo effects are not genuine indicators of ADRs for reasons discussed in the chapter. Specific excipients can be the causes of reaction; knowledge of the chemical structure of drugs with established ADRs assists in the identification of reactions; removal of patients for trials reduces the estimation of the true effects in wider populations.
6. **A, B, C and D**
   Given the macromolecular nature of these products physicochemical assessment is an insufficient indicator of product performance, unlike conventional drug products where *in vitro* evaluation can be a significant factor once the quality of the drug substance has been proven, hence answer option E is incorrect.

Eponymous equations

Make the connections between the correct boxes.

EPONYMOUS EQUATIONS I

HENDERSON–HASSELBALCH	Diffusion	$v = 2ga^2(\rho_1-\rho_2)/9\eta$
NOYES–WHITNEY	Colloid stability	$D = RT/6\pi\eta aN_A$
VAN'T HOFF	Dissolution	$\pi V = n_2 RT$
DLVO	Osmotic pressure	pH=pK_a+log[salt/acid] pH=pK_w-pK_b+log[base/salt]
STOKES–EINSTEIN	pH of buffers	$V_{total} = V_A + V_R$
STOKES LAW	Sedimentation	$dw/dt = DA(c_s-c)/\delta$

EPONYMOUS EQUATIONS II

FERGUSON'S PRINCIPLE	Diffusion	$p_i = p_i^e x_i$
FICK'S FIRST LAW	Vapour pressure liquid mixtures	$J = -D(dc/dx)$
RAOULT'S LAW	Adsorption	Thermodynamic activity & biological activity link
LANGMUIR ISOTHERM	Biological activity	$c/(x/m)=1/ab+c/a$

EPONYMOUS EQUATIONS III

FREUNDLICH EQUATION	Surface concentration of surfactant molecules	$\mu_E = \zeta\varepsilon/4\pi\eta$
GIBBS EQUATION	Adsorption on to solids	$[\eta] = KM^{\alpha}$
HENRY EQUATION	Viscosity of polymer solutions and mol. wt	$x/m = ac^{1/n}$
STAUDINGER EQUATION	Zeta potential	$\Gamma_2 = -1/xRT\,[d\gamma/2.303\,d(\log c)]$

Index

absorption, drug. *See* drug absorption
acidic drugs (weakly) and their salts
   ionisation of drugs in solution, 77
   permeability, 192
   pH-partition hypothesis, 192
acidic drugs, partitioning of drugs between
   immiscible solvents, 86
activity and activity coefficient,
thermodynamic properties of drugs in solution, 84
ADCs. *See* antibody–drug conjugates
adhesion of suspension particles to containers,162
adhesivity of dosage forms
   bioadhesivity, water-soluble polymers, 176
   in vitro assessment, 321
adsorption at the solid liquid interface
   adsorption in drug formulation, 122
   adsorption of poisons/toxins, 122
   consequences of adsorption, 247
   factors affecting adsorption, 121
   Freundlich equation, 119
   haemoperfusion, 122
   Langmuir equation, 119
   pharmaceutical applications, 122
   surfactants, 119
   taste masking, 122
adsorption of drugs
   drug interactions/incompatibilities, 247
   protein and peptide adsorption, 248
adverse events
   bioavailability, 255
   chemical photosensitivity, 270
   cross-reactivity of drugs, 261
   crystallisation, 268
   delivery devices and materials, 266
   dosage form type, 263
   drug eluting stents, 267
   E-numbers, 259
   excipient effects, 258
   eye drops, 265
   impurities, 266
   photochemical reactions, 269
   photoinduced reactions, 269
   testing for, 269
   transdermal patches, 268
aerosols
   delivery devices, 210
   drug absorption, 209
   inhalation therapy, 209
   particle size distribution, *in vitro*
   assessment, 322
   physical factors affecting deposition of
   aerosols, 209

Raoult's law, 72
   solvents, 71
aggregation
   nanosystems, 310
   proteins, 281
alginates, water-soluble polymers, 175
amorphous solids, 16
amphoteric drugs
   aerosols, 71
   ionisation of drugs in solution, 77
   partitioning of drugs between immiscible
   solvent, 86
   solubility, 75
amphoteric surfactants, 111
anionic surfactants, 112
   Sodium Lauryl Sulfate BP, 112
Arrhenius equation
   drug stability, 106
   shelf-life calculation, 106
   stability testing, 106

basic drugs, partitioning of drugs between
   immiscible solvent, 86
basic drugs (weakly) and their salts
   ionisation of drugs in solution, 78
   permeability, 192
   pH-partition hypothesis, 192
bicarbonate buffer system, 83
bile salts and fat absorption pathways, 198
bioadhesivity, water-soluble polymers, 176
biological membranes
   cholesterol, 190
   drug transport, 189
   lipophilicity and absorption, 191
   membrane structure, 189
   pH-partition hypothesis, pH at membrane
   surfaces, 194
biosimilars
   generic biologicals, 338
   Issues, 333
   monoclonal antibodies, 336
   proteins, 336
Bravais lattices, crystal structure, 11
Brønsted-Bjerrum equation, ionic strength, 102
buccal and sublingual absorption, 199
   mechanisms of absorption, 199
buffers, 81
   bicarbonate buffer system, 83
   drug stability, 100
   phosphate buffer system, 83
   physiological buffers, 83
   protein buffer system, 83

respiratory buffer system, 83
universal buffers, 82
urinary buffer system, 84

calcitonin, 288
carboxypolymethylene (Carbomer, Carbopol),
    water-soluble polymer, 174
carrier-mediated and specialised transport,
    gastrointestinal tract, 197
cation–anion interactions, drug interactions/
    incompatibilities, 243
cationic surfactants, 112
    hydrophile–lipophile balance (HLB), 114
cellulose derivatives, water-soluble polymers, 174
chelation and other forms of complexation, 244
    drug interactions/incompatibilities, 244
    ion-exchange interactions, 247
chemical breakdown of drugs. See also kinetics of
    chemical decomposition in solution
    hydrolysis, 93
    isomerisation, 94
    kinetics of chemical decomposition in
    solution, 95
    oxidation, 93
    photochemical decomposition, 94
    polymerisation, 95
chemical potential, thermodynamic properties of
    drugs in solution, 84
chitosan, water-soluble polymer, 175
cholesteric (or chiral nematic) liquid crystals, 128
cholesterol, biological membranes, 190
cloud point, temperature, 126
CMC. See critical micelle concentration
coacervation and complexation techniques,
    nanoparticle manufacturing method, 304
co-crystallisation, 16
colloid stability, 139
    classification of colloids, 140
    DLVO theory, 140
    electrolytes effect, 143
    enthalpic stabilisation, 145
    entropic effect, 144
    forces of interaction between colloidal
    particles, 140
    osmotic effect, 144
    repulsion between hydrated surfaces, 144
    Schulze-Hardy rule, 144
    steric stabilisation, 144
    Stokes' law, 139
common ion effect, 75
complex reactions, kinetics of chemical
    decomposition in solution, 99
concentration units, 69
    conversion into SI units, 71
    milliequivalents, 70

molality, 70
molarity, 70
mole fraction, 70
volume concentration, 69
weight concentration, 69
consecutive reactions, kinetics of chemical
    decomposition in solution, 99
contact angle, 18
copolymers, structure, 168
creams, semi-solid emulsions (creams, ointments),
    157
critical micelle concentration (CMC), 122
    counterions, 122
    electrolytes, 125
    factors affecting, 125
    hydrophilic group, 125
    hydrophobic group, 125
    temperature, 126
crystal habit, crystal structure, 13
crystal hydrates, 15
crystallinity, water-soluble polymers, 177
crystal structure. See also liquid crystals
    Bravais lattices, 11
    crystal habit, 13
    external appearance, 11
    Miller indices, 11
    unit cells, 11

Debye–Hückel equation, thermodynamic
    properties of drugs in solution, 84
dextran, water-soluble polymer, 175
diffusion of drugs in solution, 88
dimeticones, water-insoluble polymers, 178
dissolution of drugs
    Noyes-Whitney equation, 21
    solids, 21
dissolution testing of solid dosage forms, 317
    flow-through systems, 319
    in vitro assessment, 317
    pharmacopoeial and compendial dissolution
    tests, 319
distribution coefficient, P, partitioning of drugs
    between immiscible solvents, 87
DLVO theory, colloid stability, 140
DNA, 288
drug absorption
    aerosols, 209
    biological membranes, 189
    buccal and sublingual absorption, 199
    ear, 208
    eye, 206
    gastrointestinal tract, 195
    inhalation therapy, 209
    intramuscular and subcutaneous injection, 200
    intrathecal drug administration, 214

intravenous injection and infusion, 200
nasal route, 211
rectal route, 212
transdermal delivery, 202
vagina, 208
drug interactions/incompatibilities
adsorption of drugs, 247
cation–anion interactions, 243
chelation and other forms of complexation, 244
dilution of mixed solvent systems, 242
gastric effects, 241
intestinal absorption, 241
in vitro effects, 241
in vivo effects, 241
ion exchange interactions, 240
ion-pair formation, 244
peptide adsorption, 248
pH effects, 241
plastics, 248
precipitation of drugs *in vivo*, 242
protein adsorption, 248
protein binding of drugs, 248
solubility problems, 239
solvent effects, 242
urinary pH, 241
drugs in solution. *See also* solubility ionisation
isotonic solutions, 85
osmotic properties, 85
pH, 74
thermodynamic properties, 84
drug stability
Arrhenius equation, 106
buffers, 100
chemical breakdown of drugs, 93
excipients, 105
general acid-base catalysis, 100
ionic strength, 102
light, 105
moisture, 105
oxygen, 105
peptides, 281
pH, 100
proteins, 281
shelf-life calculation, 106
solid dosage forms, 105
solvent effects, 104
specific acid-base catalysis, 100
stability testing, 106
temperature, 102
testing, 106
drug targeting, nanosystems, 299
drug transport, biological membranes, 189

ear, drug absorption, 208
elderly patients, 231

complicating factors, 231
enteral nutrition, 232
emulsion–diffusion, nanoparticle manufacturing
method, 304
emulsions
biopharmaceutical aspects, 157
choice of emulsifier, 154
hydrophile-lipophile balance (HLB), 152
intravenous fat emulsions, 158
microbial spoilage, 158
microemulsions, 155
multiple emulsions, 154
oil-in-water emulsions stability, 151
preservative availability in emulsified
systems, 158
rheology, 158
semi-solid emulsions (creams, ointments), 157
transdermal delivery, 181
water-in-oil emulsions stability, 151
emulsion-solvent evaporation, nanoparticle
manufacturing method, 304
enthalpic stabilisation, colloid stability, 145
entropic effect, colloid stability, 144
eutectic mixtures, 23
excipients
drug stability, 105
solid dosage forms, 29
expanded monolayers, surfactants, 117
external appearance
crystal structure, 11
solids, 11
eye
aqueous humour, 207
cornea, 206
drug absorption, 206
eye drops, 207
formulation influence, 207
prodrugs, 207
reservoir systems, 208
tears, 206

Ferguson's principle, partitioning of drugs between
immiscible solvents, 87
Fick's first law
diffusion of drugs in solution, 88
water-insoluble polymers, 177
film coating, polymers, 178
first-order reactions, kinetics of chemical
decomposition in solution, 96
flocculation, suspensions, 159
foams and defoamers, 163
freeze drying, solids, 22
Freundlich equation, surfactants, 119
gaseous monolayers, surfactants, 117
gastrointestinal tract

bile salts and fat absorption pathways, 198
carrier-mediated and specialised transport, 197
drug absorption, 195
gastric emptying, motility and volume of
   contents, 198
large intestine, 197
small intestine, 196
stomach, 196
structure, 196
gels, polymer
   properties, 172
   syneresis, 173
   viscosity, 173
general acid-base catalysis
   drug stability, 100
   pH, 100
generic medicines
   equivalence, 333
   regulatory requirements, 333
   specific medical conditions, 335
geriatric patients. See elderly patients
Gibbs equation, surfactants, 114
glass transition temperature, Tg, polymers, 169
Gouy-Chapman electrical double layer, 123
   ionic surfactants, 123
   micellisation, 122
gum arabic (acacia), water-soluble polymer, 175
gum tragacanth, water-soluble polymer, 175

haemoperfusion, adsorption at the solid–liquid
   interface, 122
Henderson-Hasselbalch equation, 81
HLB. See hydrophile–lipophile balance
homopolymers, structure, 167
hydrolysis, chemical breakdown of drugs, 93
hydrophile-lipophile balance (HLB)
   calculation of, 153
   cationic surfactants, 112
   emulsions, 154
hydrophobicity
   peptides, 279
   proteins, 279
hydroxypropylmethylcellulose (hypromellose),
   water-soluble polymer, 174

immersional wetting, 20
inhalation therapy. See also aerosols, drug
   absorption
in situ polymerisation, nanoparticle manufacturing
   method, 304
insoluble monolayers, surfactants, 116
insulin
   intramuscular and subcutaneous injection, 200
   precipitation, 200
   types, 202

interactions/incompatibilities. See drug
   interactions/incompatibilities
interfacial tension, surfactants, 114
intramuscular and subcutaneous injection. See
   also transdermal delivery
   blood flow, 201
   formulation effects, 201
   insulin, 202
   site of injection, 200
   vehicles, 201
intrathecal drug administration, 214
intravenous injection and infusion, 200
in vitro assessment
   adhesivity of dosage forms, 321
   aerosols, particle size distribution, 322
   dissolution testing of solid dosage forms, 317
   In vitro-in vivo correlations, 325
   particle size distribution in aerosols, 322
   solid dosage forms, dissolution testing, 317
   suppositories, 320
   topical products, 320
   transdermal systems, 320
in vivo effects, drug interactions/
   incompatibilities, 241
ion-exchange resins, water-insoluble
   polymers, 178
ionic strength
   Brønsted–Bjerrum equation, 102
   drug stability, 103
ionic surfactants
   Gouy-Chapman electrical double layer, 123
   micellisation, 122
   Stern layer, 122
ionisation of drugs in solution, 77
   amphoteric drugs, 79
   polyprotic drugs, 79
   weakly acidic drugs and their salts, 77
   weakly basic drugs and their salts, 78
ion-pair formation, 244
ion-pair formation, drug interactions/
   incompatibilities, 244
iontophoresis, transdermal delivery, 206
isomerisation, chemical breakdown of drugs, 94
isotonic solutions, drugs in solution, 85

jet injectors, transdermal delivery, 206

kinetics of chemical decomposition in solution. See
   also chemical breakdown of drugs
   complex reactions, 99
   consecutive reactions, 99
   first-order reactions, 96
   parallel reactions, 99
   pseudo first-order reaction, 96
   reversible reactions, 99

second-order reactions, 98
zero-order reactions, 95

Langmuir equation, surfactants, 119
large intestine, structure, 197
light. *See also* photochemical decomposition
    drug stability, 105
    solid dosage forms, 48
Lipinski's rule of five, 192
lipophilicity and absorption
    biological membranes, 191
    drugs with high log P values, 192
    drugs with low log P values, 192
lipophilicity, protein binding of drugs, 249
liposomes, vesicles, 129
liquid crystals
    cholesteric (or chiral nematic), 128
    lyotropic, 126
    nematic, 128
    smectic, 128
    thermotropic, 128
Lundelius' rule, 121
lung surfactant monolayers, 118
lyophilised proteins, 286
lyotropic liquid crystals, 126

MAbs. *See* monoclonal antibodies
MAC. *See* maximum additive concentration
macrogols (polyoxyethylene glycols), water-soluble
    polymers, 175
matrices, polymers, 179
maximum additive concentration (MAC),
    solubilisation, 130
membranes. *See also* also biological membranes,
    rate-limiting membranes and devices, polymers
methylcellulose, water-soluble polymer, 174
micellisation
    counterions, 122
    critical micelle concentration (CMC), 115
    electrolytes, 125
    factors affecting, 125
    factors affecting micellar size, 125
    Gouy-Chapman electrical double layer, 123
    hydrophilic group, 123
    hydrophobic group, 125
    ionic surfactants, 125
    non-ionic surfactants, 126
    palisade layer, 123
    Stern layer, 122
    temperature, 126
microbial spoilage, emulsions, 158
microcapsules, polymers, 180
microemulsions, 155
Miller indices, crystal structure, 11
milliequivalents, concentration units, 70

moisture
    drug stability, 105
    solid dosage forms, 40
molality, concentration units, 70
molarity, concentration units, 70
molecular weight
    drug absorption, 192
    rule of five, 192
mole fraction, concentration units, 70
monoclonal antibodies, 277
monomers, structure, 168

nanocrystal formation, nanoparticle manufacturing
    method, 309
nanoparticle manufacturing methods
    coacervation and complexation
    techniques, 304
    emulsion-diffusion, 304
    emulsion-solvent evaporation, 304
    in situ polymerisation, 304
    nanocrystal formation, 309
    salting-out, 304
    solvent displacement, 303
nanosystems, 297
    aggregation, 310
    application of nanoparticles in drug
    delivery, 300
    characteristics, 300
    drug targeting, 299
    nanoparticle diffusion, 311
    nanoparticle manufacturing methods, 303
    nanoparticles as drug carriers, 302
    particle size, 301
    PEGylation, 310
    pharmacokinetics vs particokinetics, 299
    physicochemical characterisation, 298
nasal route, drug absorption, 211
natural gums and mucilages, water-soluble
    polymers, 175
nematic liquid crystals, 128
niosomes, vesicles, 130
non-aqueous suspensions, 162
non-ionic surfactants
    micellisation, 123
    palisade layer, 131
    pluronics, 114
    poloxamers, 113
    polysorbates, 113
    sorbitan esters, 113
Noyes-Whitney equation
    dissolution of drugs, 21
    particle size, 21

oil-in-water emulsions stability
    multiple emulsions, 154

ointments, semi-solid emulsions (creams,
  ointments), 157
oligonucleotides, 289
oral route. See buccal and sublingual absorption
osmotic effect, colloid stability, 144
osmotic properties of drugs in solution, 85
  van't Hoff equation, 85
osmotic pumps, polymers, 181
oxidation
  chemical breakdown of drugs, 93
  pH, 101
  proteins, 284
oxygen
  drug stability, 105
  solid dosage forms, 48

paediatric medication, 223
  appropriateness, 224
  dose, 226
  excipients, 226
  extemporaneous formulations, 225
  routes of administration, 227
palisade layer
  non-ionic surfactants, 123
parallel reactions, kinetics of chemical
  decomposition in solution, 99
particle size
  bioavailability of drugs, 156
  formulation of solid dosage forms, 17
  manufacture of solid dosage forms, 17
  nanosystems, 301
  Noyes-Whitney equation, 21
particle size distribution in aerosols, in vitro
  assessment, 322
particokinetics vs pharmacokinetics, nanosystems,
  299
partition coefficient, partitioning of drugs between
  immiscible solvents, 88
partitioning of drugs between immiscible solvents
  acidic drugs, 87
  amphoteric drugs, 75
  basic drugs, 87
  distribution coefficient, P, 87
  Ferguson's principle, 87
  partition coefficient, 88
patches and devices, transdermal delivery, 204
pectin, water-soluble polymer, 175
PEGylation, nanosystems, 310
peptide adsorption, drug interactions/
  incompatibilities, 248
peptides. See also proteins
  calcitonin, 288
  chemical instability, 283
  deamidation, 283
  defining, 277

hydrophobicity, 279
proteolysis, 284
solution properties, 277
stability, 281
structure, 277
therapeutic, 286
permeability, pH-partition hypothesis, 192
pH
  buffers, 101
  drug solutions, 74
  drug stability, 100
  general acid-base catalysis, 100
  oxidation, 284
  photochemical decomposition, 94
  specific acid-base catalysis, 100
pharmacokinetics vs particokinetics, nanosystems,
  299
pH effects, drug interactions/incompatibilities
  gastric effects, 241
  intestinal absorption, 241
  in vitro effects, 241
  in vivo effects, 241
  precipitation of drugs in vivo, 242
  urinary pH, 241
phosphate buffer system, 83
photochemical decomposition. See also light
  chemical breakdown of drugs, 95
  pH, 101
pH-partition hypothesis, 192
  complicating factors, 194
  convective water flow, 194
  discrepancies in absorption, 193
  effect of the drug, 194
  permeability, 192
  pH at membrane surfaces, 194
  quantitative application problems, 193
  unstirred water layers, 194
  variability in pH conditions, 194
physiological buffers, 83
plasma proteins, protein binding of drugs, 249
plastics, drug interactions/incompatibilities, 248
pluronics, non-ionic surfactants, 114
poloxamers, non-ionic surfactants, 113
polymerisation, chemical breakdown of drugs, 95
polymers
  alginates, 175
  application in drug delivery, 178
  carboxypolymethylene (Carbomer,
    Carbopol), 174
  cellulose derivatives, 174
  chitosan, 175
  copolymers, 168
  dextran, 175
  dimeticones, 178
  film coating, 178

gels, properties, 172
gels, viscosity, 173
glass transition temperature, Tg, 169
gum arabic (acacia), 175
gum tragacanth, 175
homopolymers, 167
Hydroxypropylmethylcellulose
(hypromellose), 174
ion-exchange resins, 178
macrogols (polyoxyethylene glycols), 175
matrices, 179
methylcellulose, 174
microcapsules, 180
monomers, 167
natural gums and mucilages, 175
osmotic pumps, 181
pectin, 175
polydispersity, 170
polyvinylpyrrolidone, 173
rate-limiting membranes and devices, 181
solution properties, 170
Staudinger equation, 171
structure, 167
transdermal delivery systems, 181
viscosity, 171
water-insoluble, 177
water-soluble, 174
polymorphic solvates, 15
polymorphism
analytical issues, 14
bioavailability differences, 15
formulation problems, 14
solids, 14
polyprotic drugs, ionisation of drugs in solution, 79
polysorbates, non-ionic surfactants, 113
polyvinylpyrrolidone, water-soluble polymer, 173
powders. *See also* solids, wetting
preservative availability in emulsified systems, 158
protein adsorption, drug interactions/
incompatibilities, 248
protein binding of drugs, 248
lipophilicity, 249
plasma proteins, 249
protein buffer system, 83
proteins. *See also* peptides accelerated stability
testing of protein formulations
aggregation, 281
beta-elimination, 284
chemical instability, 283
defining, 277
denaturation, 281
disulfide formation, 285
formulation and protein stabilisation, 281
hydrophobicity, 279
insulin, 287

lyophilised proteins, 286
oxidation, 284
physical stability, 282
polyamino acids, 286
protein formulation and delivery, 285
racemisation, 284
solution properties, 277
stability, 281
stability testing, 281
structure, 278
surface adsorption and precipitation, 281
therapeutic, 286
pseudo first-order reactions, kinetics of chemical
decomposition in solution, 96
pseudopolymorphic solvates, 15

Raoult's law, aerosols, 72
rate-limiting membranes and devices, polymers,
181
rectal route, 212
absorption from formulations, 213
drug absorption, 212
fate of drug, 213
incompatibility between base and drug, 213
rectal cavity, 213
suppositories, 212
respiratory buffer system, 83
reversible reactions, kinetics of chemical
decomposition in solution, 99
rheological characteristics of products, 321
rheological characteristics of products, *in vitro*
assessment, 321
rheology, emulsions, 158
rule of five
drug absorption, 192
molecular weight, 192

salting-out, nanoparticle manufacturing
method, 304
Schulze-Hardy rule, colloid stability, 144
second-order reactions, kinetics of chemical
decomposition in solution, 98
shelf-life calculation, 106
Arrhenius equation, 106
drug stability, 107
stability testing, 106
small intestine, structure, 196
smectic liquid crystals, 128
Sodium Lauryl Sulfate BP, 112
solid dispersions, 23
solid dosage forms. *See also* solids
amorphous solids, 16
dissolution testing, *in vitro* assessment, 317
drug stability, 105
excipients, 29

light, 48
moisture, 48
oxygen, 48
temperature, 49
solid or condensed monolayers, surfactants, 117
solids. *See also* solid dosage forms
  co-crystallisation, 16
  crystal hydrates, 15
  crystal structure, 11
  dissolution of drugs, 21
  external appearance, 11
  freeze drying, 22
  particle size, 17
  polymorphism, 14
  solid dispersions, 23
  solid solutions, 24
  sublimation, 22
  wetting, 18
solid solutions, 23
solubilisation
  factors affecting, 131
  maximum additive concentration (MAC), 130
  method of preparation of solubilised systems, 132
  pharmaceutical applications, 133
  solubilisate, 130
  surfactants, 131
  temperature, 132
solubility. *See also* drugs in solution
  additives, 73
  amphoteric drugs, 79
  basic drugs, 78
  boiling point of liquids, 73
  common ion effect, 75
  drugs, 69
  factors influencing, 73
  inorganic electrolytes, 73
  isoelectric point, 75
  melting point of solids, 73
  methods to increase, 76
  solubility product, 75
  substituents, 73
solubility problems, drug interactions/
  incompatibilities, 239
solutions, transdermal delivery, 181
solvent displacement, nanoparticle manufacturing
  method, 303
solvent effects, 104
  dilution of mixed solvent systems, 242
  drug interactions/incompatibilities, 240
  drug stability, 104
solvents, aerosols, 71
sorbitan esters, non-ionic surfactants, 113
specific acid-base catalysis
  drug stability, 100
  pH, 101

spreading coefficient, 18
spreading wetting, 18
stability, drug. *See* drug stability
Staudinger equation
  polymers, 171
  viscosity, 171
steric stabilisation, colloid stability, 144
Stern layer
  ionic surfactants, 123
Stokes-Einstein equation
  diffusion of drugs in solution, 88
  nanoparticle diffusion, 302
Stokes' law, colloid stability, 139
stomach, 196
  gastric emptying, motility and volume of
    contents, 198
  structure, 196
subcutaneous injection. *See* intramuscular and
  subcutaneous injection; transdermal delivery
sublimation, solids, 22
supercritical fluid technologies, 309
supercritical fluid technologies, nanoparticle
  manufacturing method, 309
suppositories
  in vitro assessment, 320
  rectal absorption of drugs, 212
surface tension, surfactants, 114
surfactants
  adsorption at the solid-liquid interface, 119
  amphoteric, 111
  anionic, 112
  cationic, 112
  expanded monolayers, 117
  Freundlich equation, 119
  gaseous monolayers, 117
  Gibbs equation, 114
  hydrophile-lipophile balance (HLB), 113
  insoluble monolayers, 116
  interfacial tension, 114
  ionic, 122
  Langmuir equation, 119
  lung surfactant monolayers, 118
  non-ionic, 112
  reduction of surface and interfacial tension, 114
  Sodium Lauryl Sulfate BP, 112
  solid or condensed monolayers, 117
  solubilisation, 130
  surface tension, 114
  Traube's rule, 116
  types, 111
  typical, 112
  zwitterionic, 111
surfactant vesicle, 130
suspensions
  adhesion of suspension particles to containers, 162

controlled flocculation, 161
flocculation, 159
non-aqueous, 162
stability, 159
transdermal delivery, 181
zeta potential, 141
syneresis, gels, 173

taste masking, adsorption at the solid–liquid
  interface, 122
temperature
  cloud point, 126
  critical micelle concentration (CMC), 126
  drug stability, 106
  micellisation, 122
  solid dosage forms, 52
  solubilisation, 132
thermodynamic properties of drugs in solution, 84
  activity and activity coefficient, 84
  chemical potential, 84
  Debye-Hückel equation, 84
thermotropic liquid crystals, 128
topical products, *in vitro* assessment, 320
transdermal delivery. *See also* intramuscular and
  subcutaneous injection
  drug release from vehicles, 204
  emulsions, 204
  formulations, 204
  influence of drug, 203
  in vitro assessment, transdermal systems, 320
  iontophoresis, 206
  jet injectors, 206
  patches and devices, 204
  polymers, 181
  routes of skin penetration, 202
  solutions, 204
  suspensions, 204
  ultrasound and transdermal penetration, 206
Traube's rule, surfactants, 116

ultrasound and transdermal penetration,
  transdermal delivery, 206
unit cells
  Bravais lattices, 11
  crystal structure, 11
universal buffers, 82
urinary buffer system, 84

vagina, drug absorption, 208
vesicles
  liposomes, 129
  niosomes, 130
  surfactant, 129

viscosity
  gels, 171
  polymers, 171
  Staudinger equation, 171
volume concentration, concentration units, 69

water-in-oil emulsions stability, 151
  multiple emulsions, 154
water-insoluble polymers, 177
  dimeticones, 178
  ion-exchange resins, 178
  properties, 177
water-soluble polymers, 174
  bioadhesivity, 176
  crystallinity, 177
weight concentration, concentration units, 69
wetting
  critical surface tension for spreading, 19
  immersional wetting, 20
  powders, 18
  solids, 18
  spreading coefficient, 18
  spreading wetting, 18
  Young's equation, 18

Young's equation, wetting, 18

zero-order reactions, kinetics of chemical
  decomposition in solution, 95
zeta potential, suspensions, 141
zwitterionic surfactants, 111